Evolutionary Cell Biology of the Fetal-Maternal Interface

Viviparity combined with sustained invasive placentation is a unique reproductive innovation of placental mammals (Eutheria). This fact is remarkable as viviparity, of various kinds, is a quite frequent reproductive feature of animals in general. In this book, the authors argue that sustained invasive placentation faced a number of cell biological obstacles, known as biological paradoxa. In the evolution of eutherian mammals, each paradoxon was overcome by a specific evolutionary innovation that overcame the cellular biological constraint on the evolution of mammal-like viviparity. Each of these innovations also identifies specific mechanisms that entail clinical vulnerabilities of human pregnancy. The evolution of mammalian pregnancy is thus a paradigm of a significant evolutionary novelty, and this book exemplifies the conceptual tools necessary to explain evolutionary novelties in general, as well as the importance of an evolutionary and cell biological perspective on human reproductive health.

Evolutionary Cell Biology

Published Titles

Cells in Evolutionary Biology*: Translating Genotypes into Phenotypes – Past, Present, Future*
Edited by Brian K. Hall and Sally Moody

Deferred Development: Setting Aside Cells for Future Use in Development in Evolution
Edited by Cory Douglas Bishop and Brian K. Hall

Cellular Processes in Segmentation
Edited by Ariel Chipman

Cellular Dialogues in the Holobiont
Edited by Thomas Bosch and Michael G. Hadfield

Evolving Neural Crest Cells
Edited by Daniel Meulemans Medeiros, Brian Frank Eames, Igor Adameyko

Development of Sensory and Neurosecretory Cell Types: Vertebrate Cranial Placodes, volume 1
By Gerhard Schlosser

Evolutionary Origin of Sensory and Neurosecretory Cell Types: Vertebrate Cranial Placodes, volume 2
By Gerhard Schlosser

Evolutionary Cell Processes in Primates: Bones, Brains, and Muscle, Volume I
Edited by M. Kathleen Pitirri and Joan T. Richtsmeier

Evolutionary Cell Processes in Primates: Genes, Skin, Energetics, Breathing, and Feeding, Volume II
Edited by M. Kathleen Pitirri and Joan T. Richtsmeier

The Notochord: Development, Evolution and contributions to the vertebral column
Eckhard P. Witten and Brian K. Hall

Evolution of Neurosensory Cells and Systems: Gene regulation and cellular networks and processes
Edited by Bernd Fritzsch and Karen L. E. Thompson

The Evolution of Multicellularity
Edited by Matthew D. Herron, Peter Conlin, and William C. Ratcliff

Phenotypic Plasticity & Evolution: Causes, Consequences, Controversies
Edited By David W. Pfennig

Hox Modules in Evolution and Development
Edited By David E. K. Ferrier

Odontodes: The Developmental and Evolutionary Building Blocks of Dentitions
Edited By Donglei Chen

Evolutionary Cell Biology of the Fetal-Maternal Interface: Reflections on Evolutionary Innovation
By Günter P. Wagner and Mihaela Pavličev

For more information about this series, please visit: www.crcpress.com/Evolutionary-Cell-Biology/book-series/CRCEVOCELBIO

Evolutionary Cell Biology of the Fetal-Maternal Interface

Reflections on Evolutionary Innovation

Günter P. Wagner and Mihaela Pavličev

CRC Press
Taylor & Francis Group
Boca Raton London New York

CRC Press is an imprint of the
Taylor & Francis Group, an **informa** business

Designed cover image: Image is from figure 166 in Grosser (1909), Vergleichende Anatomie und Entwicklungsgeschichte der Eihäute und der Placenta. Braumüller, Vienna.

First edition published 2027
by CRC Press
2385 NW Executive Center Drive, Suite 320, Boca Raton FL 33431

and by CRC Press
4 Park Square, Milton Park, Abingdon, Oxon, OX14 4RN

CRC Press is an imprint of Taylor & Francis Group, LLC

ISBN: 978-1-032-71045-7
ISBN: 978-1-032-71776-0
ISBN: 978-1-032-71777-7

DOI: 10.1201/9781032717777

Typeset in Times LT STD
by Deanta Global Publishing Services, Chennai, India

Gratefully dedicated to our mentors who introduced us into the world of reproductive medicine: Professor Dr. Roberto Romero and Professor Dr. Lou Muglia.

Contents

About the Authors

Günter P. Wagner is the Alison Richard Professor Emeritus of Ecology and Evolutionary Biology. After undergraduate education in chemical engineering, he studied zoology and mathematical logic at the University of Vienna, Austria. He finished his PhD in theoretical population genetics in 1979 and conducted postdoctoral research at Max Planck Institutes in Göttingen and Tübingen, as well as at the University of Göttingen. He began his academic career as Assistant Professor in the Theoretical Biology Department of the University of Vienna. He then moved to Yale University as Full Professor of Biology and has served as the First Chair of Yale's Department of Ecology and Evolution. The focus of Wagner's work is on the evolution of complex characters. His research utilizes both the theoretical tools of population genetics and experimental approaches in evolutionary developmental biology. He has contributed substantially to the current understanding of evolvability of complex organisms, the origin of novel characters, and modularity. He is a recipient of numerous awards, among them the prestigious MacArthur Prize, and the Humboldt Research Prize. He was Gomperz Lecturer, University of California, Berkeley; Koopmans Distinguished Lecturer, IIASA Vienna; Sewall Wright Speaker, University of Chicago, IL. He is also a corresponding member of the Austrian Academy of Sciences, a Fellow of the American Association for the Advancement of Science, and a Fellow of the American Academy of Arts and Sciences. He was elected to the National Academy of Sciences in 2018, and Hagler Fellow of the Institute for Advanced Study at Texas A&M University in 2023. In 2021 he retired from the faculty at Yale and now is teaching and conducting research at the University of Vienna as lecturer and senior research fellow.

Mihaela Pavličev, Univ.-Prof. Mag. Dr., is Deputy Head of the Department of Evolutionary Biology and Head of the Unit for Theoretical Evolutionary Biology at the University of Vienna. Her research focuses on the organismal features that enable evolvability of complex organisms. She seeks to understand phenotypic evolution, patterns of heritable phenotypic variation in the developmental/physiological systems, and the consequences of specific patterns of variation over short terms under selection and drift.

Preface

Neither of us had the plan to become a reproductive biologist, and perhaps we still are not, but rather evolutionary biologists who at some point in our careers chanced upon issues of mammalian reproduction. For GPW, it was the chance discovery of an accelerated rate of amino acid substitution in the mammalian lineage of the transcription factor HoxA11 (Chiu et al. 2000). Initially, we studied this protein because of its role in limb development and evolution (Blanco et al. 1998). As it happens, the increase in the rate of evolution in the mammalian lineage was intriguing, as it was already known that HoxA11 is essential for the development of the endometrial stromal cells and hence for female reproduction (Hsieh-Li et al. 1995). The evolution of the HoxA11 protein seemed to be associated with the origin of placental reproduction. The natural question was whether the amino acid differences are functionally relevant to the biology of endometrial stromal cells, which we ultimately could answer experimentally to be the case (Lynch et al. 2004, Nnamani et al. 2016). With that discovery, the engagement and interest in the evolution of placental reproduction deepened and was ultimately irreversible. For MP, the engagement with reproductive biology started with a job offer as a research professor at the Cincinnati Children's Hospital in a group spearheading the study of the causes of premature birth and the regulation of pregnancy length in humans. It became clear that understanding the pathological deviations in human pregnancy length required understanding the regulation of the human healthy pregnancy length in the first place. One powerful way to approach that is to trace its evolution, that is, by comparative work across mammals. It wasn't clear to us at all at the time how complex a task this was, pulling us into first identifying the fundamental questions of mammalian pregnancy. As evolutionary biologists, we brought our perspective to the study of mammalian reproduction, which led to a commitment to view female reproductive function under an evolutionary perspective.

In the meantime, and coincidentally with our own turn toward reproductive biology, evolutionary studies in female reproductive biology blossomed. We are thus living in a time when an evolutionary perspective on the biology of female reproduction is re-emerging, informed by the progress in molecular and phylogenetic biology, as well as conceptual changes in evolutionary biology itself. The latter led to a then-new branch of evolutionary biology under the heading of "Developmental Evolutionary Biology," and our approach to reproduction is deeply influenced by the ideas of developmental evolution. We thus feel that a synthesis of the ideas on the evolution of mammalian reproduction could be of value. We are grateful to Gerhard Schlosser, editor in chief of the book series on Evolutionary Cell Biology, for suggesting publishing this book in this series, as our aim was truly to bring the evolutionary cell biology approach to the table.

We acknowledge that the perspective offered in this book is, to a large extent, idiosyncratic, reflecting our personal journey into evolutionary reproductive biology, down to the species we had the privilege to study over the years, i.e., opossums, armadillos, spiny mice, gerbils, guinea pigs, and most recently pigs thanks to a collaboration with Texas A&M researchers, Fuller Bazer and Greg Johnson. A comprehensive and disinterested summary of the whole field needs to be written by another person. But we believe that the benefit, if any, the book can offer to the scientific community has to be found in its deviations from mainstream consensus. The decision whether this approach offers value is not in our hands, but in the hands of the next generation of scientists and scholars. With that, we dedicate this book to the further development of the science of female reproduction.

None of what we report here could have been developed without the input, encouragement, and help from a large number of friends, colleagues, and collaborators. We particularly want to mention our mentors that opened to us the world of human reproductive medicine in particular Roberto Romero from the Eucine Kennedy Shriver NI of Child Health and Human Development of the NIH, Lou Muglia and Ge Zhang, then at the Cincinnati Children's Hospital, Jan Brosens from the University of Warwick Medial School, and Errol Norwitz from the Tufts University Clinical and Translational Science Institute. Most recently we have been privileged to learn and work on large animal reporduction thanks to the generosity of our collaborators at Texas A&M University, Fuller Bazer and Greg Johnson. The biggest impact on us, naturally, came from the close collaboration with extraordinary students and postdocs: Chi-hua Chiu, Vincent Lynch, Oliver Griffith, Mauris Nnamani, Deena Emera, Arun Chavan, Daniel Stadtmauer, Cong Liang, and Jacob Musser to only mention those former members of the Yale lab directly involved in reproductive biology research and cell type evolution, as well as Caitlin McDonough Goldstein and Silvia Basanta at the University of Vienna. Special acknowledgement is reserved for Jamie Maziarz, who was GPW's fearless and reliable companion in all experimental work done in the last ten-plus years at Yale. Equally important, though maybe unexpected for a scientific enterprise, is our collaboration on conceptual issues of evolutionary biology with a group of outstanding philosophers of science, in particular Laura Nuño de la Rosa, Arantza Etxeberria, Alan Love, and James DiFrisco. Finally, we want to acknowledge the benefit we derived from conversations and collaborations with colleagues at Yale and the University of Connecticut: Stephen Stearns, Richard Prum, Ruslan Medzhitov, Andre Levchenko, Kshitiz, Casey Dunn, Erika Edwards, Kurt Schwenk, and Michael Donoghue. We are deeply grateful for the chance and privilege to interact and work with all these and other extraordinary individuals.

REFERENCES

Blanco, M. J., B. Y. Misof and G. P. Wagner (1998). "Heterochronic differences of Hoxa-11 expression in Xenopus fore- and hind limb development: evidence for a lower limb identity of the anuran ankle bones." *Dev Genes Evol* **208**: 175–187.

Chiu, C.-H., D. Nonaka, L. Xue, C. T. Amemiya and G. P. Wagner (2000). "Evolution of Hoxa-11 in lineages phylogenetically positioned along the fin-limb transition." *Mol Phylogen Evol* **17**: 305–316.

Hsieh-Li, H., D. Witte, M. Weinstein, W. Branford, H. Li, K. Small and S. Potter (1995). "Hoxa 11 structure, extensive antisense transcription, and function in male and female fertility." *Development* **121**(5): 1373–1385.

Lynch, V. J., J. J. Roth, K. Takahashi, C. W. Dunn, D. F. Nonaka, G. F. Stopper and G. P. Wagner (2004). "Adaptive evolution of HoxA-11 and HoxA-13 at the origin of the uterus in mammals." *Proc Roy Soc B: Biol Sci* **271**(1554): 2201–2207.

Nnamani, M. C., S. Ganguly, E. M. Erkenbrack, V. J. Lynch, L. S. Mizoue, Y. Tong, H. L. Darling, M. Fuxreiter, J. Meiler and G. P. Wagner (2016). "A derived allosteric switch underlies the evolution of conditional cooperativity between HOXA11 and FOXO1." *Cell Rep* **15**(10): 2097–2108.

1 Introduction

Scientific disciplines and their scholarly counterparts develop in waves, with rapid progress in some decades, and relative stagnation before and after. This pattern also seems to hold in particular for evolutionary reproductive biology. In the 20th century, there was rapid progress and excitement after the early discoveries of endocrine control of reproductive functions, such as the pioneering work of Eugen Steinach (1861–1944), Ludwig Haberlandt (1885–1932), and Frank R. Lillie (1870–1947), which initiated the causal analysis of reproductive functions and their translational application. This work was performed in a culture of comparative zoology, so that the evolutionary and comparative research was also rapidly advancing in parallel with physiological research up to the 1960s, as exemplified by the work of Otto Grosser (1873–1951), Harland W. Mossman (1898–1991), Elizabeth M. Ramsey (1906–1993), Allen C. Enders, and Anthony Carter. After that, work in reproductive biology increasingly shifted from broad comparative approaches to a focus on human reproduction, as well as work on model species such as the mouse, rat, and guinea pig. In parallel, excellent work was done in animal science on the reproduction of cattle, sheep, pigs, and horses. An example of the latter is the pioneering work on maternal recognition of pregnancy in farm animals by Fuller Bazer, R. Michael Roberts and Rodney Geisert. The comparative tradition has continued, but it was less dynamic compared to that in the first half of the 20th century. To mention is the work by Marilyn Renfree and her colleagues on marsupial reproduction, as well as Daniel G. Blackburn, James R. Stewart, Michael B. Thompson, and others on lizards, who were bucking the trend toward work on model organisms and advanced knowledge on reptilian reproduction. Since the 2000s, however, there has been an increase in the number of investigators working on the evolution of reproduction, in particular on the evolution of viviparity. Given this trend, it might be useful to present a perspective on the evolution of viviparity for researchers and students entering the field. This is what this book aims to do, i.e., provide an intellectual and conceptual context for the exciting work made possible by recent advances in research technology, such as genomics and single-cell sequencing, and others.

VIVIPARITY IS NOT A SIMPLE TRAIT

There are not many concepts in biology that are as clearly defined and unambiguous as the notion of viviparity: that is, giving rise to live offspring, in contrast to egg laying and incubation outside the body of the mother. This contrasts with many concepts in biology that are difficult to define and are only understood after extensive study and research, such as "the gene," "cell type," "species," "homology," and others. These concepts have attracted ample attention from biologists and philosophers of biology to unravel their meaning and role in scientific investigations. Naturally, concepts like viviparity have received less attention, primarily because of their perceived clarity and simplicity. Yet, simplicity can be deceptive and, in its deceptiveness, can have insidious consequences for the practice of biology. The simplicity of the notion of viviparity, as we will see later, hides a vast amount of biological complexity and heterogeneity. This in itself might not seem to be a big problem, because one of the most successful heuristic strategies of science is abstraction, i.e., ignoring irrelevant detail and focusing on the salient properties of an object or process. While this is true, not every case of abstraction is equally successful and legitimate. Note that successful abstractions ignore *irrelevant* detail, not relevant complexity, and the difference is not always obvious at the outset. It is always good to remember the quote attributed to Albert Einstein: "In science we shall make everything as simple as possible, but not more so." As I will argue, the notion of viviparity is

DOI: 10.1201/9781032717777-1

an example of "more so," i.e., a simplification that goes beyond what is scientifically warranted. – Why could this be a problem?

The main reason why oversimplified concepts are problematic is that they invite generalizations that are bound to fail. For instance, an investigator who studies viviparity and its genetic and cell biological bases in a particular species (there is no alternative to doing an experimental study on a particular species) may feel justified to claim that he or she has discovered "the genetic basis of viviparity." If the investigator is lucky, she may have discovered the genetic basis of the form of viviparity that is present in this species. But how far can this insight be generalized? Obviously, the best chance for successful generalizations is projecting this knowledge to other species that have the same kind (i.e., homologous) form of viviparity, i.e., all those species that derive their form of reproduction from a common ancestor and have not undergone additional major innovations (Figure 1.1). Generalizations beyond that range are not unthinkable if strong similarities can be expected in evolutionarily independent origins of viviparity. But whether such a generalization is warranted remains an empirical question, as all instances of generalization remain subject to potential falsification. Hence, the tendency of concepts like viviparity to oversimplify is problematic because they invite premature abstraction and unwarranted generalization.

For some reason, reproductive biology has many concepts of deceptive simplicity. Placentation is another such overgeneralized concept, and even the relatively detailed concepts of forms of placentation introduced by Otto Grosser (hemochorial, epitheliochorial … placentation) are not free of problematic generalizations (Grosser 1909). This becomes a problem when species are classified according to these concepts, and the so-generated data matrix of "species x (times) character states" (placental vs non-placental) is analyzed on a phylogenetic tree to trace the evolution of this mode of reproduction. We acknowledge that research has to start at the point where knowledge is at the

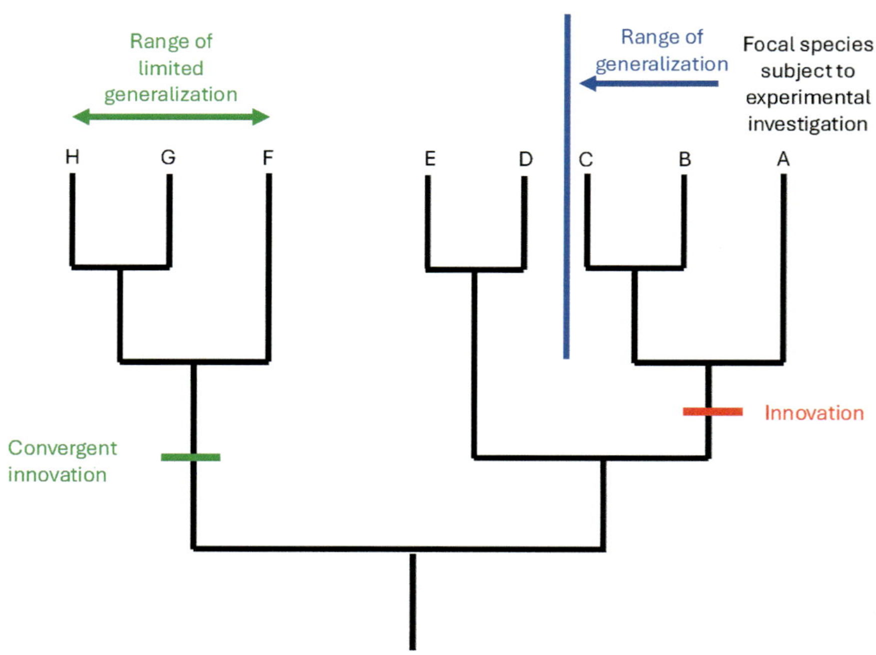

FIGURE 1.1 Example of how phylogenetic relationships affect the range of possible generalizations in biology. If we investigate a character in species A, which arose before the common ancestor of the clade (A,(B,C)), the range of generalization is limited to this clade, and nothing can be said about species D and E. On the other hand, if there is a convergent innovation that arose in the stem lineage of the clade (F,(G,H)), some limited generalization also extends to this clade. (Image generated by GPW.)

beginning of an investigation, and we need to do what is possible at the time. This is true, and no practicing scientist would say otherwise. But what is expected is that, after all is said and done, one should ask questions about whether the phylogenetic inferences lead to biologically plausible insights. For instance, it is well established that marsupials and hoofed animals (among others) are similar as their placentation remains superficial and are thus often lumped into "epithelio-chorial placental." Yet the reasons for that anatomical similarity in opossums and sows are fundamentally different. In one case, the opossum, the invasive placentation is not tolerated by the mother, leading to birth after a short period of fetal-maternal contact, giving birth to highly immature neonates. In contrast, the sow (for instance) actively prevents the fetus from invading but maintains a long gestation until the fetus is quite mature at birth.

This book is written to unpack the phenomenon of the fetal-maternal relationship and aid in eventually finding the level of abstraction that supports the most productive generalizations. The elaboration of this topic will be heavily biased toward research on amniote vertebrates and, in particular, mammals, as those are the areas in which the authors have the most experience and also the largest number of published results is available. As comparative biologists, however, the authors do hope that this treatment will inspire similar efforts in other animal groups, from cnidarians to insects, to unpack the diverse biologies that characterize different types of organisms.

UNDERSTANDING REPRODUCTION THROUGH DEVELOPMENTAL EVOLUTION

There are three broadly accepted theoretical approaches to explain the outcomes of evolutionary change. One is the model of natural selection, where the evolutionary outcome is explained as the result of the preferential reproduction of individuals with the derived character or character state, either due to a survival or a reproductive advantage caused by this new trait or character. The survival advantage is also called "fitness," where fitness is understood as a measure of the competitive advantage of one phenotype or gene over another (Wagner 2010). The results of natural selection are then called adaptations. This mode of explanation, of course, goes back to the ideas of Charles Darwin (1809–1882) and Alfred Russel Wallace (1823–1913) in the mid-19th century and was mathematically articulated by Ronald Fisher (1890–1962) and Sewall Wright (1889–1988) (Provine 1971). A second mode of evolutionary change is that of random genetic drift (Kimura 1983), where variants that do not affect the fitness of the organism become fixed in the population because of random effects in finite populations. This mode of explanation is mostly associated with the name of Motoo Kimura (1924–1994) and plays a major role in explaining the evolution of molecular features of the genome (see also Lynch 2007). A variant of natural selection explanations is the so-called conflict theories, which play a major role in the explanation of reproductive traits (Haig 1993). Conflicts are situations where the fitness of an individual depends on the traits of other individuals, as is the case in the fitness consequences of fetal-maternal interactions. This theory was largely developed by David Haig, and we will discuss it in various contexts later in the book. These are the main modes of explanation used in evolutionary biology and, by implication, in the biology of reproduction. However, this monograph assumes a different perspective, one that arose from the field of evolutionary developmental biology (evo devo), or, as we prefer to call it, developmental evolutionary biology (devo-evo). The latter term more accurately reflects the nature of the model used here, i.e., a branch of evolutionary biology that uses insights from developmental and cell biology to explain evolutionary outcomes.

The explanatory model of developmental evolutionary biology (DEB) differs from the other three mentioned above by its focus on the mechanistic changes that were necessary to reach a particular evolutionary result. While the classical models assume that relevant genetic variation is either present or likely to occur in short order, the mechanistic nature of these mutations is rarely articulated, or at least does not play a major explanatory role, since natural selection or selective forces generated by the interactions among individuals are the main explanatory modes. In contrast, the model of developmental evolution focuses on the nature of the changes to the development and functioning of organisms (Wagner, Chiu et al. 2000). At the surface, this perspective seems to be a simple complement to the population genetic models of explanations (selection or drift). But assuming this perspective also changes the very nature of evolutionary explanations. I will illustrate this point with an example from outside reproductive biology. The rest of the book will provide more detailed examples directly related to the evolution of reproduction.

One of the simplest traits to evolve seems to be body size. There seems to be no need for specific innovations to evolve a larger body size. A larger body is just more of the same, or so it seems. In most species where body size has been investigated, the heritability (the fraction of variance explained by additive genetic effects) is high, between 0.63 and 0.72 in humans (Mook-Kanamori, van Beijsterveldt et al. 2012). Quantitative genetic theory thus predicts that body size change of several percent per generation is easily attainable, and in fact, body size evolution has been documented in the fossil record to be fast (Caron and Pie 2024). The body size of mammals, for instance, can vary from 1.8 grams in the Etruscan shrew (*Suncus etruscus*) to 200 tons in the case of the blue whale, a 10^8-fold difference. Case closed! Or is it? – Recent developments in evolutionary cancer biology tell a different story. For one, increased body size, in most but not all cases,[1] implies that the larger body also has more cells and thus the cells of the body have to undergo additional cell divisions. Additional cell divisions increase the risk of mutations in the somatic cells and thus increase the risk of cancer. In fact, mathematical models of cancer risk show that large mammals should succumb to cancer as soon as they reach adulthood, assuming cancer-causing mutations occur at a rate as in humans. The reason is that the number of cell divisions necessary to reach their body size increases the mutational target for the origin of tumorigenic mutations. That the cancer risk is not scaling with body size has been called "Peto's Paradox" (Caulin and Maley 2011), although there is substantial variation in cancer mortality risk among mammals (Vincze, Colchero et al. 2022). What then explains Peto's paradox? The emerging story is that certain levels of body size can only be achieved if "Peto's Constraint" is overcome by the evolution of mechanisms that decrease the rate of tumorigenic mutations to an acceptable level. What exactly these mechanisms are is still subject to intense research, but some candidate mechanisms are emerging (Nagy 2007, Sulak, Fong et al. 2016).

To evolve a larger body size is not as simple as it appears when one only looks at the population genetic parameters, like heritability and selection strength. The reason is that the evolutionary change in body size is subject to cell biological constraints, such as the link between the number of cell divisions, mutation rate, and cancer risk. The conceptual pattern arising from this example, and others discussed later in this book, is one where certain (but not all) evolutionary changes are subject to constraints due to mechanistic side effects, and these evolutionary changes only become possible if and when these constraints are somehow overcome, usually by some molecular or cell biological innovations. The explanatory model of developmental evolution is thus one of the dialectic of constraints and innovations, or the explanandum "how to overcome this constraint" and the explanans "this innovation overcame this constraint" (Wagner and Müller 2002). The constraints define the kind of innovations that are necessary to allow an evolutionary transformation, and identifying the innovations that did that is the actual explanation (explanans). Interesting evolutionary constraints are often recognized as a kind of paradoxon, i.e., the realization that a certain evolutionary outcome seems to be incompatible with another piece of biological knowledge. We have seen this above in the case of Peto's paradox, that is, the seeming incompatibility of known somatic mutation rates and the number of cell divisions necessary to grow a large mammalian body. Reproductive biology is full of evolutionary paradoxes, the best known is the immunological paradox proposed by Paul Medawar (1953; see Chapter 4). Explaining how these paradoxa have been solved by evolution is the core DevoEvo explanatory strategy. Wherever the necessary information is available, we will follow this mode of explanation in the rest of the book.

One heuristic benefit of this model is that it explains why, in many cases, we still have species around that have not followed the pathway to "functional perfection," as one would have to expect if natural selection is the all-powerful driver of evolutionary change. At this point, it is important to note that the perspective advanced here does not deny the validity of models of natural selection as such but recognizes that evolutionary outcomes are influenced and perhaps prevented or enabled by the pleiotropic effects of mutations that affect the focal trait (Galis and Metz 2007). In other words, predictions based on models focusing on only a focal trait are vulnerable to the influence of organismal integration. *The heuristic argument is that a mechanistic understanding of how, rather than why, an evolutionary transformation was achieved is a way to identify the complex web of pleiotropic effects and interactions shaping the outcome of evolution.* Such an approach also allows one to realize that the way a particular outcome is achieved, such as viviparity, can be lineage specific, i.e., different in mammalian viviparity than in lizard viviparity. This is not to diminish the importance of studying lizard viviparity, but recognizing the richness of biological diversity and avoiding flattening our understanding and appreciation of biological complexity.

THE COMPLEMENTARITY OF ADAPTATIONIST AND CELL BIOLOGICAL APPROACHES

While in the previous section we made a case for an approach to evolutionary explanations that is different from the standard selectionist explanations, it is still important to discuss the relationship these two perspectives can have for understanding reproductive biology, in particular, the evolution of female reproduction. We think that these two perspectives are complementary rather than competing attempts to explain evolution. The complementarity, however, is of a particularly structured kind. For instance, the timing and extent of embryonic diapause in mammals is most likely explained by the details of the reproductive ecology of the species, i.e., when is the best time in the year for mating, and when is the best time for giving birth and raising offspring. The cell and developmental approach outlined above has little to say about these questions. On the other hand, the difference between marsupial and eutherian gestational timing, i.e., how much time during gestation is spent before and after the establishment of direct fetal-maternal contact, is not subject to an adaptive explanation, or at least that is what we will argue later in this book. It is important to understand why this is the case.

Natural selection is acting on heritable variation, which is produced within the constraints of a particular "body plan," broadly speaking (Pavličev 2025), which determines what kinds of variations are easily accessible by the majority of mutations occurring in the genome. Gestational diapause can readily evolve because stopping embryonic development at the blastocyst stage before implantation seems to be relatively easy.[2] On the other hand, the timing difference of "implantation" between marsupials and eutherians is due to the fact that only eutherians, and to some limited extend macropods (Dudley, Renfree et al. 2024), have "invented" a way to sustain direct fetal maternal contact for a longer time, a degree of freedom that most marsupials do not have to their adaptive disposal (see Chapter 4). Hence, models of adaptive explanations are most readily applicable within a clade of species that share a common developmental/cell biological configuration with its associated adaptive degrees of freedom and variational and functional constraints.

We are now ready to turn our attention to evolutionary reproductive biology, in particular, the evolution of viviparity, which will occupy our attention for most of this book.

THE PLAN

There are many excellent reviews and monographs about the diversity and evolution of the placenta, that is, in the majority interpretation, the strictly fetal part of the fetal-maternal interface (Grosser 1909, Mossman 1937, Ramsey 1982, Wooding and Burton 2008, Geisert and Spencer 2021). There are many reasons why research has focused on the placenta rather than the interaction with the female body. For one, the placenta can be studied as an isolated organ delivered into the hands of investigators, often in one piece, after birth, at least in the case of many mammals. On the other hand, studying the maternal side requires more determination, as it involves sacrificing the animal or removing the uterus from the body of the mother. The endometrium, the principal maternal tissue of the fetal-maternal interface, is anatomically less striking than the placenta, in particular in those animals where the placenta is a distinct organ, like in primates and rodents. These coincidental facts, we believe, have led to an unconscious bias in favor of the biology of the placenta, leading to such offensive language as "the fetus educating the uterus," as if the maternal body requires "education" from a few hours old ball of cells. Yes, there is signaling between the blastocyst and the maternal body, but that signaling is going both ways, and the success of the fetal signals depends on the maternal preparation to receive these signals and react accordingly. The same bias is visible in the influential literature about fetal-maternal conflict (Haig 1993), coloring much of our theoretical and evolutionary understanding of viviparity. More will be said about the role of genomic conflict in the evolution of viviparity later in the book, but only this should be said here: conflict likely exists, but it arises and is recognizable as such as a deviation from a base of cooperation. For that reason, conflict theory, however much it otherwise explains, plays a minor role in understanding the origin of viviparity, and will thus play a minor role in the story to be told in this book. The reason for this should also be obvious, namely, the fetus has at least half of its genes from the mother, and thus there is still a maternal "Darwinian interest" served in bringing the fetus into life (Haig 2015).

Of course, there is also an extensive research literature on the biology of the uterus and the endometrium in particular, but in the evolutionary and broad biological perspective, this literature seems to be underappreciated. In this book, we want to advance a perspective on the evolution of viviparity that focuses on the interactive nature of the relationship between fetus and mother, and thus the title of the book is on the evolutionary cell biology of the fetal-maternal relationship and not on the evolution of the placenta per se or even viviparity as such. In fact, looking over the chapter outline, the perspective advanced here has an emphasis on the evolution of the maternal biology that made viviparity and the placenta possible. This bias may be excusable given the extensive and excellent works published on the fetal side of the story. But beyond that, a deeper biological fact justifies this bias in our approach. A detailed review of the likely evolutionary steps necessary to establish a sustainable fetal-maternal unit shows that many of the initial innovations are maternal. Maternal innovations enable the subsequent elaboration of the placenta, a fact that leads us to conclude that maternal innovations are the primary drivers that enabled the evolution of eutherian pregnancy with its extensive gestational period and sustained fetal-maternal relationship (Stadtmauer and Wagner 2020).

With that said, the book will first provide a short overview of the phylogenetic, anatomical, and developmental background for the evolution of mammalian female reproduction. This will be the subject of Chapters 2 and 3. Chapters 2 and 3 can be skipped by readers familiar with vertebrate phylogeny and reproduction. The conceptual core of the essay is developed in Chapter 4, where we review the so-called paradoxa of mammalian pregnancy (*sensu lato*), which in fact identifies cell biological constraints on the evolutionary origin of the mammalian fetal-maternal unit. Furthermore, the fact that mammalian pregnancy is biologically paradoxical also identifies evolutionary innovations that overcame them, which leads to the pivotal role of the decidua for the evolution of placentation. Chapter 5 is then dedicated to the "natural history" of the decidua, that is, the taxonomic distribution, its role in different species, its cellular composition, etc. Chapter 6 is dedicated to a synthetic scenario of the evolutionary origin of the decidual cell type. This is the most speculative part of the book, but perhaps also the most important, as it aims at defining the research agenda that could lead to revealing the mechanistic innovations specific to decidual cell differentiation. In Chapter 7, we turn our attention to the integration of pregnancy into the physiology of the mother, a process called "maternal recognition of pregnancy." Chapter 8 turns to the diversity on the fetal side, arguing that the term "placenta" represents a diversity of organs of fetal-maternal communication. Some of them are true organs, like those of humans and rodents, while others are little more than slightly modified extra-embryonic tissues, fully homologous to those of oviparous amniotes. Chapter 9 deals with biological phenomena that are likely secondary consequences of the evolution of the fetal-maternal unit, namely menstruation and the consequences of placental biology for cancer malignancy. The final chapter returns to the topics raised in this introduction and is an attempt to summarize and generalize the conceptual implications of the previous chapters. We also reflect upon the metaphors people develop around human female reproductive biology and offer an alternative narrative.

What is not adequately covered, if at all, are other important dimensions of viviparity, like the evolution of hormonal regulation of ovarian function necessary for the evolution of viviparity, or the behavioral adaptations that are associated with viviparity. The role of ovarian regulation is covered in part in Chapter 7 and more comprehensively in a recent review (Basanta and Pavlicev 2025). The behavioral dimensions of viviparity reach far beyond the expertise of either of us and can be found in other books, such as the monograph by Hayssen and Orr (2017). We feel that these and other aspects of viviparity are too broad and go too far beyond the cell biology of viviparity to be covered in one relatively short book. We apologize for these shortcomings, but do not want to raise expectations we are not intending to meet.

NOTES

1. The other way to increase the size of the body is to increase the size of the cells but keep the number of cells the same. That can be achieved by increased DNA amount, which automatically increases cell size.
2. There are other forms of diapause, where either the fertilization is delayed, or post-implantation embryo development is slowed down or stopped (for a discussion see Hayssen and Orr 2017), but these forms are rarer than pre-implantation diapause.

REFERENCES

Basanta, S. and M. Pavlicev (2025). "The shifting role and regulation of the corpus luteum in vertebrate reproduction: a synthetic review." Q Rev Biol **100**(3): 189–231.

Caron, F. S. and M. R. Pie (2024). "The evolution of body size in terrestrial tetrapods." *Evol Biol* **51**: 283–294.

Caulin, A. F. and C. C. Maley (2011). "Peto's paradox: evolution's prescription for cancer prevention." *Trends Ecol Evol* **26**(4): 175–182.

Dudley, J. S., M. B. Renfree, G. P. Wagner and O. W. Griffith (2024). "The extension of mammalian pregnancy required taming inflammation: independent evolution of extended placentation in the tammar wallaby." *Proc Natl Acad Sci U S A* **121**(42): e2310047121.

Galis, F. and J. A. Metz (2007). "Evolutionary novelties: the making and breaking of pleiotropic constraints." *Integr Comp Biol* **47**(3): 409–419.

Geisert, R. D. and T. Spencer (2021). *Placentation in Mammals: Tribute to E.C. Amoroso's Lifetime Contributions to Viviparity*. New York etc., Springer.

Grosser, O. (1909). *Vergleichende Anatomie und Entwicklungsgeschichte der Eihäute und der Placenta*. Vienna, W. Braumüller.

Haig, D. (1993). "Genetic conflicts in human pregnancy." *Q Rev Biol* **68**(4): 495–532.

Haig, D. (2015). Fertil soil or no man's land: cooperation and conflict in the placental bed. *Placental Bed Disorders*. R. Rijneborg, I. Brosens and R. Romero. Cambridge, Cambridge University Press**:** 165–173.

Hayssen, V. D. and T. Orr (2017). *Reproduction in Mammals: The Female Perspective*. Baltimore, Johns Hopkins University Press.

Kimura, M. (1983). *The Neutral Theory of Molecular Evolution*. New York, Cambridge Univeristy Press.

Lynch, M. (2007). *The Origins of Genome Architecture*. Sunderland, MA, Sinauer Associates.

Medawar, P. (1953). Some immunological and endocrinological problems raised by the evolution of viviparity in vertebrates. pp. 320-338 n R. Brown and J. F. Danioelli (eds.) Evolution, New York, NY, Academic Press.

Mook-Kanamori, D. O., C. E. van Beijsterveldt, E. A. Steegers, Y. S. Aulchenko, H. Raat, A. Hofman, P. H. Eilers, D. I. Boomsma and V. W. Jaddoe (2012). "Heritability estimates of body size in fetal life and early childhood." *PLoS One* **7**(7): e39901.

Mossman, H. W. (1937). "Comparative morphogenesis of the foetal membranes and accessory uterine structures." *Contr Embyol* **26**: 129–246.

Nagy, J. D. (2007). "Why don't all whales have cancer? A novel hypothesis resolving Peto's paradox." *Integr Comp Biol* **47**: 317–328.

Pavlicev, M. (2025). "Cracking open the blackbox of genotype-phenotype map: crossing the explanatory gap between micro- and macroevolution." *Evolution.* **80:** 301–311.

Provine, W.-B. (1971). *The Origins of Theoretical Population Genetics.* Chicago, University of Chicago Press.

Ramsey, E. M. (1982). *The Placenta. Human and Animal.* Santa Barbara, CA, Praeger Inc.

Stadtmauer, D. J. and G. P. Wagner (2020). "The primacy of maternal innovations to the evolution of embryo implantation." *Integr Comp Biol.* **60:** 742–752.

Sulak, M., L. Fong, K. Mika, S. Chigurupati, L. Yon, N. P. Mongan, R. D. Emes and V. J. Lynch (2016). "TP53 copy number expansion is associated with the evolution of increased body size and an enhanced DNA damage response in elephants." *Elife* **5**. e11994.

Vincze, O., F. Colchero, J. F. Lemaitre, D. A. Conde, S. Pavard, M. Bieuville, A. O. Urrutia, B. Ujvari, A. M. Boddy, C. C. Maley, F. Thomas and M. Giraudeau (2022). "Cancer risk across mammals." *Nature* **601**(7892): 263–267.

Wagner, G. P. (2010). "The measurement theory of fitness." *Evolution* **64**(5): 1358–1376.

Wagner, G. P., C.-H. Chiu and M. Laubichler (2000). "Developmental evolution as a mechanistic science: the inference from developmental mechanisms to evolutionary processes." *Am Zool* **40**: 819–831.

Wagner, G. P. and G. B. Müller (2002). "Evolutionary innovations overcome ancestral constraints: a re-examination of character evolution in male sepsid flies (Diptera: Sepsidae)." *Evol Dev* **4**: 1–6.

Wooding, F. B. P. and G. J. Burton (2008). *Comparative Placentation.* Berlin and Heidelberg, Springer.

2 Phylogenetic and Developmental Context

BRIEF RECAP OF VERTEBRATE PHYLOGENY

This is not the place to review in any detail the phylogeny and body plan diversity of vertebrates. There are many excellent monographs and textbooks that do that, and the amount of information to cover would outstrip the size of this book. What we do want to do, however, is to provide readers less familiar with vertebrate evolution a reference about the major phylogenetic divisions of vertebrates, since taxonomic precision in communication about evolution is absolutely essential. Too often, one finds statements about "vertebrates" that are actually referring to traits shared among the jawed vertebrates (gnathostomes) only and not to the cyclostomes, which are also vertebrates, or statements about the reproduction of "mammals" that really pertain only to eutherian (placental) mammals, but not to marsupials and monotremes. Precision in taxonomic reference helps prevent flattening the complexity of evolutionary history and also points to research opportunities that arise from the comparison between, say, the placental mammals and marsupials. Needless to say, our fellow vertebrate biologists will find nothing surprising in this section and are encouraged to skip it and go to the next section, which explores less well-developed issues. It will be helpful to at least know what we think are the relevant, though not uncontroversial, facts.

Vertebrates are metazoan (= multicellular) bilaterian animals and are members of a group called chordates belonging to the deuterostomes (Figure 2.1A and B). Chordates share membership in the deuterostome clade with two highly diverged groups, the echinoderms (sea urchins, sea stars, etc.) and the acorn worms. The echinoderm body plans are so derived that the comparison between vertebrates and extant adult echinoderms is of limited value. The acorn worms are a little bit more interesting for comparative biology, as they do share some features with chordates, such as gill slits, and are thus more similar to the likely common ancestor of deuterostomes than extant echinoderms. Nevertheless, for reproductive biology, the comparisons with acorn worms are not too enlightening. Outgroup comparisons for vertebrates are thus limited to other chordates, and on those we want to focus on here.

The chordates consist of three groups: the cephalochordates (the lancelets, Amphioxus, etc.), the tunicates (including sea squirts and other highly derived groups), and the vertebrates (Figure 2.1C). Traditionally, and based on overall similarity, it was thought that cephalochordates should be the sister group of vertebrates and the tunicates the most basally branching lineage. However, molecular evidence firmly places the tunicates as the sister taxon of vertebrates (Satoh, Rokhsar et al. 2014), and the lancelets as the most basally branching lineage of chordates, as reflected in the tree in Figure 2.1C.

The cephalochordates are a small group of interesting marine invertebrates (about 25 species), the survival of which is a happy accident for comparative biology. It was through the investigation of these animals in the 19th and early 20th century that allowed Alexander Kowalevsky (1840–1901), Eli Metchnikoff (1845–1916), Berthold Hatschek (1854–1941), and others to demonstrate how the highly derived vertebrates can be understood as derived from a process of stepwise evolution from the bewildering diversity of invertebrates.

The cephalochordates display a number of features that they share with vertebrates, and which, in vertebrates, are core characters of their body plan (for the notion of "body plan" as used here see DiFrisco and Wagner 2022) (Figure 2.2A). These are a central nervous system that consists of

DOI: 10.1201/9781032717777-2

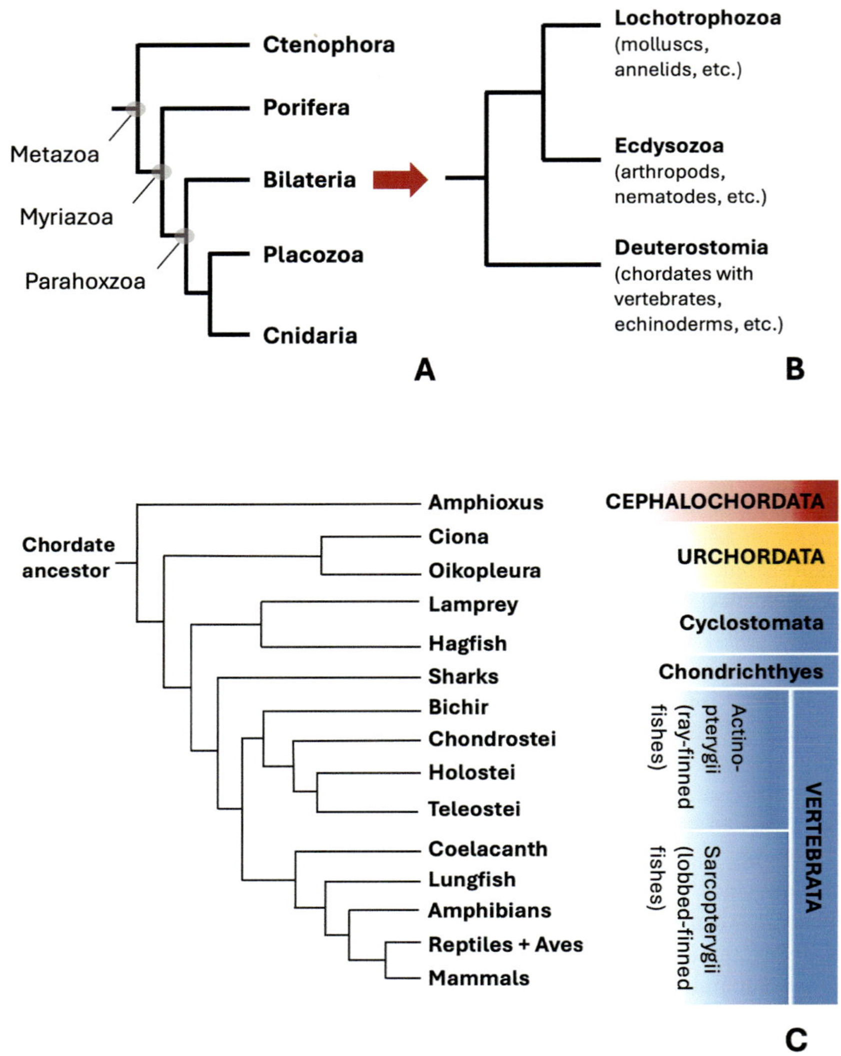

FIGURE 2.1 Simplified overview phylogeny of (A) basally branching lineages of animals (Metazoa) (after figure 4 of Schultz, Haddock et al. (2023), CC BY). (B) Simplified overview phylogeny of Bilateria (GPW). (C) Overview phylogeny of chordate animals (after figure 1 Pascual-Anaya, D'Aniello et al. (2022), CC BY).

a neural tube, a chorda dorsalis (a connective/muscular tissue rod supporting the body axis) ventral to the central nervous system, gill slits, a postanal extension of the body axis, colloquially called a "tail," segmented body musculature, as well as some less obvious characters: a homologue of the thyroid gland (the endostyle, which produces mucus to trap food particles) and a homologue of the adenohypophysis (a part of the pituitary developmentally derived from the embryonic mouth roof) which in amphioxus is called Hatschek's pit. See (Schlosser 2021) for an in-depth discussion of this character. Of course, there are many characters that are added to this basis to yield the body plan of vertebrates. The most important are: a stratified epidermis, bone tissue, a muscular heart and gut, distinct kidneys, the differentiation of the brain into the five canonical segments of vertebrate brains (telencephalon, diencephalon, mesencephalon, metencephalon, and myelencephalon), and others.

The actual sister taxon of vertebrates are the tunicates, which, in their adult anatomy, are all highly derived. These include the ascidians (sea squirts), the thaliaceans, and the larvacaeans.

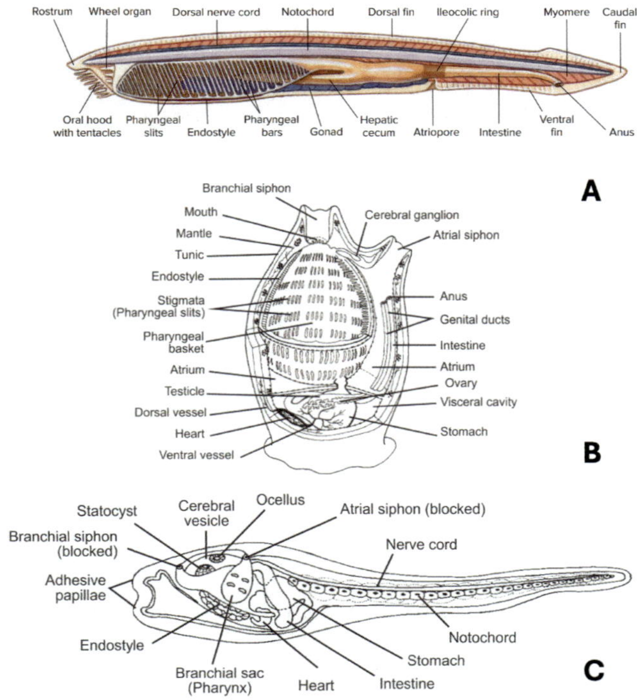

FIGURE 2.2 Overview of chordate body plans. (A) The main body parts of Amphioxus, a representative member of the Cephalochordata (Systematicist, CC BY-SA 4.0 <https://creativecommons.org/licenses/by-sa/4.0>, via Wikimedia Commons). (B) Adult body plan of an adult ascidian, a member of the Urochordata (Jon Houseman, CC BY-SA 3.0 <https://creativecommons.org/licenses/by-sa/3.0>, via Wikimedia Commons). (C) Body composition of an ascidian larva, including the larval tail, which contains a notochord and a neural tube, and segmented muscles, as is typical also for the body axis of cephalochordates and vertebrates. These traits are absent in the adult ascidian body (Jon Houseman, CC BY-SA 3.0 <https://creativecommons.org/licenses/by-sa/3.0>, via Wikimedia Commons).

Among them, the largest group are the ascidians, which, as adults, are sessile and, for that reason, assume an adult body plan that is very different from that of vertebrates and cephalochordates (Figure 2.2B). The morphological affinity of the ascidians to the other two chordate groups is only visible in their larval stage, which is pelagic and has a somewhat simplified tail with a neural tube, a notochord, and segmented musculature (Figure 2.2C). This tail, however, is lost during metamorphosis to the adult, such that the adult is much unlike any other chordate.

The other two tunicate groups, the thaliaceans and the larvacaeans, are both pelagic, i.e., are free swimming. The larvacaeans are easiest characterized as permanent ascidian larvae with a motile tail, while the thaliaceans can be thought of as "swimming ascidians" as they form a free-floating colony. Both are highly specialized for their filter-feeding pelagic lifestyle and are not particularly informative about the evolutionary origin of vertebrates.

When we now turn to the phylogeny of vertebrates we need to observe a number of major phylogenetic divisions: that between cyclostomes and jawed vertebrates (gnathostomes); that between the cartilaginous fishes (chondrichtyes) and the bony fish (or better "bony vertebrates," Osteichthyes); within Osteichthyes that between the ray-finned fishes (Actinopterygia) and the lobed (fleshy) finned fishes (Sarcopterygia) (Figure 2.3A). Within the Sarcopterygia, the main group are the tetrapods, which are joined with two minor groups, the lungfish (Dipnoi) and the two species of Coelacanths (*Latimeria chalumnae* and *L. menadoensis*). Within the tetrapods, the important split is between amphibians and amniotes (Figure 2.3B). Of note here is the fact that taxonomic terms can be

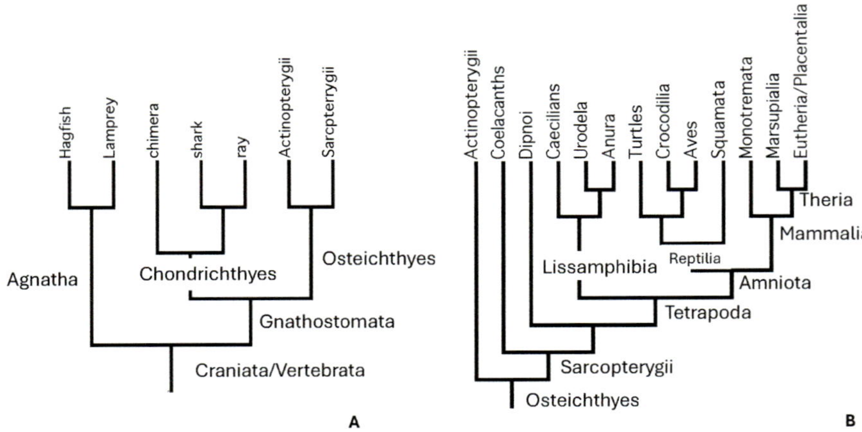

FIGURE 2.3 Overview of phylogenetic trees of the main vertebrate groups. (A) The major groups of vertebrates and their phylogenetic relationships (by GPW, CC BY). (B) The major groups of the bony vertebrates (Osteichthyes) and their phylogenetic relationships (by GPW, CC BY).

confusing. For instance, the bony fishes include all the descendants of the most recent common ancestor of ray-finned and lobed finned "fishes," and these include tetrapods, including humans; yes, my reader, you are a bony fish and a lobed finned body fish for good measure, technically speaking.

Of all these major groups, the amniotes play a special role in our exploration of the fetal-maternal relationship, since this clade encompasses the two groups with the most extensive research on viviparity and placentation, the mammals and the squamate reptiles.

In most chordates and "lower" vertebrates (meaning "fishes" and amphibians), the fertilized egg more or less directly develops into the embryo, and that into the free-living organism. There are no tissues other than the embryo itself and the yolk sac in animals where the yolk cannot be directly incorporated into the body of the embryo. For instance, frogs have a relatively large egg with a good amount of yolk, but during gastrulation, the yolk-bearing cells are nevertheless incorporated into the body of the embryo. In contrast, in many fishes, the embryo develops on top of the yolk mass, which is kept outside the body and surrounded by extra-embryonic tissue, the so-called yolk sac. The latter serves as the organ to mobilize the nutrients in the yolk to be used by the embryo. Most of the oviparous amphibians and "fishes" have their eggs develop in the water. In contrast, the amniotes are the vertebrate group that emancipated themselves from the need to have their eggs develop in water and also have evolved a complicated system of additional extra-embryonic tissues, which also became important in the evolution of reptilian and mammalian viviparity. These include a protective tissue bubble around the embryo, called the amnion, which also gave the name to the taxon. The other extraembryonic tissues will be described further down in this chapter.

The group of amniotes is divided into two major clades, called Reptilia and Mammalia. The reptiles include the Lepidosauria (tuataras and squamates, i.e., lizards, snakes, and amphisbaenians) and the Archosauria (turtles, crocodilians, and birds) (Figure 2.3B). The mammals consist of three major clades: the monotremes (the egg-laying mammals), the marsupials (aka Metatheria; opossums, koalas, kangaroos, and their relatives), as well as the eutherian mammals, also sometimes called placental mammals (all the species that evolved from the most recent common ancestor of humans and elephants (Figure 2.3C)). We will avoid the term placental mammals because marsupials also, technically, have placentas.

Monotremes are a group of only five species, found in Australia and the neighboring islands, such as New Zealand and New Guinea (Griffiths 1978). The two body types are the Platypus, one species, and four species of hedgehog-like echidnas. Biologically, they represent a combination of reptilian and mammalian characteristics. The plesiomorphic characters include egg laying and a rather reptilian shoulder girdle, yet they have hair, like all the other mammals, three middle ear bones, and they lactate. The latter, though, is not through nipples or teats; rather their milk is secreted broadly from specialized hair organs into the belly fur, where the young are licking it off the hair of the mother (Renfree and Shaw 2002). Milk secretion is thought to have evolved initially as a way to keep the eggs moist during incubation and was taken up by the young after hatching and thus transformed from moistening to a nutritional role. Unfortunately, research on monotreme reproduction is limited in part because of their highly protected status, even though they are not particularly rare.

Marsupials and eutherians form the clade of therians, i.e., are sister taxa (Hunsaker 1977). Most of the 334 extant marsupial species live in Australia and the neighboring islands. The other area of diversification is the Americas, with most species in South and Middle America and one species in North America (the Virginia Opossum, *Didelphis virginiana*). They share live birth with eutherians, although their female reproductive biology is different in important and highly informative ways (Renfree and Shaw 2002, Renfree 2010). The comparison between marsupials and mammals will play a major role in the discussion of the evolution of eutherian reproduction and will be discussed in the next chapter.

The eutherian mammals include all the descendants of the most recent common ancestor of humans and elephants and comprise the largest share of mammalian diversity, with estimates of species numbers between 4,000 and 5,000 species. The eutherian mammalian lineage diverged from the marsupial lineage between 143 and 178 million years (Reilly and White 2003, Luo, Yuan et al. 2011), and with the marsupial most recent common ancestor at about 74 to 89 million years, and for eutherians about 84 million years ago (Meredith, Westerman et al. 2008). That means that we have for both the marsupials and the eutherians about 100 million years long stem lineages. The additive divergence between the most recent common ancestors of marsupials and eutherians is about 200 million years, which is a long evolutionary history that is not accessible through comparison of extant species, which affects our ability to understand the steps in the evolution of the respective reproductive modes.

Among the eutherians, the deepest split is between the clades of the Atlantogenata and the Boreoeutheria (Figure 2.4). The former contains the Afrotheria with elephants as the most charismatic species, but also includes hyrax, the dugong, tenrecs, and others. In addition, the sister taxon of Afrotheria within the Atlantogenata is the Xenarthra, with armadillo as the best-known species, and including also anteaters and sloths, for example. The Boreoeutheria, on the other hand, contains all of the better-known groups of mammals, such as primates, rodents, bats, carnivores, and the hoofed animals known as "farm animals" (cattle, sheep, pigs, etc.). To learn about the very early stages of eutherian evolution, a comparison between Boreoeutheria and Atlantogenata is essential. Most reproductive biology is known from humans and very few rodents, in addition to a deep literature on farm animals, with comparatively little on carnivore reproductive biology. In contrast, there is very limited molecular and cell biological literature on the reproduction of Atlantogenata, as there is no laboratory model species available. Work on elephants, dugongs, and similar species is difficult, to say the least. It will require special efforts in the coming decades to fill these knowledge gaps. Some hope comes from tenrecs, which are small enough to be held in laboratories, but still are far from ideal laboratory animals. The nine-banded Armadillo is an abundant nuisance species in the United States and thus at least accessible to field collecting. There is a limited literature on tenrecs (Carter, Enders et al. 2004, Stadtmauer, Basanta et al. 2025), which belong to the Afrotheria, as well as on armadillos (e.g., Enders 1960, Rezende, Barbeito et al. 2012, Chavan and Wagner 2016), which belong to Xenarthra.

Although all extant eutherian species have the same amount of evolution under their belt, at least in terms of their cumulative evolutionary history, Afrotheria nevertheless include species with clearly primitive characteristics. For instance, the tenrec *Echinops telfairii* has a classical cloaca, like reptiles and birds (Riedelsheimer, Unterberger et al. 2007). A broader taxon sampling of

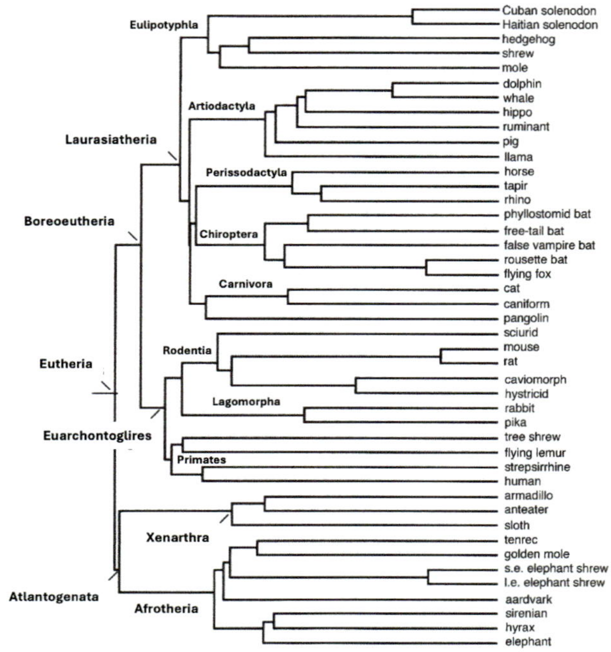

FIGURE 2.4 Phylogenetic relationships among the main lineages of eutherian mammals. (Image is figure 6 of Murphy, Pringle et al. (2007) published under CC BY-NC license, modified by relabeling the main clades.)

Atlantogenata species would thus be highly informative of the early stages of eutherian reproductive biology.

The above brief summary is meant as a point of orientation for the meaning of the taxonomic names used in this book. If the reader wants to know more about what distinguishes each of these groups, I refer them to textbooks of vertebrate biology (Kardong 2014, Linzey 2020).

A SURVEY OF FEMALE REPRODUCTIVE TRACT ANATOMY OF VERTEBRATES

The genital tract of any animal has at least two fundamental tasks: producing the sex cells (gametes, egg cells, or sperm), and releasing them from the body. These two functions suffice for animals where fertilization is happening outside the body, and consequently, the development of the offspring also occurs outside the body of the female, including mouth brooding and placentation in the pouch of male sea horses. Internal fertilization and eventually viviparity necessitate additional complications of the genital tract. But let us first consider the anatomical and developmental situation for vertebrates with external fertilization, such as "fishes" and other vertebrates, all the way to amphibians.[1] Before we do that, we have to mention another functional system that in vertebrates is closely related to and entangled with the genital tract: the excretory system, i.e., the system that produces urine and has as its primary function the elimination of nitrogenous waste as well as osmoregulation. The excretory system is similar to the reproductive system in that it produces a "product" (urine) that has to find a way out of the body.

As it happens, in vertebrates, both the reproductive system and the excretory system, use the same anatomical substrate to achieve the elimination of their "products" from the body, which is also related to the embryonic origin of their sites of "production," i.e., the gonads (ovary and testis) and the kidney (or better the glomeruli where blood filtration happens). Both the gonads and the kidney differentiate in the same region of the embryonic body, at the dorso-medial region of the splanchnic coelom, i.e., the secondary body cavity around the abdominal organs. These are the

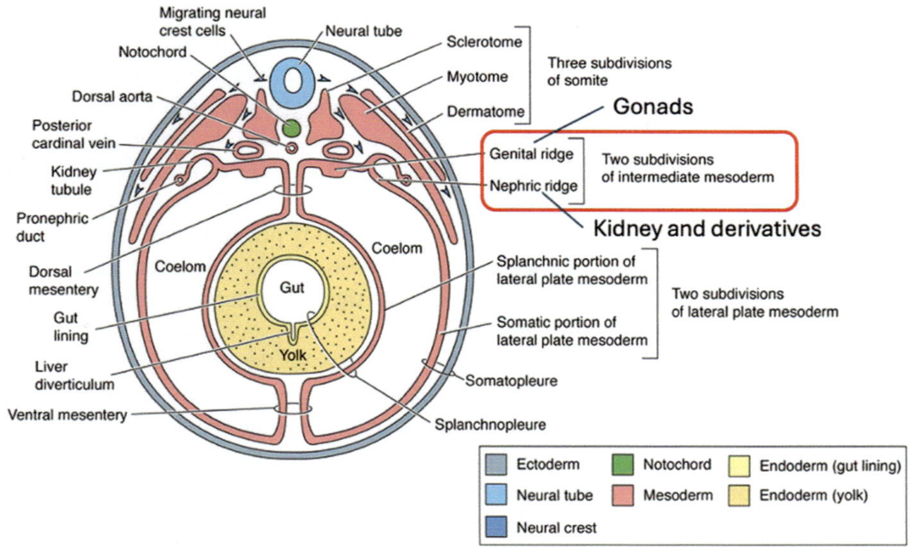

FIGURE 2.5 Schematic cross section of an amphibian larva at the stage where the somites separate from the lateral plate mesoderm. At that stage, we see at the dorsal end of the lateral plate mesoderm, the so-called intermediate mesoderm, consisting of the genital ridge and the nephric ridge. The genital ridge gives rise to the gonads, ovaries, and testicles, and the nephric ridge gives rise to the kidney. (From Liem, Bemis et al. (2000), with permission ©Willy Bemis 2025.)

genital ridge and the nephric ridge, respectively (Figure 2.5). Putting a large amount of comparative anatomical and phylogenetic evidence to work suggests that both gonads and "kidneys" ancestrally released their products into the splanchnic coelom (i.e., the abdominal body cavity) and from there somehow outside. This is, for instance, the case with lampreys (cyclostome), where the gametes are released into the coelom and then released via a *coelomoporus* into the end of the gut. Also, the space into which the glomeruli filtrate is released is in open communication with the coelom (Romer and Parsons 1997, Richardson, Admiraal et al. 2010). This is the reason why, in vertebrates, we speak of the urogenital system, i.e., a system where excretory and reproductive functions are deeply intertwined. Much of the evolution of the urogenital system is the evolution of more efficient and secure ways to lead urine and gametes out of the body, and much of what we call the genital tract is the product of an evolutionary cooption of parts of the urinary system.

It seems that the excretory system took the lead in evolving ways, beyond coelomoporus, to eliminate its product from the body cavity, and the evolution of the genital tract consists in coopting these anatomical innovations for reproductive functions. To make this plausible, let us consider the situation in the lamprey, a member of the most basally branching lineage of vertebrates (see above). As mentioned above, in lamprey, the gametes are released into the abdominal cavity and then exported through a coelomoporus that opens between the body cavity and the end of the gut. This means that the lamprey only has gonads but no specialized reproductive ducts, like oviduct or uterus. Similarly, the primary filtrate (aka the primary urine) in lamprey is also released into the abdominal cavity and is then streamed by ciliary action into a separate opening in the body cavity and led into a urinary canal which ends close to the opening of the gut. That means that the transport of urine already has a dedicated structure, while the gametes do not.

In contrast to the situation in lamprey, all gnathostomes have specialized ducts for the transport of sperm or egg cells or early embryos.[2] The variation revealed by the comparative anatomy of the urogenital system of vertebrates is very interesting and complex and goes beyond what we can cover here (Major, Estermann et al. 2022). In brief, the ray-finned fishes have genital tubes and structures that seem to have arisen independently from those of cartilaginous fishes and tetrapods. In tetrapods, the female reproductive tract is derived from a tube that runs in parallel to the urinary tract and is either called the para-mesonephric tract or Müllerian tract (named after Johannes Peter Müller, 1801–1858). This is likely a coopted urinary tract, as it also opens into the body cavity and picks up the gametes just as primitively the urinary tracts open into the body cavity and pick up the primary urine of the glomerulus (Major, Estermann et al. 2022). In fact, the oviduct of human females, which differentiates from the Müllerian duct, still opens into the body cavity and picks up the egg cell and transports it into the uterus. This is a remarkably primitive trait that makes humans vulnerable to abdominal cavity pregnancies and endometriosis. This is in contrast to, for example, mice, which managed to permanently fuse the oviduct to the ovary, permanently closing the opening between the coelomic cavity and the outside world.

There is a similar duct in elasmobranchs (sharks and relatives) that has been hypothesized to be homologous to the Müllerian duct of tetrapods. It shows a similar embryonic development as the Müllerian duct in tetrapods, but the number of characters connecting the shark structure with that of tetrapods is low (Felix and Bühler 1906). The difficulty is also that the ray-finned fishes do not seem to have a structure similar to the Müllerian duct, and it is thus possible that the sharks have an independently evolved a "Müllerian duct" analog, rather than having the same structure as tetrapods. It is also thinkable that the ray-finned fishes lost the Müllerian duct and replaced it with a different structure, but that would require one to understand why such a transition would happen. At this point, it is more likely that the sharks have an independently derived paramesonephric duct that is not homologous to the Müllerian duct of tetrapods (Major, Estermann et al. 2022).

The Müllerian duct eventually differentiates, in parallel with the reproductive mode and thus with the roles that it fulfills: either only internal fertilization, combined with forming a shell for the fertilized egg, or incubating the embryo, to name just familiar modes. Up to five different segments are known in tetrapods (Schatten and Constantienscu 2007): the opening or infundibulum, which forms also the opening of the duct to the body cavity, which has the task of capturing the ovulated egg cell; then the oviduct,[3] in which, in many species, fertilization occurs, and which leads the ovum to the uterus. The uterus is demarcated toward the posterior by the cervix, a barrier structure between the uterus and the vagina. The cervix exists in many but not all tetrapods. For instance, armadillos and tenrecs do not have a distinct cervix, but a utero-vaginal canal. This is often the case in species where the male is ejaculating into the uterus or even the oviduct and thus would not be able to do so in the presence of a cervix. Caudal to the cervix comes the vagina, the anterior part of which is derived from the Müllerian duct and developmentally different from the posterior part of the vagina that eventually opens into the urogenital sinus or the remnant of it, the vestibulum (see Pavličev, Herdina et al. (2022) for an overview of mammalian external genitalia).

Embryologically, the Müllerian duct is a paired structure, as are the ovaries (Felix and Bühler 1906). Hence ancestrally, and retained in many mammalian species, the Müllerian duct derivatives are also paired. For instance, the opossum has two oviducts (as all other amniotes that retain two ovaries, which is not the case in birds and snakes, for instance), two uterine tubes, and two cervices (Tyndale-Biscoe and Renfree 1987). Such a situation is called uterus duplex, a complete pair of uteri. In most eutherian mammals, however, at least the cervix is fused into a single structure, and often also the posterior part of the uterus. This is called a bi-cornuate uterus. An example of such anatomy is present in the laboratory mouse: a uterus with a small unpaired segment, called the uterine body, and paired uterine "horns." In a smaller number of species, the uterus completely fuses, forming a triangular "uterus simplex" as is known for humans and many other primates. This situation is, however, not limited to primates, as the armadillos also evolved a uterus simplex. A casual examination of the phylogenetic relationships among placental mammals (Figure 2.3C) convinces us that the uterus simplex in armadillos has to be independently derived from that in primates. The different degrees of fusion of the uterine and cervical structures as seen among species are paralleled by anatomical variation in humans. Although most women have a uterus simplex, there are rare cases of women with a complete duplication, a uterus duplex, or a bi-cornuate uterus (Verkauf 1993).

Oviparous amniotes also differentiate their Müllerian ducts into specialized segments, as the therian mammals do (Lombardi 1998). In birds, the different segments are specialized in providing different vestments to the egg, like albumin or the calcified eggshell in birds. In the chicken, one distinguishes five segments: the infundibulum, the magnum where the egg receives its albumin (egg-white), the isthmus, the shell gland, and the utero-vaginal junction, followed by the so-called vagina. There is some evidence that the magnum and isthmus correspond to the oviduct, the shell gland to the uterus, and the utero-vaginal junction to the cervix of viviparous amniotes.

The Müllerian duct is the maternal anatomical substrate for the evolution of viviparity in amniotes. The other substrates are the extraembryonic tissues provided by the embryo that, eventually together with the derivatives of Müllerian duct, will form the fetal-maternal unit. We will next briefly summarize the various extraembryonic vestments of the amniote embryo.

THE EXTRA-EMBRYONIC STRUCTURES

As mentioned in the first section of this chapter, when we introduced the clade of amniotes, the most widely distributed extra-embryonic tissue is the yolk sac, which is found in vertebrate embryos with large endowments of yolk, i.e., when the amount of yolk is too large to fit into the body of the gastrulating embryo. As such, the yolk sac is a bulge of the embryonic gut and thus is composed of embryonic endoderm covered by ectoderm (Figure 2.6). The yolk sac is not only the organ that stores the yolk and mobilizes it for embryo use, but is also the primary location for the development of blood cells (hematopoiesis) and vascular endothelial cells (angiogenesis) (Carlson 2014), and where the germ cells are set aside. For that reason, the yolk sac is also found in species where the egg has no

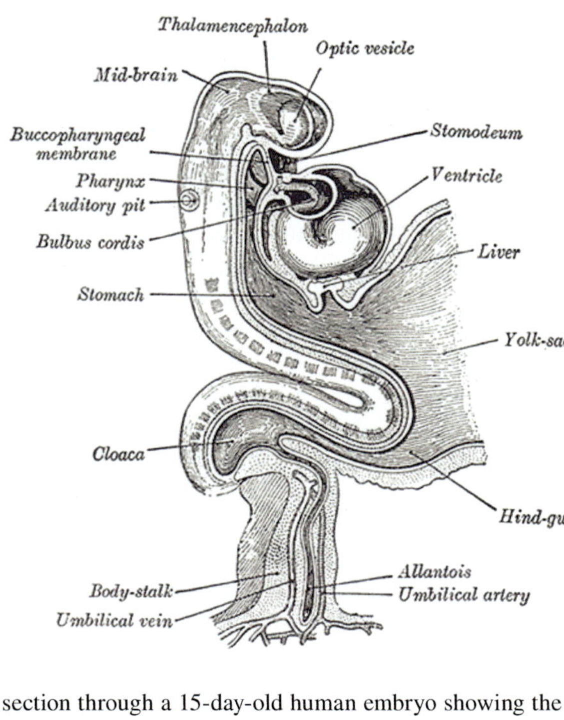

FIGURE 2.6 Sagittal section through a 15-day-old human embryo showing the attachment of the yolk sac to the embryonic gut. Hence, the yolk sac is an outpocketing of the embryonic gut. A second outpocketing of the gut is the allantois, which is visible posterior to the yolk sac. The allantois gives rise to the placenta and the umbilical cord in humans. (Image by Henry Vandyke Carter, Public domain, via Wikimedia Commons.)

yolk at all, like in all eutherian species. The function of the yolk reservoir has been replaced by the placenta, but its role for hematopoiesis, angiogenesis and germ cell differentiation still requires the development of the yolk sac, a classic case of a developmental constraint due to "burden" (*sensu* Riedl 1978), a structure cannot be lost because it retained some developmental function even after its apparent "primary" function was lost.

As an organ specialized for the mobilization and uptake of nutrients, the yolk sac is also an ideal anatomical substrate for the evolution of a placenta, i.e., an organ of fetal-maternal exchange and communication. In fact, some shark species, after exhausting the yolk, attach with their empty yolk sac to the uterine wall and form a placenta, as one in a bewildering variety of ways in which viviparous sharks nourish their developing feti (Wourms 1977, Hamlett 1989).

In amniotes, the yolk sac is joined by two other types of extraembryonic organs: the amnion and the allantois (Carlson 2014). The amnion, giving the name to the clade, develops as a fold of the peri-embryonic ectoderm that gradually grows over the embryo and eventually surrounds it, forming a protective bubble. At least that is the sequence of events one can see in the development of the chicken embryo and other reptiles. In eutherians, an amnion also exists but develops differently, as described further below.

The allantois is, like the yolk sac, also an out-pocketing of the embryonic gut, originating more toward the posterior end of the gut than the yolk sac (Figure 2.6). It grows out toward the surface of the extraembryonic cover and performs two functions. On the one hand, it is the storage structure for the embryo's urine[4] (the chicken cannot go to the bathroom while in the eggshell), and postnatally, the urinary bladder develops from internal structures continuous with the allantois. On the other hand, it is highly vascularized and functions as an extra-embryonic lung. The latter fact also predisposes the allantois to become the main form of placenta for oxygen, nutrients, and waste exchange.

All through the development of these three extra-embryonic organs, the outermost cover of the amniote embryo forms, which is called the chorion. It is a composite structure of extra-embryonic ectoderm and mesoderm that surrounds the whole embryo, including the extra-embryonic organs. In placental species, it is the surface that is in direct contact with maternal tissues and thus the locus of various innovations to manage the fetal-maternal relationship. Its fusion with underlying extra-embryonic membranes (yolk sac and/or allantois) provides the chorion with extensive vasculature and enables the feto-maternal exchange of viviparous amniotes.

The short summary of the various extraembryonic tissues, as viewed from an avian and reptilian perspective, is relatively logical in its topology and developmental sequence (see Ramsey 1982). However, this mode of development is not what one sees in the development of a eutherian species such as mice and humans (Carlson 2014). One could speak of an eutherian revolution when it comes to early embryonic developmental processes. While in the chicken egg, the first steps are the formation of the embryo and then the stepwise addition of extra-embryonic structures; the eutherian embryo has completely reorganized the sequence of events. After fertilization and cleavage divisions, the embryo transforms into a so-called blastocyst. The blastocyst consists of an outer cell layer that harbors a fluid-filled cavity and a so-called inner cell mass. The outer cell layer is called the trophoblast or trophectoderm and eventually forms the outer layer of the chorion, and the inner cell mass is the source of cells for the other extra-embryonic membranes and the embryo proper. Hence, the very first cell fate decision in the eutherian development is that between one part of the extra-embryonic membranes, the trophoblast, and all the rest. Next, the yolk sac and the amnion form, but still no proper embryo. The embryo finally forms from the contact zone between the amnion and the yolk sac. This happens through a form of gastrulation. This radical re-organization of the first steps in embryogenesis (better even: extra-embryogenesis) makes it so hard to understand and compare eutherian early development with that of other amniotes. On the side, it should be noted that the early marsupial embryo is similar to the eutherian, except that the first embryo is a hollow ball, and the cells of the inner cell mass segregate from that ball a little later by immigrating into the lumen of the blastula-like ball of cells (Tyndale-Biscoe and Renfree 1987).

With this brief overview, let us dive into the subject matter of viviparity in the next chapter.

NOTES

1. Notably, in this range of species, i.e., "fish" to amphibians, includes various lineages where internal fertilization and viviparity have evolved independently.
2. The "chicken egg" is, if fertilized, actually an embryo.
3. In much of the literature, the term "oviduct" is used interchangeably with the whole Müllerian duct. We find this terminology confusing and inaccurate and limit the term oviduct to that segment of the Mullerian duct which communicates between the ostium and the uterus.
4. At least this is the traditional interpretation. However, this theory has been challenged by investigations of the composition of the sheep allantoic fluid (see Bazer, F. W. (1989). Allantoic fluid: regulation of volume and composition. *Fetal and Neonatal Body Fluids.* R. A. Brace. Cornell, NY, Perinatology Press: 135–157.). This is interesting but does not exclude the possibility that the ancestral function in oviparous species was in fact waste storage.

REFERENCES

Bazer, F. W. (1989). Allantoic fluid: regulation of volume and composition. *Fetal and Neonatal Body Fluids.* R. A. Brace. Cornell, NY, Perinatology Press**:** 135–157.

Carlson, B. M. (2014). *Human Embryology and Developmental Biology.* Philadelphia, Elsevier.

Carter, A. M., A. C. Enders, H. Kunzle, D. Oduor-Okelo and P. Vogel (2004). "Placentation in species of phylogenetic importance: the Afrotheria." *Anim Reprod Sci* **82–83**: 35–48.

Chavan, A. R. and G. P. Wagner (2016). "The fetal-maternal interface of the nine-banded armadillo: endothelial cells of maternal sinus are partially replaced by trophoblast." *Zoological Lett* **2**: 11.

DiFrisco, J. and G. P. Wagner (2022). "Body plan identity: a mechanistic model." *Evol Biol* **49**(2): 123–141.

Enders, A. C. (1960). "Development and structure of the villous haemochorial placenta of the nine-banded armadillo (Dasypus novemcinctus)." *J Anat* **94**: 34–45.

Felix, W. and A. Bühler (1906). Entwicklung der Ableitungswege der beiden Keimdrüsen. *Handbuch der vergleichenden Entwicklungslehre der Wirbeltiere.* O. Hertwig. Jena, Germany, Verl. Gustav Fischer. **3 part 1:** 742–820.

Griffiths, M. (1978). *The Biology and Monotremes.* San Diego, CA, Academic Press.

Hamlett, W. C. (1989). "Evolution and morphogenesis of the placenta in sharks." *J Exp Zool*: 35–52.

Hunsaker, D. (1977). *The Biology of Marsupials.* New York, Academic Press.

Kardong, K. (2014). *Vertebrates: Comparative Anatomy, Function, Evolution.* New York, McGraw-Hill.

Liem, K., W. Bemis, W. F. Walker and L. Grande (2000). *Functional Anatomy of the Vertebrates: An Evolutionary Perspective.* Independence, KY, Cengage Learning.

Linzey, D. W. (2020). *Vertebrate Biology: Systematics, Taxonomy, Natural History, and Conservation.* Baltimore, Maryland, Johns Hopkins University Press.

Lombardi, J. (1998). *Comparative Verbebrate Reproduction.* Boston, Kluwer Academic Publishers.

Luo, Z. X., C. X. Yuan, Q. J. Meng and Q. Ji (2011). "A Jurassic eutherian mammal and divergence of marsupials and placentals." *Nature* **476**(7361): 442–445.

Major, A. T., M. A. Estermann, Z. Y. Roly and C. A. Smith (2022). "An evo-devo perspective of the female reproductive tract." *Biol Reprod* **106**(1): 9–23.

Meredith, R. W., M. Westerman, J. A. Case and M. S. Springer (2008). "A phylogeny and timescale for marsupial evolution based on sequences for five nuclear genes." *J Mamm Evol* **15**(1): 1–36.

Murphy, W. J., T. H. Pringle, T. A. Crider, M. S. Springer and W. Miller (2007). "Using genomic data to unravel the root of the placental mammal phylogeny." *Genome Res* **17**(4): 413–421.

Pascual-Anaya, J., S. D'Aniello and S. Bertrand (2022). "Editorial: new approaches in Chordate and vertebrate evolution and development." *Front Cell Dev Biol* **10**: 917101.

Pavlicev, M., A. N. Herdina and G. Wagner (2022). "Female genital variation far exceeds that of male genitalia: a review of comparative anatomy of clitoris and the female lower reproductive tract in Theria." *Integr Comp Biol* **62**(3): 581–601.

Ramsey, E. M. (1982). *The Placenta. Human and Animal.* Santa Barbara, CA, Praeger Inc.

Reilly, S. M. and T. D. White (2003). "Hypaxial motor patterns and the function of epipubic bones in primitive mammals." *Science* **299**(5605): 400–402.

Renfree, M. and G. Shaw (2002). Reproduction in monotremes and marsupials. *Encyclopedia of Life Sciences.* New York, Wiley and Sons**:** 1–5.

Renfree, M. B. (2010). "Marsupials: placental mammals with a difference." *Placenta* **31**: S21–S26.

Rezende, L. C., C. G. Barbeito, P. O. Favaron, A. Mess and M. A. Miglino (2012). "The fetomaternal interface in the placenta of three species of armadillos (Eutheria, Xenarthra, Dasypodidae)." *Reprod Biol Endocrinol* **10**: 38.

Richardson, M. K., J. Admiraal and G. M. Wright (2010). "Developmental anatomy of lampreys." *Biol Rev Camb Philos Soc* **85**(1): 1–33.

Riedelsheimer, B., P. Unterberger, H. Künzle and U. Welsch (2007). "Histological study of the cloacal region and associated structures in the hedgehog tenrec Echinops telfairi." *Mamm Biol* **72**(6): 330–341.

Riedl, R. (1978). *Order in Living Organisms: A Systems Analysis of Evolution*. New York, Wiley.

Romer, A. S. and T. S. Parsons (1997). *The Vertebrate Body*. New York, Harcourt Brace Jovanovich College Publishers.

Satoh, N., D. Rokhsar and T. Nishikawa (2014). "Chordate evolution and the three-phylum system." *Proc Biol Sci* **281**(1794): 20141729.

Schatten, H. and G. H. Constantienscu (2007). *Comparative Reproductive Biology*. Ames, Iowa, Blackwell Pub.

Schlosser, G. (2021). *Development of Sensory and Neurosecretory Cell Types: Vertebrate Cranial Placodes, Volume 1 (Evolutionary Cell Biology)*. Boca Raton, FL, CRC Press.

Schultz, D. T., S. H. D. Haddock, J. V. Bredeson, R. E. Green, O. Simakov and D. S. Rokhsar (2023). "Ancient gene linkages support ctenophores as sister to other animals." *Nature* **618**(7963): 110-117.

Stadtmauer, D. J., S. Basanta, J. D. Maziarz, A. G. Cole, G. Dagdas, G. R. Smith, F. van Breukelen, M. Pavlicev and G. P. Wagner (2025). "Cell type and cell signalling innovations underlying mammalian pregnancy." *Nat Ecol Evol* **9**: 1469–1486.

Tyndale-Biscoe, C. H. and M. B. Renfree (1987). *Reproductive Physiology of Marsupials*. Cambridge, UK, Cambridge University Press.

Verkauf, B. S. (1993). *Congenital Malformations of the Female Reproductive Tract and their Treatment*. Appleton & Lange.

Wourms, J. P. (1977). "Reproduction and development in chondrichthyan fishes." *Amer Zool* **17**: 379–410.

3 The Many Faces of Viviparity

Viviparity, as mentioned in Chapter 1, is one of these biological concepts that has a simple meaning but hides tremendous biological complexity and diversity (or rather "disparity" to be precise). It simply means that the offspring leaves the maternal body as a free-living animal, a larva or a juvenile, rather than encased in an egg covering. But this simple and even operational definition does not mean that "viviparity" is a unitary biological trait. In fact, it is not a trait at all, but a collection of biologically different modes of female reproduction. In this chapter, we will put some substance to this claim in order to prevent over-simplified "explanations" of "viviparity as such."

DIMENSIONS, MODES, AND CATEGORIES IN FEMALE REPRODUCTION

Here, we first want to situate viviparity within the wide variety of female reproductive modalities. To get a handle on this variation, it is useful to introduce concepts that both capture the scope and provide structure to this variation. First are "dimensions." Dimensions are ranges of biological conditions that "structurally" vary independently of each other. Structural independence does not imply statistical independence but only means that all combinations of the states of the two dimensions are biologically possible and realized. The most important dimensions, as conceptualized by Blackburn, are (1) the way the embryo and the fetus are provisioned with nutrients, and (2) in what form the reproductive product leaves the body of the mother, i.e., either an egg or a free-living individual (Blackburn 1992, 2000, 2015). Let us consider these two dimensions in turn.

Fetal provisioning spans the range between full lecitotrophy to full matrotrophy. In the case of lecitotrophy, all the nutritional resources are provided in the egg yolk, i.e., are invested into the egg cell before fertilization. On the other hand, matrotrophy is any provisioning of the developing offspring by the mother after fertilization. Most often, this term is used for maternal provisioning during the prenatal period, which could be called fetal or prenatal matrotrophy. Of course, in many animals, maternal provisioning continues after birth or hatching by other means. In mammals, it takes the form of lactation, whereas in birds it takes the form of feeding of nestlings. It can also include specialized secretions in birds that are not coming from structures homologous to mammary glands, such as the crop milk of pigeons. In this chapter, however, we will limit ourselves to prenatal matrotrophy.

Lecitotrophy and matrotrophy are extremes of a range of possibilities rather than categorical alternatives. It is easy to see that it is possible to have an egg with yolk, but which is insufficient to support development all the way to hatching (after oviposition) or parturition. In this case, the resources available to the fetus need to be supplemented by matrotrophy in one way or another. One could thus easily envision different degrees of lecitotrophy and matrotrophy combined in one species. For mammals, a striking example is the monotremes, which are oviparous but start with an egg that has less biomass than the eventual hatchling. It is thus clear that the female reproductive tract must be producing secretions that can diffuse through the egg covering and be taken up by the fetus, increasing its resource base that lasts through to the post-oviposition period of incubation.

While the relative amount of matrotrophic resources provided is a one-dimensional range from 0% to 100% matrotrophy, the modes of matrotrophic provisioning include at least two categorical alternatives (Blackburn 2015). On the one hand, there is phagotrophy,[1] on the other, there is placentotrophy. One can also say that placentotrophy is a direct maternal-fetal transfer of material to the fetal bloodstream, while phagotrophy is indirect, where the fetus is actively acquiring and ingesting resources in one way or another.

DOI: 10.1201/9781032717777-3

Phagotrophy includes oophagy, the feeding of a fetus on additionally ovulated eggs. This is nicely documented for the shortfin mako sharks (*Isurus oxyrinchus*) and the porbeagle (*Lama nasus*).[2]. A more violent variety of phagotrophy is "embryophagy," also sometimes called "adelphophagy" or "siblicide," and consists of eating siblings while inside the mother's body (Gilmore et al. 2005). This is known to occur, for instance, in the gray nurse shark (*Carcharias taurus*), which eventually gives birth to two large neonates, only one from each uterus. Phagotrophy also includes actively ingesting parts of maternal tissue or maternal secretions.

Placentotrophy, in contrast, consists of the transfer of nutrients from the mother to the embryo via direct contact between fetal and maternal tissues. A widely used and broad definition of a placenta is that of Mossman: "an intimate apposition or fusion of fetal organs to the maternal (or paternal, in the case of seahorses) tissues for physiological exchange" (Mossman 1937). While very general and aiming to cover a wide variety of fetal-maternal relationships, it is also not entirely satisfactory. One reason is that it is inconsistent with the usual notion of a placenta, as representing only the fetal part of the fetal-maternal unit. There are other uses of the term "placenta" which include fetal as well as maternal structures, but those are minority positions. The other problem is the ambiguous notion of "fusion" in Mossman's formulation. What constitutes a fusion? Does this require cell fusion, as is the case in the sheep or bandicoots? In what sense is the destruction of part of the maternal endometrium, so common in eutherian pregnancy, a fusion?

Given these difficulties, one may be tempted to slightly modify Mossman's definition by saying: "a placenta is a fetal structure that is integrated into a biological unit with maternal or paternal structures dedicated to the physiological exchange of nutrients, oxygen, and waste products." This re-formulation avoids the ambiguous notion of fusion by replacing it with "integration." The inclusion of "paternal" tissues is intended to cover examples of male pregnancies, such as in seahorses and pipe fishes (Wilson et al. 2001). The integration in this definition individualizes a phenomenon, which underwent the main diversification. The type of integration is therefore the most pressing to understand. Integration can be only physiological without structural integration, or it can include major remodeling of the maternal tissue, as in the case of the human placental bed. Physiological integration without structural integration covers cases where the fetal and maternal cells are engaged in an exchange of cell-cell signals and provisioning of nutrients and oxygen, but only via apposition with each other. An example is the wallaby placenta, which consists of fetal membranes in apposition with the luminal epithelium of the uterus.

Cell biological integration would be true attachment of fetal epithelia and maternal uterine epithelia, mediated via a molecular bridge connecting fetal and maternal cells. An example is the placenta of the pig, which is connected to the luminal epithelium via integrin–osteopontin bridges (Johnson et al. 2021). Another form of cell biological integration is the formation of heterokaryons, i.e., the fusion of maternal and fetal cells as described in the sheep (Wooding and Burton 2008).

Finally, the most radical integration of fetal and maternal tissues consists of the invasive, hemochorial placentae of eutherian mammals. In this case, the maternal tissue is greatly remodeled from the mucosal covering of the uterine cavity into the "decidua" and integrated with an often highly derived placental organ. The latter consists of novel structural arrangements forged from parts of the fetal membranes. Examples are the mouse and human placentae, where the fetal membranes are transformed into a distinct organ with a highly specialized internal structure (Figure 3.1A and B). A less radical form a fetal-maternal integration is exemplified by the situation in ruminants (e.g., cattle and sheep), where the uterus has preformed tissue structures, called caruncles, which during pregnancy interdigitate with parts of the fetal membranes forming multiple placentomes (Ramsey 1982, Wooding and Burton 2008).

The other dimension of female reproductive variety we mentioned is the nature of the reproductive product leaving the maternal body: either an egg, i.e., oviparity, or a free-living individual, i.e., viviparity. This dimension of female reproductive modes seems to be categorical, either an egg or a free neonate. Yet this definition nevertheless hides a continuum of possibilities. The point is that

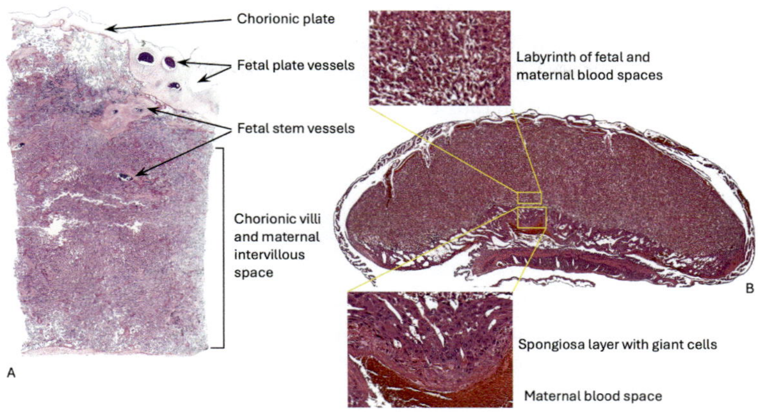

FIGURE 3.1 (A) Section of part of the human placenta. The placental surface consists of treelike branched extensions, called villi, that extend into a space filled with maternal blood (from Harvey Kliman, Yale University, with permission). (B) Cross section through a spiny mouse placenta, Acomys caharensis. The structure of the rodent placenta is more complex than that of the human placenta. It consists of a junctional zone composed of so-called spongio-trophoblast cells without fetal blood vessels and a labyrinth, which is a tight interdigitation of the maternal blood space and the trophoblast with fetal vessels (image by GPW CC BY-NC).

viviparity can be realized with different degrees of egg retention and complementary, with very different amounts of fetal-maternal contact.

In oviparous species, embryonic and sometimes fetal development inside the mother happens inside an egg covering and continues for various periods after oviposition. If the developmental period post-oviposition gets shorter, and the hatching occurs either immediately at or even shortly before oviposition, this mode naturally blends, technically, into viviparity. The distinction between oviparity and viviparity that is based solely on the form of the reproductive product in such cases deals merely with the short period before and after oviposition/parturition, at which hatching from the egg coverings happens. At this point, the distinction between oviparity and viviparity becomes biologically devoid of meaning. This situation could be distinguished and called "ovoviviparity," although this term fell out of favor (Wourms 1981, Blackburn 2000, Lode 2012).

THE CONTROVERSY ABOUT THE TERM "OVOVIVIPARITY" AND ITS RESOLUTION

As outlined above, there is a natural transition between oviparity and viviparity when the amount of time an egg is incubated after oviposition shrinks to zero. However, there is another continuum emerging after oviparity technically becomes viviparity, and that is when the fetus sheds the egg covering while inside the reproductive tract of the mother. Then the fetus could be (living as a free individual and) engaging in phagotrophy or placentotrophy as discussed above. Hence, there are various forms of female reproduction that bridge the gap between proper oviparity and viviparity with extensive placentotrophy, as in eutherian mammals. To intuitively capture these transitional forms of female reproduction, the term "ovoviviparity" was introduced. Blackburn has provided a history of its use (Blackburn 1994). The term fell out of favor when attempts to clearly define ovoviviparity failed due to increasing knowledge about various types of matrotrophy, in particular the existence of extensive matrotrophy of the egg-laying mammals (Monotremes; Griffiths 1978). Matrotrophy is thus not exclusive to viviparous species, and distinguishing viviparity with and without matrotrophy became meaningless. As a consequence, definitions of ovoviviparity became confused and confusing, leading to the rejection of the concept as a whole.

Based on a historical survey of the uses of the term ovoviviparity (Wourms 1981, Blackburn 1994, 2000), it can be inferred that the problem arises from assumptions about which aspect of the fetal-maternal relationship is critical for what is perceived as "a fully developed form of viviparity."[3] Somewhat naturally, the older literature sought to distinguish "lesser" forms of viviparity from more advanced ones by referring to the extent and mode of matrotrophy. For instance, Balinsky (1975)[4] defined ovoviviparity as "bearing of young developed from eggs which have been retained in the body of the mother but without the maternal organism providing additional nourishment for the embryo." Balinsky goes on requiring that "viviparity" be called a mode of reproduction in which "the embryo establishes a direct connection with the maternal body, so that nutrition can pass from the mother to the embryo without the intermediate state of being dissolved in the uterine fluid." It is clear that Balinsky and other authors, such as Mackie (Mackie 1978), confounded the kind of product (egg or neonate) with the mode of nutrition provisioning. As already mentioned above, this became absurd when it was realized that there is substantial matrotrophy in the egg-laying mammals. This problem was solved by Blackburn's two-dimensional classification, where the mode of provisioning and the kind of partition product are understood as two structurally independent dimensions of reproductive modalities. As discussed above, we also follow this way of thinking. However, there are other aspects of the fetal-maternal relationship, other than nutrition, that have an important bearing on the biology of this relationship. These are cell biological and immunological issues, like the control of inflammation and attack by the adaptive immune system, the suppression of wound healing in species with embryo implantation (see Chapter 4 for a more in-depth discussion). The cell biology of the fetal-maternal interface radically changes with the loss of separation between fetal and maternal tissues, i.e., when the egg covering is lost while the fetus is still inside the body of the mother (Griffith and Wagner 2017). Because of the importance of these issues, it seems wise to acknowledge the differences in the nature of the fetal-maternal relationship by reflecting it in the terminology. We are thus inclined to modify the notion of ovoviviparity to read: *ovoviviparity is a form of viviparity (sensu Blackburn 1994) in which fetal and maternal tissues remain separated by an egg covering during the whole period of gestation.*

Before we leave this topic, let us reflect more generally about the arguments put forward in favor of abandoning the term "ovoviviparity." Blackburn's rejection of the term "ovoviviparity" is based on the inconsistent and confusing way that term was used in the past, going back to the 18th and 19th centuries. However, the same argument applies to the term "viviparity" as also documented by Blackburn (2000), i.e., the question of whether the definition of viviparity should include certain forms of matrotrophy. Does this mean we have to abandon the term "viviparity" as well? Obviously not, as Blackburn continues to use this term in his two-dimensional classification of reproductive modes. Many terms refer to complicated concepts that were used inconsistently in the past, and we would have little to talk about in biology (and in all the sciences, for that matter) if we used this criterion as sufficient to abandon these terms. Imagine abandoning the notion of "species," "cell type," or "gene" only because these terms were used inconsistently in the past. And they have been used inconsistently for much of the 19th and 20th centuries. Even in the physical sciences, concepts have a confusing history; such as the notion of "acid" in chemistry, ranging from Aristotle's "sharp taste" to Lavoisier's idea that "oxygen" causes acidity, to the sophisticated concepts of acid-base reactions by Gilbert N. Lewis (1875–1946) based on electron transfer. In spite of these changes in specific meaning, the modern concepts of species, genes, acids, etc., are still in use, because they describe meaningful, and with time better defined, categories. We just have to live with the fact that scientific concepts are the product of historical developments, which are not always entirely logical or even rational. The historical continuity and changes in the definitions of these terms are part of the cultural fabric of science. They should be acknowledged by maintaining the names rather than obscuring them by inventing new terms whenever a concept is modified by new discoveries. The name of a scientific concept then refers to the historically continuous idea that is undergoing occasional modification.

We think, therefore, that there is a strong case to be made to reinstall the term "ovoviviparity" to denote a situation where viviparity is achieved solely by egg retention without a period of fetal life in the maternal body outside the egg coverings. This means it would be helpful to divide the term viviparity into cases of *ovoviviparity* (only egg retention) and viviparity with an "uncovered" fetus, which can include cases of both phagotrophic and placentotrophic viviparity. Note that this distinction is not about matrotrophy per se, either phagotrophy or placentotrophy, both of which assume intra-maternal hatching from egg covers, i.e., an "uncovered" fetus interacting directly with the uterus. As mentioned above, the strong case for reintroducing the concept of ovoviviparity derives from the biological implications of direct fetal-maternal contact. The removal of the egg covering leads to a host of biological changes and challenges (see Chapter 4) that need to be acknowledged rather than hidden under the umbrella term "viviparity." Viviparity in the sense of Blackburn (1994, 2000) retains its validity even when subdivided into different forms of viviparity. In the next section, we want to discuss a lizard, which has attracted a lot of attention as a paradigm of the evolution of viviparity because it represents one of the few cases of reproductive polymorphism within a species. In particular, this is a paradigm of ovoviviparity as we will see.

THE COMMON LIZARD PARADIGM OF OVOVIVIPARITY (*ZOOTOCA VIVIPARA*)

Zootoca vivipara is a small palearctic lizard (Figure 3.2A) with a very wide geographic distribution, from southwestern Europe to Japan and from the sub-Mediterranean to the Arctic Circle in Scandinavia (Figure 3.2B). It is considered one of the most widely distributed squamates and is particularly interesting for evolutionary reproductive biology. The majority of *Z. vivipara* populations are viviparous, as the name already indicates. Most exciting, though, is the fact that two populations of *Z. vivipara* were found to be oviparous, which makes *Z. vivipara* polymorphous with respect to reproductive mode (Heulin et al. 1993, Heulin et al. 1999). It is one of three species with a polymorphic mode of reproduction. The others are two skink species, *Saiphos equalis* (Smith and Shine 1997) and *Lerista bouigainvillii* (Fairbairn et al. 1998), both from Australia.

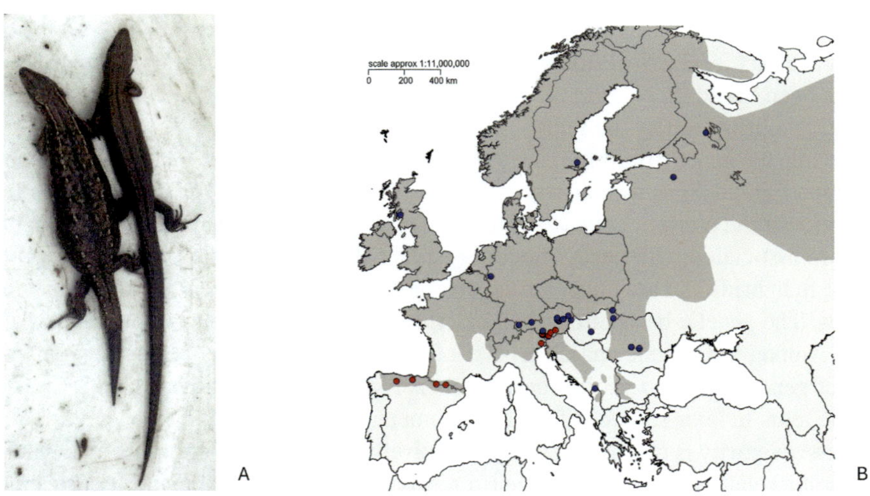

FIGURE 3.2 (A) Female (left) and male (right) specimen of *Zootoca vivipara*. Note regenerated tail section of the female (by Волков Владислав Петрович – Own work, CC BY-SA 3.0, https://commons.wikimedia.org/w/index.php?curid=20062633). (B) Geographic distribution of *Zootoca vivipara* in Europe. Red dots indicate the location of oviparous populations and blue dots the locations of viviparous populations included in the study of Recknagel and collaborators (2018) (image is figure 2 in Recknagel et al. (2018), with permission CC BY).

One cluster of oviparous *Z. vivipara* populations is found in Southwest Europe, that is, the Pyrenees and areas in the Basque Country as well as southern France. These populations are called *Z. vivipara-louislantzi* (Arribas 2009). A second, eastern, population was discovered in Slovenia's Snežnik mountains (Mayer et al. 2000). This population extends into southern Austria (Carinthia) and north-east Italy, called *Z. vivipara-carniolica*. Hence, *Z. vivipara* is divided into three subspecies: the viviparous *Z. vivipara-vivipara,* and two oviparous subspecies, *Z. vivipara-louislantzi* and *Z. vivipara-carniolica*.

Viviparity evolved within this species from oviparous populations (Surget-Groba et al. 2001) related to the eastern oviparous population *Z. v.-carniolica*. The western European population has reverted to oviparity (Surget-Groba et al. 2006, Cornetti et al. 2015, Recknagel et al. 2018). Some genetic evidence suggests that *Z. v.-carniolica* is in the state of incipient speciation from *Z. vivipara-vivipara* (Cornetti et al. 2015, Sandberger-Loua et al. 2017). Nevertheless, natural hybridization has been found between *Z. v.-carniolica* and *Z. v.-vivipara* (Recknagel et al. 2021). In contrast, the western oviparous populations are geographically isolated, and we know of no report of natural hybridization between them and the viviparous populations. In the laboratory, however, hybrid offspring can be produced (Heulin and Guillaume 1989, Arrayago et al. 1996). The fact that both oviparous populations are found at the southern extreme end of the distribution area of *Z. vivipara* tempts one to speculate that *Z. v.-carniolica* may be derived from a refuge population from the last glaciation period, since it is geographically close to the inferred refuge based on phylo-geographic evidence (Cornetti et al. 2015).

From the discovery of a polymorphic reproductive mode, the exciting possibility arises for studies of the genetic causes of viviparity (Recknagel et al. 2021). More on this below. But before we discuss the genetic studies, let us consider the kind of viviparity that *Z. v.-vivipara* represents. The published evidence clearly shows that *Z. v.-vivipara* is an example of ovoviviparity, as conceived in the previous section. There are no differences in the structure and development of the extra-embryonic membranes between oviparous and viviparous populations, probably reflecting the relatively recent origin of viviparity in this species as well as the lack of direct fetal-maternal contact during gestation (Stewart et al. 2004). Neonates hatch from the egg coverings either shortly before birth or up to two days after oviposition and, as such, represent exactly the situation where oviparity blends into viviparity, as defined by the reproductive output according to Blackburn (1994). Nutrition is reported to be entirely lecitotrophic (Panigel 1956) based on radioactive tracer experiments (see also Shine 2005, Stewart 2013). Nevertheless, evidence for direct calcium transport from the uterus to the fetus has been found (Stewart et al. 2009), instead of deposition of calcium in the eggshell and its subsequent mobilization by the fetus.

To investigate the genetic basis for parity mode and its consequences, genome sequence comparisons (Cornetti et al. 2018) as well as whole-genome association study (GWAS), supplemented with transcriptomics of the uterine tissue (Recknagel et al. 2021), have been performed. Two phenotypic characters are associated with parity mode: eggshell calcification and gestational length. Both are intermediate in hybrids and are under strong divergent selection between populations with different parity modes. The genetic basis of eggshell calcification is considerably simpler than that of gestation length. Among the genetic characteristics of the viviparous uterus during pregnancy is higher expression of genes related to angiogenesis. This is likely related to the need for increased oxygen supply to the fetus in later stages of fetal development. In this context, it is interesting to note that even squamate oviparity is characterized by a relatively long period of egg retention, where egg laying happens at a relatively advanced stage (in terms of embryo development, it corresponds to the limb bud paddle stage), compared to other reptiles, including birds. The extent of egg retention in squamates is likely limited by the increasing oxygen demand after this stage of fetal development (Blackburn 2015). Hence, increased uterine vascularization could be the key innovation for the transition from oviparity to ovoviviparity.

There are many more genes associated with parity mode as discovered by Cornetti et al. (2015) and Reckenagel et al. (2021), but their functional significance is currently difficult to assess. As always with genetic association studies, the genes so detectable do not represent the full pathways underlying a trait but reflect only those genes in a physiological pathway that happen to be polymorphic in that population, or in this case, divergent between populations. At best, genes identified by GWAS are indicative of the pathways that could be involved. As an example for human gestational length, compare the GWAS results of (Zhang et al. 2017) and the mechanistic follow-up in (Pavlicev et al. 2024). This second step, from GWAS allele discovery to mechanistic understanding, requires a great deal of biological intuition and experimental skill and is not at all straightforward.

FACULTATIVE VIVIPARITY: PLASTICITY AND THE TRANSITION TO VIVIPARITY

The example of the common lizard shows that differences in parity mode are genetically determined even among closely related populations. However, there are also cases reported in the literature where parity mode is a plastic trait. One example is the South African tortoise *Chersina angulata*. *Ch. angulata* is usually oviparous, as most other turtles, although oviposition happens at a much later stage of embryonic development than in other turtles (Kuchling and Hofmeyr 2023), and egg retention can vary between 23 and 212 days (Hofmeyr 2004). It has been reported that in very hot summers, the females delay oviposition until the sand temperature is favorable for embryo development, and in some summers, the females delay oviposition until a fully developed hatchling is born (Kuchling and Hofmeyr 2023). High summer temperatures can thus induce facultative ovoviviparity in this species (Kuchling and Hofmeyr 2022).

Another case of facultative viviparity has been reported from the Australian skink *Saiphos equalis* (aka yellow-bellied three-toed skink) (Laird et al. 2019). *S. equalis* is a squamate with bimodal reproduction. The 2019 report is based on observations on a single individual in captivity, but still demonstrates the possibility of plasticity with respect to parity mode.

It is an interesting question to ask whether some or all the cases of viviparity via egg retention documented in squamates evolved via a stage of facultative, environment-dependent viviparity. A possible test for this idea could be attempts to induce viviparity by manipulating the environment of pregnant females, in an oviparous species closely related to a viviparous species.

A SQUAMATE PLACENTOTROPHIC PARADIGM: THE *CHALCIDES* SKINKS

Chalcides is a clade of mostly Mediterranean skinks. The Reptile Database lists 33 species,[5] including the two model species *Ch. chalcides* and *Ch. ocellatus*. This genus is remarkable as it includes species with advanced forms of epithelio-chorial placentation and a variety of body forms from standard quadrupedal lizard body shape, e.g., *Ch. ocellatus,* to elongated forms with digit-reduced morphologies, e.g., *Ch. chalcides* (Caputo et al. 1995, Caputo et al. 2000, Young et al. 2009). In fact, *Ch. chalcides* was the first species in which reptilian placentation was discovered by Cesare Studiati (1821–1894) and published in 1855 (cited after Blackburn et al. 2015). Coincidentally, *Ch. chalcides* turned out to be one of the most advanced forms of placentation, only surpassed by the discovery of placentation in *Mabuya heathi*, the Brazilian Mabuya[6] (Blackburn et al. 1984).

Ch. chalcides is also called the "three-toed Italian skink" or "*luscengola*" in Italian, is a skink of 100–150 mm snout-vent length (SVL) in females and produces small ova of about 2.5 to 3 mm diameter, with a small amount of yolk (Figure 3.3A). *Ch. chalcides* females produce 4 to 15 neonates (average 7.8; Caputo et al. 2000) of about 94 mm, after a pregnancy of three months. The placenta is epitheliochorial, made from the chorioallantois and interdigitates with folds of the uterus on the mesometrial side of the uterus, but does not directly attach to the luminal epithelium (Blackburn 1993, Blackburn and Callard 1997). Both sides of the fetal-maternal contact are well vascularized. The yolk sac is small and forms a vestigial vitelline placenta. Given how advanced and in many respects mammal-like the *Ch. chalcides* placentation is, the early development is surprisingly conservative, i.e., the development of the extra-embryonic tissues follows the same trajectories as seen

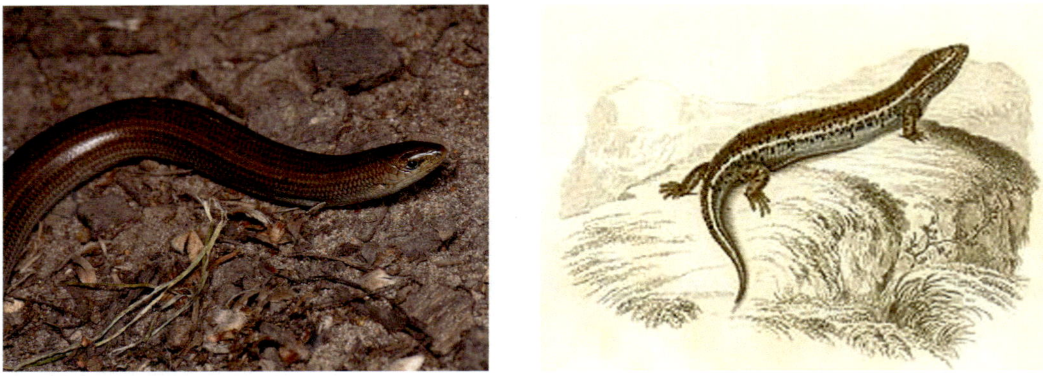

FIGURE 3.3 (A) The three-toed Italian skink, *Chalcides chalcides* (photo by Paolo Mazzei, CC BY-NC 4.0). (B) The ocellated skink, *Chalcides ocellatus*. (Image from Charles Orbigny, Dictionnaire D'Histoire Naturelle. 1849; public domain. Downloaded from https://commons.wikimedia.org/wiki/File:Gongylus_occelatus.jpg?uselang=en#Licensing).

in other reptiles (Blackburn and Callard 1997), rather than the radically altered sequence of events seen in eutherian mammals (see Chapter 2).

An intriguing aspect of *Ch. chalcides* pregnancy is its endocrine regulation. As expected, after ovulation and during the first half of pregnancy, the corpus luteum (CL) produces progesterone. However, at mid-pregnancy, the CL degenerates. This in itself is not surprising, since progesterone is not necessary for the maintenance of pregnancy in its full length in many viviparous lizards (Norris and Lopez 2024) and even marsupials (Tyndale-Biscoe and Renfree 1987). What is surprising, however, is that after the CL degenerates, progesterone is still produced by the endometrium of the placental contact zone (Guarino et al. 1998). This has been shown by progesterone production in explant culture and the immunolocalization of 3β-hydroxysteroid dehydrogenase (3β-HSD), the enzyme catalyzing the last step in progesterone synthesis.[7] This is highly reminiscent of the shift in progesterone production to extraovarian sources in several mammalian species (placenta in human, guinea pig), where, after the CL degenerates, the progesterone production is taken over by other tissues. The difference being that in luteo-placental shift, the fetal cells of the placenta are producing the hormone, while in *Ch. Chalcides,* it is the maternal tissue.

An instructive contrast can be drawn with a congeneric viviparous skink, the ocellated skink or "*gongylus*" (*Chalcides ocellatus*) (Figure 3.3B). *Ch. ocellatus* is a quadrupedal skink that also develops a placenta, but that placenta is much less developed than that of *Ch. chalcides,* in the sense that the allantoic placenta is not dominant relative to the vitelline placenta (Giacomini 1906, cited after (Blackburn et al. 2017)). The eggs are comparatively large, with a diameter of 11 mm compared to the <3 mm of *Ch. chalcides,* which amounts to a 50-fold larger egg volume. Hence, embryo provisioning is mostly lecitotroph, rather than matrotroph. Vincenzo Caputo and colleagues noted a curious trend within the *Chalcides* clade that links body elongation with the decrease of egg size, elaboration of placental structure, and increase in placentotrophy (Caputo et al. 2000). The authors show that despite the decreased body cross-section, the litter size remains the same and even increases at extreme ends of the range of body elongation. Vincenzo Caputo and colleagues argue that adaptively driven change in body shape might have affected the size and number of eggs that can be kept in the body of the mother, leading to a compensatory decrease in yolk mass and thus egg size and driving a higher need for a more effective and elaborate placentation. This is an intriguing idea and suggests that the evolution of placentation could be primarily driven by evolutionary changes outside the female reproductive tract, i.e., represent compensatory evolution rather than direct adaptation of female reproductive biology.[8]

The genus *Chalcides* is a paradigm for the evolution of complex reptilian placentation with a number of important messages for the general biology of viviparity. Effective complex placentation, as in *Ch. chalcides*, can evolve without major reorganization of early development, which raises the question of why eutherian mammals have so radically re-arranged the early developmental events. An effective epitheliochorial placenta is possible without direct attachment between the chorion and uterine epithelium, suggesting that the ability of embryo attachment was a non-trivial innovation in mammals (see Chapter 4). Finally, the evolution of highly effective and complex placentation might have been driven by evolutionary changes outside the female reproductive tract, for instance, by evolutionary changes in body shape and mode of locomotion (quadrupedal locomotion to snake-like "grass swimming").

ANURAN VIVIPARITY: THE NIMBA TOAD

While viviparity is common in urodeles, such as *Salmadra atra*, and universal in Gymnophiones, viviparity is rare in anurans (frogs and toads) (Wake 2015). In this context, the example of the Nimba toad, *Nimbaphrynoides occidentalis*, is a remarkable exception (Sandberger-Loua et al. 2017).[9] The Nimba toad is a small 15–27 mm SVL anuran from the Nimba mountain range located in the Guinea, Ivory Coast, and Liberia tri-border region (Figure 3.4). The females produce small eggs with very little yolk, a parallel to the small yolk-poor eggs of eutherian mammals and the placentotrophic squamates. The animals give birth to fully developed, postmetamorphic froglets after a gestation of 9 months. The neonate is about 200-fold heavier than the egg, and thus there has to be a substantial matrotrophic contribution. Nevertheless, there is no placentation, and matrotrophy is provided by uterine secretions, "uterine milk" consisting of mucoproteins and glycogen. The hypothesis of phagotrophy is supported by the observation that the fetuses have a functioning gut and develop labial papillae, supposedly helpful in acquiring uterine milk from the uterine wall.[10] Parturition occurs by behaviorally restricting the movement of the fetus rather than expulsion by uterine contraction. The myometrium is very thin and apparently not able to expel the fetus. Nimba toad fetuses do not express typical larval characters such as gills, spiracles, or a coiled gut and thus seem to skip the larval stage completely.

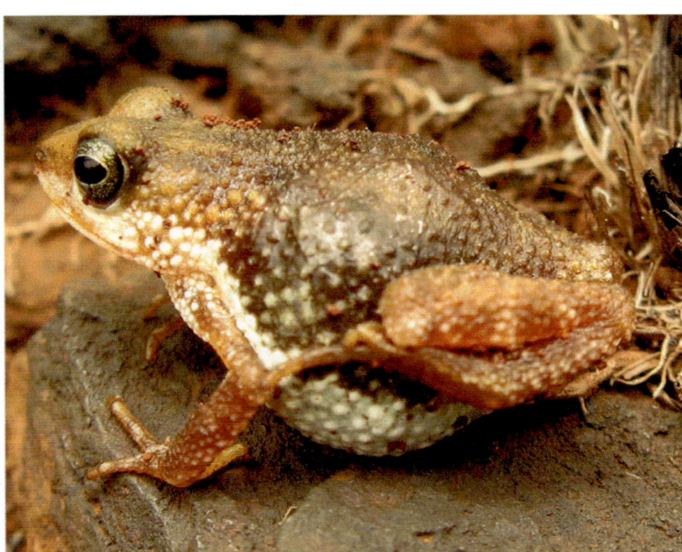

FIGURE 3.4 A pregnant female of the Nimba toad, *Nimbaphrynoides occidentalis*. (Image from figure 3 of Sandberger-Loua et al. (2017) published under CC BY license.)

For an anuran, this is a remarkably advanced form of viviparity. To start with, viviparity is only known from 17 species from five genera out of > 6,500 anuran species (0.26%). And even among these 17 species, the Nimba toad is unique as it is the only species with predominant matrotroph nutrition. The reproduction of its closest relative, *Didynamipus sjostedti,* is not well understood, but the consensus seems to be that it is directly developing oviparous (Gonwouo et al. 2013). It shares a common ancestor with *Nimbaphrynoides* about 13 Mio years ago. The next outgroup is *Altiphrynoides* (Liedtke et al. 2016), which is also oviparous and indirectly developing and has a common ancestor with *Nimbaphrynoides* about 23 Mio years ago. Nevertheless, fertilization is terrestrial and internal in *Altiphrynoides malcolmi* (Wake 1980) and *A. osgoodi* (Grandison 1978), a prerequisite for later evolving viviparity. This phylogenetic distribution suggests that within 23 Mio years the Nimba toad lineage lost its larval stage, lost almost all of its yolk, and evolved a 9-month-long pregnancy, although no placentation.

PHYLOGENETIC PATTERNS OF FEMALE REPRODUCTIVE MODES

Among vertebrates, almost every major clade has evolved some cases and forms of viviparity, including sharks, teleost fish, amphibians, many reptiles, and, of course, mammals (Blackburn 2015). Viviparity requires fertilization to occur in the body of the female and thus excludes groups with exclusively external fertilization, such as lamprey and hagfish. The other major exception are birds, which do have internal fertilization, and are species-rich (>9,000 species), but nevertheless, not a single case of viviparity has been reported. The reason for this is still obscure. Many theories have been published, but all of them have fatal flaws (see review and critique by Blackburn and Evans 1986). In the same paper, Blackburn and Evans proposed a theory based on arguments on the inferred fitness benefits of intermediate stages between oviparity and viviparity during the evolutionary transition to viviparity. This is a subtle argument and too detailed to be covered here, but we encourage interested readers to consult that paper. The absence of avian viviparity is a problem that will challenge the creativity of biologists for years to come.

The clade with the largest number of inferred independent origins of viviparity is the squamate reptiles, lizards, and snakes (Tinkle and Gibbons 1977). The exact estimate of independent origins depends on the accuracy of the phylogenetic reconstruction and the methods of ancestral state reconstruction (Griffith et al. 2015). In one study, the authors even came to the conclusion that viviparity in squamates only evolved once and was many times reverted to oviparity (Pyron and Burbrink 2014). Returns to oviparity do happen, e.g., in sand boas *Eryx jajakari* (Lynch and Wagner 2010). Nevertheless, the consensus is that there are about 115 cases of independent origination of viviparity and 8 to 9 cases of likely reversions to oviparity (Blackburn 2015). A comparative genomic and transcriptomic study of the endometrium from closely related agamids, *Phrynocephalus przewalskii* and *P. vlangalii* (toad-headed agamids), where *P. przewalskii* is oviparous, and *P. vlangalii* is viviparous, revealed that the majority of genetic differences are cis-regulatory, suggesting that reversion from viviparity to oviparity is genetically easily reversible (Gao et al. 2019).

The vast majority of viviparous squamates are cases of ovoviviparity, i.e., cases of extended egg retention. As already mentioned above, this high rate of origination of ovoviviparity in squamates is correlated with relatively extensive egg retention even in oviparous squamates (Blackburn 2015), making this group particularly "close" to undergoing hatching before oviposition. As mentioned above, the reason that egg retention is limited to paddle or earlier stages is likely due to constraints on oxygen availability to the fetus in utero, without additional maternal adaptations such as increased vascularization. Remember that one of the differences between oviparous and viviparous populations of the common lizard (*Zootoca vivipara*, see above) is the expression of genes related to vascularization (Recknagel et al. 2021).

In contrast, the number of squamate species with placentotrophy is small (four to five species), and even smaller is the number of species with some degree of invasive placentation (one species). Examples of squamates with complex placentation are the species of the genus *Chalcides*, a clade of skinks mostly found in the Mediterranean (see above). Another prominent example is *Mabuya,* a genus of skinks that is found in Brazil and the Caribbean (Blackburn et al. 1984). *Mabuya* placenta is organized into highly folded placentomes surrounded by a para-placenta specialized in the uptake of nutrients secreted by uterine glands. *Mabuya* eggs are essentially yolk-free, with a diameter of 1 mm, implying that *Mabuya* exclusively relies on placentotrophy. Gestation is very long and lasts between 8 and 12 months.

Invasive placentation has been described in the Central African skink *Trachylepis ivensii*[11] (Blackburn and Flemming 2012). This species also ovulates very small eggs and thus is almost completely placentotroph (Flemming and Blackburn 2003). The eggshell is shed early in gestation, similar to the shedding of the zona pellucida in eutherian mammals.[12] At the placental-uterine interface, the luminal epithelium is stripped from the basal membrane and undergoes degeneration, but no stromal invasion has been detected, making it a desmochorial placental type according to the classification of Grosser, a descriptive term rarely used today (Grosser 1909). The fact that this degree of invasiveness has only been described once in squamates is testimony to the fact that the evolution of placentation that involves partial destruction and modification of the maternal tissue is hard to evolve. Unfortunately, the chances to learn more about the cell biology of embryo implantation in this species are currently slim. It lives in some of the least hospitable areas of Africa,[13] and is rarely found in museums.

Viviparity and matrotrophy are also documented in a wide array of invertebrate animals, all the way from cnidarians to insects (Ostrovsky et al. 2016). Among the 36 recognized animal phyla, only 12 do not have reports of matrotrophy or viviparity. The invertebrate groups with the highest fraction of matrotrophic species are Platyhelmints, Arthropoda, and Bryozoa. A particularly interesting case is the viviparity of the Sea Star *Cryptasterina hystera.* Viviparity is rare in echinoderms, and in this species the embryo develops within the gonads (Byrne 2005).

Overall, it is estimated that matrotrophy evolved between 140 and 145 times, with 29 to 31 times in Arthropoda alone (Ostrovsky et al. 2016), with a wide array of locations in the maternal body where matrotrophy is happening. Examples are viviparous aphids, as well as velvet worms (a relative of arthropods). In terms of placental structures, the invertebrate placentas are less complex but more diverse (for details, see Ostrovsky et al. 2016).

The patterns revealed from the comparative study of matrotrophy and viviparity show an astonishing tendency to matrotrophic and viviparous modes of female reproduction, with a wide array of anatomical and physiological ways these reproductive modes are achieved, a clear sign of massive convergent evolution. It is unlikely that a common ecological or selective reason exists for the evolution of viviparity in general. For instance, in squamates, there is strong evidence that lower temperature environments are associated with higher incidences of viviparous species (Tinkle and Gibbons 1977, Shine 1995). But this thermal factor is unlikely to explain the frequent evolution of viviparity in aquatic species (Ostrovsky et al., 2016). In the aquatic environment, pelagic species seem to be more likely to evolve viviparity. For a pelagic species, the "problem" driving viviparity or other associations with the mother could be related to the lack of structures to deposit the eggs on and not lose them to the deep recesses of the ocean or deep lakes. In this respect, the rather unusual form of teleost "placentation" in some rice fishes is interesting. In general, rice fishes use adhesion fibers of the eggshell to attach their eggs to vegetation. However, they also have the ability to attach the eggs to the body of the female, either to the distal segment of the gonoduct or the anal fin (Iwamatsu et al. 2007, Hilgers et al. 2022). The latter form of brood care is preferentially found in species that live in a pelagic environment, where there is precious little substrate to attach their eggs to.[14] Hence, it is also conceivable that other forms of vivipary or on-body-brooding of aquatic species are driven by the same consideration, the lack of egg deposit sites in pelagic environs.

CONCLUSION

Viviparity, brooding, and matrotrophy are reproductive traits that are widespread among animals, with a massive number of convergent origins. They are also diverse in nearly every respect, i.e., in terms of fetal nutrition, anatomical location of fetal development, kind of fetal-maternal contact, etc. Hence, the term viviparity covers a vast array of biological situations, and there is neither a unitary evolutionary cause for the evolution of viviparity and matrotrophy, nor is there a unitary genetic basis for viviparity among a wider range of species. This assertion does not exclude the cooption of similar or even homologous genes and cell biological pathways involved in various forms of matrotrophy, as has been demonstrated in squamates (Brandley et al. 2012, Gao et al. 2019, Recknagel et al. 2021). These similarities are expected with respect to vascularization of the uterus for oxygen and nutrient exchange, the reduction of expression or loss of genes related to yolk and eggshell production, the expression of transporter proteins or even inflammatory mediators, and others. The expression of these genes, however, does not amount to a unitary, trans-species, genetic "explanation" of viviparity. What they reflect are convergent functional needs. Explanation of placentotrophic viviparity, however, will likely differ for each individual case, i.e., the genetic changes that caused the origin of viviparity in each separate lineage.

One way to view the viviparity-oviparity dualism is to de-emphasize it in the large scope of vertebrate evolution. Instead, it seems that the key evolutionary steps were the evolution of internal fertilization (which enabled any kind of internal embryo development) and then the evolution of implantation, which leads to the direct maternal-fetal interface. The stages in between these two key innovations mostly lead to oviposition but can result in apparent live birth when hatching predates oviposition (i.e., egg retention and ovoviviparity). The next reproductive key transition then is implantation, which introduces a qualitatively new form of maternal-embryo interaction, which, in all species with implantation, obligatorily results in live birth. Thus, the contrast of viviparity vs. oviparity in terms of the form of reproductive product is an obvious, but not as biologically crucial a distinction. One way to deal with this, as suggested above, is to maintain the term "ovoviviparity" for the cases of apparent viviparity based on egg retention, without implantation.

NOTES

1. Phagotrophy is a term that is also used in cell biology with a more specialized meaning, i.e., ingestion via a vesicle, better called phagocytosis. Here, the term is used to simplify terminology by covering a number of very similar modes of matrotrophic provisioning where the fetus ingests various products via the mouth rather than via transfer from maternal tissue to extra-embryonic tissues. These are oophagy, adelphophagy, ingesting uterine epithelial cells or secretions.
2. See https://australian.museum/learn/animals/fishes/oophagous-sharks/.
3. Of course, what is considered a "fully developed form of viviparity" is essentially a human or at least eutherian perspective on reproduction, which could be challenged given the variety of female reproductive modes that exist for instance in "fishes" (Wourms 1981) or even invertebrates (Ostrovsky et al., 2016).
4. Cited after Wourms 1981.
5. https://reptile-database.reptarium.cz/advanced_search?genus=Chalcides&exact%5B0%5D=genus&submit=Search. Accessed 06/06/2025.
6. *Mabuya heathi* is listed as *Brasiliscincus heathi* in the Reptile database: https://reptile-database.reptarium.cz/species?genus=Brasiliscincus&species=heathi
7. 3β-HSD is not only involved in progesterone synthesis but also catalyzes the last step of testosterone synthesis and is thus not definite proof but combined with the explant culture its expression in the luminal epithelium of the incubation chamber is highly suggestive.
8. The scenario of Caputo and colleagues is an example of a broader pattern called "Selection, Pleiotropy and Compensation" or SPC (see Pavlicev, M. and G. P. Wagner (2012). "A model of developmental evolution: selection, pleiotropy and compensation." Trends Ecol Evol **27**(6): 316–322).
9. All the facts noted in this paragraph are from the cited review by Sandberger-Loua and colleagues, as well as information compiled in https://amphibiaweb.org, in addition to the cited references.

10. Or stimulate the uterine wall to increase secretion dependent on the activity of the fetus.
11. This species is listed in the Reptile database as *Lubuya ivensii*, https://reptile-database.reptarium.cz/species?genus=Lubuya&species=ivensii.
12. Note that the *zona pellucida* of the eutherian ovum is the product of follicular cells, while eggshells and egg coats are secreted by parts of the Müllerian duct, either in the oviduct or in parts of the uterus.
13. This statement reflects the political situation at the time this book was written and, hopefully, may be wrong in the future.
14. Interestingly, attachment of the eggs to the maternal body involves similar inflammatory processes as those activated during mammalian implantation (Hilgers et al., 2022).

REFERENCES

Arrayago, M. J., A. Bea and B. Heulin (1996). "Hybridization experiment between oviparous and viviparous strains of *Lacerta vivipara*: a new insight into the evolution of viviparity in reptiles." *Herpetologica* **52**: 333–342.

Arribas, O. J. (2009). "Morphological variability of the Cantabro-Pyrenean populations of Zootoca vivipara (JACQUIN, 1787) with description of a new subspecies." *Herpetozoa* **21**: 123–146.

Balinski, B. I. (1975). An Introduction to Embryology. W. B. Saunders Co., Philadelphia, PA.

Blackburn, D. G. (1992). "Convergent evolution of vivipary, matrotrophy, and specializations for fetal nutrition in reptiles and other vertebrates." *Amer Zool* **32**(2): 313–321.

Blackburn, D. G. (1993). "Histology of the late-stage placentae in the matrotrophic skink Chalcides chalcides (Lacertilia; Scincidae)." *J Morphol* **216**(2): 179–195.

Blackburn, D. G. (1994). "Discrepant usage of the term 'ovoviviparity' in the herpetological literature." *Herpetol J* **4**: 62–72.

Blackburn, D. G. (2000). "Classification of the reproductive patterns of amniotes." *Herpetol Monogr* **14**: 371–377.

Blackburn, D. G. (2015). "Evolution of vertebrate viviparity and specializations for fetal nutrition: a quantitative and qualitative analysis." *J Morphol* **276**(8): 961–990.

Blackburn, D. G. (2015). "Evolution of viviparity in squamate reptiles: reversibility reconsidered." *J Exp Zool B Mol Dev Evol* **324**: 473–486.

Blackburn, D. G., A. M. Avanzati and L. Paulesu (2015). "Classics revisited. History of reptile placentology: Studiati's early account of placentation in a viviparous lizard." *Placenta* **36**(11): 1207–1211.

Blackburn, D. G. and I. P. Callard (1997). "Morphogenesis of placental membranes in the viviparous, placentotrophic lizard Chalcides chalcides (Squamata: Scincidae)." *J Morphol* **232**(1): 35–55.

Blackburn, D. G. and H. E. Evans (1986). "Why are there no Viviparous Birds?" *Am Nat* **128**(2): 165–190.

Blackburn, D. G. and A. F. Flemming (2012). "Invasive implantation and intimate placental associations in a placentotrophic African lizard, Trachylepis ivensi (scincidae)." *J Morphol* **273**(2): 137–159.

Blackburn, D. G., L. Paulesu, A. M. Avanzati and M. Roth (2017). "History of reptile placentology, part III: Giacomini's 1891 histological monograph on lizard placentation." *Placenta* **60**: 93–99.

Blackburn, D. G., L. J. Vitt and C. A. Beuchat (1984). "Eutherian-like reproductive specializations in a viviparous reptile." *Proc Natl Acad Sci U S A* **81**(15): 4860–4863.

Brandley, M. C., R. L. Young, D. L. Warren, M. B. Thompson and G. P. Wagner (2012). "Uterine gene expression in the live-bearing lizard, Chalcides ocellatus, reveals convergence of squamate reptile and mammalian pregnancy mechanisms." *Genome Biol Evol* **4**(3): 394–411.

Byrne, M. (2005). "Viviparity in the sea star Cryptasterina hystera (Asterinidae) – conserved and modified features in reproduction and development." *Biol Bull* **208**(2): 81–91.

Caputo, V., F. M. Guarino and F. Angelini (2000). "Body elongation and placentome evolution in the scincid lizard genus Chalcides (Squamata, Scincidae)." *Ital J Zool* **67**: 385–391.

Caputo, V., B. Lanza and R. Palmieri (1995). "Body elongation and limb reduction in the genus Chalcides Laurenti 1768 (Squamata Scincidae): a comparative study." *Trop Zool* **8**: 95–152.

Cornetti, L., G. F. Ficetola, S. Hoban and C. Vernesi (2015). "Genetic and ecological data reveal species boundaries between viviparous and oviparous lizard lineages." *Heredity (Edinb)* **115**(6): 517–526.

Cornetti, L., O. W. Griffith, A. Benazzo, A. Panziera, C. M. Whittington, M. B. Thompson, C. Vernesi and G. Bertorelle (2018). "Candidate genes involved in the evolution of viviparity: a RAD sequencing experiment in the lizard Zootoca vivipara (Squamata: Lacertidae)." *Zool J Linn Soc* **183**: 196–207.

Fairbairn, J., R. Shine, C. Moritz and M. Frommer (1998). "Phylogenetic relationships between oviparous and viviparous populations of an Australian lizard (Lerista bougainvillii, scincidae)." *Mol Phylogenet Evol* **10**(1): 95–103.

Flemming, A. F. and D. G. Blackburn (2003). "Evolution of placental specializations in viviparous African and South American lizards." *J Exp Zool A Comp Exp Biol* **299**(1): 33–47.

Gao, W., Y. B. Sun, W. W. Zhou, Z. J. Xiong, L. Chen, H. Li, T. T. Fu, K. Xu, W. Xu, L. Ma, Y. J. Chen, X. Y. Xiang, L. Zhou, T. Zeng, S. Zhang, J. Q. Jin, H. M. Chen, G. Zhang, D. M. Hillis, X. Ji, Y. P. Zhang and J. Che (2019). "Genomic and transcriptomic investigations of the evolutionary transition from oviparity to viviparity." *Proc Natl Acad Sci U S A* **116**(9): 3646–3655.

Gilmore, R. G., O. Putz and J. W. Dodrill (2005). Oophagy, intrauterine cannibalism and reproductive strategy in lamnoid sharks. *Reproductive Biology and Phylogeny of Chondrichthyes.* W. C. Hamlett. Enfield, NH, USA, Science Publishers INC**:** 435–462.

Gonwouo, A. Ndeh, W. Tapondjou and B. Noonan (2013). "Amphibia, Bufonidae, Didynamipus sjostedti Andersson, 1903: new records and a review of geographic distribution." *Check List* **9**(4): 780–782.

Grandison, A. G. C. (1978). "The occurrence of Nectophrynoides (Anura: Bufonidae) in Ethiopia. A new concept of the genus with a description of a new species." *Monit Zool Ital* **11**(6): 119–172.

Griffith, O. W., D. G. Blackburn, M. C. Brandley, J. U. Van Dyke, C. M. Whittington and M. B. Thompson (2015). "Ancestral state reconstructions require biological evidence to test evolutionary hypotheses: a case study examining the evolution of reproductive mode in squamate reptiles." *J Exp Zool B Mol Dev Evol* **324**(6): 493–503.

Griffith, O. W. and G. P. Wagner (2017). "The placenta as a model for understanding the origin and evolution of vertebrate organs." *Nat Ecol Evol* **1**(4): 72.

Griffiths, M. (1978). *The Biology and Monotremes.* San Diego, CA, Academic Press.

Grosser, O. (1909). *Vergleichende Anatomie und Entwicklungsgeschichte der Eihäute und der Placenta.* Vienna, W. Braumüller.

Guarino, F. M., L. Paulesu, A. Cardone, L. Bellini, G. Ghiara and F. Angelini (1998). "Endocrine activity of the corpus luteum and placenta during pregnancy in Chalcides chalcides (Reptilia, Squamata)." *Gen Comp Endocrinol* **111**(3): 261–270.

Heulin, B. and C.-P. Guillaume (1989). "Expe´rience d'hybridization entre les souches ovipare et vivipara du le´zard Lacerta vivipara." *Rev Ecol* **44**: 39–45.

Heulin, B., C.-P. Guillaume, A. Bea and M. J. Arrayago (1993). "Interpre´tation bioge´ographique de la bimodalite de reproduction du le´zard Lacerta vivipara—Jacquin—(Sauria, Lacertidae): un modele pour l'etude de l'evolution de la viviparite." *Biogeographica* **69**: 3–13.

Heulin, B., Y. Surget-Groba, A. Guiller, C. P. Guillaume and J. Deunff (1999). "Comparisons of mitochondrial DNA (mtDNA) sequences (16S rRNA gene) between oviparous and viviparous strains of Lacerta vivipara: a preliminary study." *Mol Ecol* **8**(10): 1627–1631.

Hilgers, L., O. Roth, A. W. Nolte, A. Schuller, T. Spanke, J. M. Flury, I. V. Utama, J. Altmuller, D. Wowor, B. Misof, F. Herder, A. Bohne and J. Schwarzer (2022). "Inflammation and convergent placenta gene co-option contributed to a novel reproductive tissue." *Curr Biol* **32**(3): 715–724.e714.

Hofmeyr, M. D. (2004). "Egg production in Chersina angulata: an unusual pattern in a Mediterranean climate." *Herpetology* **38**: 172–179.

Iwamatsu, T., H. Kobayashi, Y. Shibata, M. Sato, N. Tsuji and K. Takakura (2007). "Oviposition cycle in the oviparous fish Xenopoecilus sarasinorum." *Zoolog Sci* **24**(11): 1122–1127.

Johnson, G. A., F. W. Bazer and H. Seo (2021). "The early stages of implantation and placentation in the pig." *Adv Anat Embryol Cell Biol* **234**: 61–89.

Kuchling, G. and M. D. Hofmeyr (2022). "Too hot to nest? In a hot summer the tortoise *Chersina angulata* can switch from nesting to facultativen viviparity." *Front Ecol Evol* **9**: 788764.

Kuchling, G. and M. D. Hofmeyr (2023). "Facultative embryonic diapause and a transitional stage between oviparity and viviparity in the South African Tortoise *Chersina angulata*." *Chelonian Conserv Biol* **22**(1): 3–12.

Laird, M. K., M. B. Thompson and C. M. Whittington (2019). "Facultative oviparity in a viviparous skink (*Saiphos equalis*)." *Biol Lett* **15**(4): 20180827.

Liedtke, H. C., H. Muller, M. O. Rodel, M. Menegon, L. N. Gonwouo, M. F. Barej, V. Gvozdik, A. Schmitz, A. Channing, P. Nagel and S. P. Loader (2016). "No ecological opportunity signal on a continental scale? Diversification and life-history evolution of African true toads (Anura: Bufonidae)." *Evolution* **70**(8): 1717–1733.

Lode, T. (2012). "Oviparity or viviparity? That is the question." *Reprod Biol* **12**(3): 259–264.

Lynch, V. J. and G. P. Wagner (2010). "Did egg-laying boas break Dollo's law? Phylogenetic evidence for reversal to oviparity in sand boas (Eryx: Boidae)." *Evolution* **64**(1): 207–216.

Mackie, G. L. (1978). "Are spaeriid clams ovoviviparous or viviparous?." *Nautilus* **92**: 145–147.

Mayer, W., W. Böhme, F. Tiedemann and W. Bischoff (2000). "On oviparous populations of Zootoca vivipara (JACQUIN, 1787) in south-eastern Central Europe and their phylogenetic relationship to neighbouring viviparous and South-west European oviparous populations." *Herpetozoa* **13**: 59–69.

Mossman, H. W. (1937). "Comparative morphogenesis of the foetal membranes and accessory uterine structures." *Contr Embyol* **26**: 129–246.

Norris, D. O. and K. H. Lopez (2024). *Hormones and Reproduction of Vertebrates, Volume 3: Reptiles*. San Diego, CA, Academic Press.

Ostrovsky, A. N., S. Lidgard, D. P. Gordon, T. Schwaha, G. Genikhovich and A. V. Ereskovsky (2016). "Matrotrophy and placentation in invertebrates: a new paradigm." *Biol Rev Camb Philos Soc* **91**(3): 673–711.

Panigel, M. (1956). "Contribution a l'e´tude de l'ovoviviparite´ chez les reptiles: gestation et parturition chez le lezard vivipare Zootoca vivipara." *Ann Sci Nat Zool Biol Anim* **18**: 569–668.

Pavlicev, M., C. E. McDonough-Goldstein, A. M. Zupan, L. Muglia, Y. C. Hu, F. Kong, N. Monangi, G. Dagdas, N. Zupancic, J. Maziarz, D. Sinner, G. Zhang, G. Wagner and L. Muglia (2024). "A common allele increases endometrial Wnt4 expression, with antagonistic implications for pregnancy, reproductive cancers, and endometriosis." *Nat Commun* **15**(1): 1152.

Pavlicev, M. and G. P. Wagner (2012). "A model of developmental evolution: selection, pleiotropy and compensation." *Trends Ecol Evol* **27**(6): 316–322.

Pyron, R. A. and F. T. Burbrink (2014). "Early origin of viviparity and multiple reversions to oviparity in squamate reptiles." *Ecol Lett* **17**(1): 13–21.

Ramsey, E. M. (1982). *The Placenta. Human and Animal*. Santa Barbara, CA, Praeger Inc.

Recknagel, H., M. Carruthers, A. A. Yurchenko, M. Nokhbatolfoghahai, N. A. Kamenos, M. M. Bain and K. R. Elmer (2021). "The functional genetic architecture of egg-laying and live-bearing reproduction in common lizards." *Nat Ecol Evol* **5**(11): 1546–1556.

Recknagel, H., N. A. Kamenos and K. R. Elmer (2018). "Common lizards break Dollo's law of irreversibility: genome-wide phylogenomics support a single origin of viviparity and re-evolution of oviparity." *Mol Phylogenet Evol* **127**: 579–588.

Sandberger-Loua, L., H. Müller and M.-O. Rödl (2017). "A review of the reproductive biology of the only known matrotrophic viviparous anuran, the West African Nimba toad, *Nimbaphrynoides occidentalis*." *Zoosyst. Evol.* **93**: 105–133.

Shine, R. (1995). "A new hypothesis for the evolution of viviparity in reptiles." *Am Nat* **145**(3): 809–823.

Shine, R. (2005). "Life-history evolution in reptiles." *Annu Rev Ecol Evol* **36**: 23–46.

Smith, S. A. and R. Shine (1997). "Intraspecific variation in reproductive mode within the scincid lizard Saiphos equalis." *Aust J Zool* **45**: 435–445.

Stewart, J. R. (2013). "Fetal nutrition in lecithotrophic squamate reptiles: toward a comprehensive model for evolution of viviparity and placentation." *J Morph* **274**: 824–843.

Stewart, J. R., T. W. Ecay and B. Heulin (2009). "Calcium provision to oviparous and viviparous embryos of the reproductively bimodal lizard *Lacerta* (*Zootoca*) *vivipara*." *J Exp Biol* **212**: 2520–2524.

Stewart, J. R., B. Heulin and Y. Surget-Groba (2004). "Extraembryonic membrane development in a reproductively bimodal lizard, Lacerta (Zootoca) vivipara." *Zoology* **107**: 289–314.

Surget-Groba, Y., B. Heulin, C.-P. Guillaume, M. Puky, D. Semenov, V. Orlova, L. Kupriyanova, I. Ghira and B. Smajda (2006). "Multiple origins of viviparity, or reversal from viviparity to oviparity? The European common lizard (*Zootoca vivipara*, Lacertidae) and the evolution of parity." *Biol J Linn Soc* **87**: 1–11.

Surget-Groba, Y., B. Heulin, C. P. Guillaume, R. S. Thorpe, L. Kupriyanova, N. Vogrin, R. Maslak, S. Mazzotti, M. Venczel, I. Ghira, G. Odierna, O. Leontyeva, J. C. Monney and N. Smith (2001). "Intraspecific phylogeography of *Lacerta vivipara* and the evolution of viviparity." *Mol Phylogenet Evol* **18**(3): 449–459.

Tinkle, D. W. and H. W. Gibbons (1977). *The Distribution and Evolution of Viviparity in Reptiles*. Ann Arbor, MI, Museum of Zoology, University of Michigan.

Tyndale-Biscoe, C. H. and M. B. Renfree (1987). *Reproductive Physiology of Marsupials*. Cambridge, UK, Cambridge University Press.

Wake, M. H. (1980). "The reproductive biology of *Nectophrynoides malcolmi* (Amphibia: Bufonidae), with comments on the evolution of reproductive modes in the genus Nectophrynoides." *Copeia* **1980**(2): 193–209.

Wake, M. H. (2015). "Fetal adaptations for viviparity in amphibians." *J Morphol* **276**(8): 941–960.

Wilson, A. B., A. Vincent, I. Ahnesjo and A. Meyer (2001). "Male pregnancy in seahorses and pipefishes (family Syngnathidae): rapid diversification of paternal brood pouch morphology inferred from a molecular phylogeny." *J Hered* **92**(2): 159–166.

Wooding, F. B. P. and G. J. Burton (2008). Comparative Placentation. Berlin and Heidelberg, Springer.

Wourms, J. P. (1981). "Viviparity – the maternal-fetal relationship in fishes." *Amer Zool* **21**(2): 473–515.

Young, R. L., V. Caputo, M. Giovannotti, T. Kohlsdorf, A. O. Vargas, G. E. May and G. P. Wagner (2009). "Evolution of digit identity in the three-toed skink *Chalcides chalcides*: a new case of digit identity frame shift." *Evol Dev* **11**(6): 647–658.

Zhang, G., B. Feenstra, J. Bacelis, X. Liu, L. M. Muglia, J. Juodakis, D. E. Miller, N. Litterman, P. P. Jiang, L. Russell, D. A. Hinds, Y. Hu, M. T. Weirauch, X. Chen, A. R. Chavan, G. P. Wagner, M. Pavlicev, M. C. Nnamani, J. Maziarz, M. K. Karjalainen, M. Ramet, V. Sengpiel, F. Geller, H. A. Boyd, A. Palotie, A. Momany, B. Bedell, K. K. Ryckman, J. M. Huusko, C. R. Forney, L. C. Kottyan, M. Hallman, K. Teramo, E. A. Nohr, G. Davey Smith, M. Melbye, B. Jacobsson and L. J. Muglia (2017). "Genetic associations with gestational duration and spontaneous preterm birth." *N Engl J Med* **377**(12): 1156–1167.

4 Evolutionary Paradoxa On the Way To the Fetal-Maternal Unit

How wonderful that we have met with a paradox. Now we have some hope of making progress.[1]

- Niels Bohr

When reflecting about the biology of human pregnancy, that is, implantation and placentation, a number of authors have identified "biological paradoxa" that make pregnancy appear biologically rather unlikely. These paradoxa, of course, do not only apply to human pregnancy, i.e., they are not human-specific, but apply to all mammalian species with sustained hemochorial placentation. The oldest concept along these lines is the immunological paradox proposed by Peter Medawar (Medawar 1953). The 1953 paper is the founding document of reproductive immunology, even though Medawar himself never actually worked on this problem. The immunological paradox is this: why is the fetus, which, in most cases, is immunologically different from the mother, not attacked by the maternal adaptive immune system (more on this below)? Another was pointed out by Hans-Werner Denker, which he called the cell biological paradox of implantation (Denker 1993). It consists of the recognition that embryo attachment requires an interaction between two epithelia, that of the uterine luminal epithelium and the trophoblast. Attachment between two epithelia should not happen, given that epithelia are constructed such that they do not stick to each other. Finally, in the lab of one of us (GPW), we proposed the "inflammation paradox" stating that, by embedding, the embryo is causing an endometrial injury and should lead to the activation of the innate (non-adaptive) immune system causing inflammation and eventually embryo destruction (Chavan et al. 2017), a phenomenon that one could call "nidatory inflammation." Later in this section, we will add another one, the tissue biological paradox of hemochorial placentation.

What are we going to make of the notion of biological paradoxa identified in human and mammalian pregnancy? Before we go into details, it may be helpful to reflect on what we mean when we talk about biological paradoxa, in particular with respect to the initiation of pregnancy and the evolution of evolutionary innovations in general.

Paradox is a Greek word meaning "contrary opinion," i.e., an opinion that goes contrary to common understanding.[2] In biology, a paradox can be understood as a *situation, feature, or character that exists in spite of generally accepted biological principles that should prevent the development of such features.* For instance, the presence of an allogenic organism or tissue in the human body should elicit an adaptive immune response. Since this is manifestly not the case during human pregnancy, placentation is thus a biological paradox and requires special explanation. The other paradoxa mentioned above and discussed in detail below follow the same kind of logic. What is implied in *the notion of biological paradoxa is that the existence of a paradoxical trait implies the evolution of special mechanisms to make them possible.* Recognizing a biological fact as paradoxical is an invitation to ask what kind of evolutionary novelty made it possible in spite of its paradoxical nature. Obviously, something is paradoxical only if simple modifications of the intensity or expression of the ancestral physiological pathways are not sufficient to explain that phenomenon. Some rather radical and unlikely evolutionary changes were necessary to make the paradoxical biological fact a species characteristic.

With that, we arrive at a definition of an evolutionary novelty: *a biological structure, process, or feature that is incompatible with the physiology of the ancestral organisms* (inferred from

DOI: 10.1201/9781032717777-4

investigating outgroup species). This notion is closely related to the idea that evolutionary novelties are evolutionary transformations that overcome a developmental or physiological constraint (Wagner and Müller 2002). Understanding biological paradoxa, as those that we will discuss here, is a stepping stone toward understanding how evolutionary novelties arise.

Another consequence of the resolution of a biological paradox is that the mechanisms necessary for overcoming these constraints provide an opportunity for regulating biological processes. For instance, since hemochorial placentation requires maternal accommodation of the invasive placenta, withdrawing this support is a way for the female body to terminate pregnancy. Note also that being able to withdraw or offer support makes this trait an individuated evolutionary trait. In the following, we will discuss the biological paradoxa in the order in which they appear during the natural establishment of pregnancy, from attachment to placentation, rather than in the historical order of their discovery.

INTERLUDE: FETAL-MATERNAL CONFLICT OR PARADOXA – WHAT IS THE DIFFERENCE?

Before we focus on the biological paradoxa of mammalian pregnancy, it is necessary to clarify the relationship between paradoxa and evolutionary conflict. There are at least two scientific communities concerned with the biology of the fetal-maternal relationship. One is molecular reproductive biology and reproductive medicine; the other is evolutionary biology, focusing on the evolutionary forces shaping the interaction between the fetus and the mother. Naturally, there is a (partial) overlap between these two areas of research, but otherwise they are independent fields of knowledge. Nevertheless, there is some terminological spillover that has led to conceptual misunderstandings. In the present context, one particular such misunderstanding needs to be addressed.

In the molecular and biomedical literature, the term "fetal-maternal conflict" is sometimes used to refer to one of the paradoxa that we want to describe below. Most often, this term is applied to what Peter Medawar called the immunological paradox, since it is also the most widely recognized example. The immunological paradox is the result of the natural function of the adaptive immune system in the context of an evolutionarily novel situation, i.e., the implantation of the embryo into the maternal tissue. One can think of this situation as a "conflict," namely a conflict between two evolutionary "objectives." That of defense against infection (function of the immune system) and that of supplying the embryo with oxygen and nutrients (function of the placenta). But this "conflict" is not what in evolutionary biology has been conceptualized as a conflict (Haig 1993).

The population genetic conflict theory, in contrast to the physiological "conflicts," considers situations where the fitness advantage of the fetus and that of the mother are in conflict, i.e., where a fitness increase for the fetus (the paternal genome) leads to a fitness decrease for the mother or vice versa (more on this in Chapter 10). For instance, increased extraction of nutrients from the mother benefits the fetus but could hurt the lifetime reproductive success of the mother because of lower chances for future pregnancies. From that perspective, it is clear that the immunological paradox of mammalian pregnancy is not an instance of evolutionary conflict, but rather a paradox as we are using the term here, and how Peter Medawar has defined it. If the mother's adaptive immune system attacks the fetus, this is not only bad for the fetus but also bad for the reproductive success of the mother, i.e., the fitness of both is decreased. Hence, the possibility of an immune attack on the embryo is not an evolutionary conflict since preventing it is in the fitness interest of both the mother and the fetus. It is thus important to clearly distinguish between reproductive paradoxa and evolutionary conflicts.

ATTACHMENT: THE CELL BIOLOGICAL PARADOX

The establishment of pregnancy is a multistage process, starting with fertilization, apposition, attachment, implantation, and proceeding to placentation.[3] Here we talk about one of the very early stages, where the embryo is establishing the first firm contact with the mother, i.e., an attachment to the uterine lining, rather than just an apposition, meaning the juxtaposition of the embryo and the luminal epithelium. That attachment is a biological paradox due to the nature of epithelia.

The epithelium is the fundamental form of tissue organization in animals (Figure 4.1), with the partial exception of sponges. This is the reason that, in the past, sponges were called Parazoa, meaning they are not "real" metazoans (multicellular animals), like all the other animals are. In its paradigmatic form, an epithelium is a two-dimensional array, a sheet, of polarized cells. Cell polarization here means that the cells have clearly distinct "ends," the apical side and the basal side. The apical side is facing an open space, and the basal side is covered with a thin layer of extracellular matrix, called the basal membrane.[4] Usually, the basal side faces a space filled with mesenchymal cells and extracellular matrix. The open space can be the outside of the body, i.e., the skin, or a cavity, like the lumen of blood vessels or a body cavity (e.g., a coelomatic cavity).[5] This side of the epithelium is called the apical side, while the other is called the basal side. For the apical side of the epithelium to maintain an open space, it is made "non-sticky," mostly through the presence of a glycoprotein called mucin. Mucins are membrane-bound proteins that are linked to copious amounts of highly hydrophilic carbohydrates, which makes the apical surface "slimy" and thus hard to attach to. Other cells and objects are kept away from the apical cell membrane, where they could interact with cell surface receptors, by a thicket of polysaccharides attached to the mucin anchor. In the older histological literature, this layer was called the "glycocalyx." Supporting the notion that the luminal epithelium as such is not readily interacting with the blastocyst is the fact that the uterus allows attachment of the blastocyst only during a limited period of time, the so-called window of implantation or window of receptivity. In the mouse, this is between the fourth and the fifth day after mating. Embryos artificially inserted in a mouse uterus outside that period are unable to attach and are aborted. In humans, the window of implantation is in the middle of the secretory phase of the menstrual cycle (days 19 to 23).

Having argued that embryo attachment is paradoxical because of the nature of epithelia, H.-W. Denker suggested that the window of implantation is realized by a partial loss of epithelial polarity of the luminal epithelial cells, i.e., a loss of the apical identity of the epithelial cells (Figure 4.2)

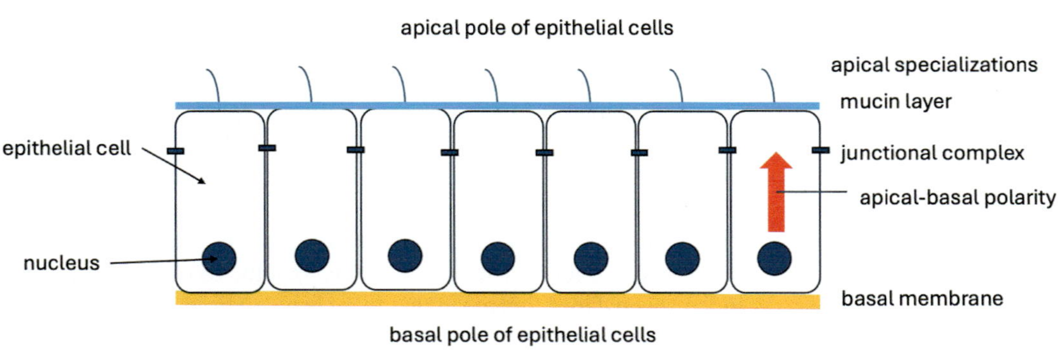

FIGURE 4.1 Schematic representation of an epithelium. A simple epithelium consists of a sheet of cells arrayed on a sheet of extracellular matrix called the basal membrane. The cells have a polarity between an apical pole facing an open space and the basal pole facing the basal membrane. The apical pole often shows some specializations, such as cilia or microvilli. The apical pole is covered by a layer of mucin, a highly hydrophilic muco-polypeptide which keeps the apical pole "non-sticky," i.e., avoids sticking to other surfaces in the body or at the surface of the body. The epithelial cells are interconnected by a number of different attachment devices called the junctional complex. (Image by GPW, CC BY--NC.)

(Denker 1993).[6] This model is confirmed by the observation that the expression of E-cadherin is reduced during the window of implantation. E-cadherins are molecules that mediate attachment among neighboring epithelial cells. Also, the typical apical actin network of epithelial cells is reduced and moved more basally. At the site of implantation, the mucin cover is also reduced under the influence of progesterone. Mucin is lost mostly due to the activity of proteases (in particular ADAM17[7] and MT1-MMP) produced by the luminal epithelial cells (Thathiah et al. 2003, Thathiah and Carson 2004). These enzymes cleave off the cytoplasmic segment of mucin, leading to the shedding of the extracellular portion of the molecule. Pre-implantation embryos also secrete trypsin-like proteases (Brosens et al. 2014), but, to our knowledge, whether these enzymes play a role in stripping the mucin coat at the site of attachment has not been directly addressed (Figure 4.2).

After the mucin coat is reduced and proper attachment becomes possible, the embryo-endometrial interaction is mediated by αβ-integrins expressed at both the luminal epithelium and the trophoblast cells (Dey et al. 2004, Aplin and Ruane 2017). A link between these two cell layers is mediated by bridging ECM molecules, to which the integrins attach. A well-characterized extracellular molecule is osteopontin (OPN, also called SPP1), but also include fibronectin, hyaluronic acid, and others. These receptor-ligand interactions trigger intracellular signal transduction in the luminal epithelial cells that finally lead to apoptotic cell death and the opening of the implantation site. Hence, the luminal epithelial (LE) cells undergo partial epithelial-to-mesenchymal transformation, but instead of turning into mesenchymal cells, they die. This is what is documented in the mouse and is also inferred to be the case in humans.

Interestingly, the attachment-induced cell death of LE cells is not a passive consequence of the impact of the embryo but actively regulated by and dependent on the activity of the LE cells themselves and is thus a permissive maternal mechanism. This has been most convincingly shown by S. K. Dey and collaborators (Cha et al. 2012, Sun et al. 2012) with a uterine-specific knock-out (KO) of KLF5, a transcription factor that is itself downstream of estrogen and progesterone signaling. In KLF5 -/- endometrium, the LE cells do not all die after embryo attachment, and the implantation, therefore, fails. The need for maternally expressed regulatory genes for implantation is an example supporting the inference, suggested at the beginning of this chapter, that a paradoxical biological phenomenon to occur requires the evolution of a dedicated biological mechanism. In this case, it is the maternally controlled EMT necessary for the physical contact between the embryo and the mother and the consequent loss of the epithelium.

The above narrative is almost exclusively based on experimental work on mouse implantation, as well as some descriptive work on humans (reviewed in Aplin and Ruane 2017]) From an evolutionary point of view, two questions present themselves: (1) Is proper attachment a general feature of eutherian pregnancy, despite the different kinds of fetal-maternal interface architectures realized in eutherian mammals (hemochorial vs epitheliochorial placentation)? (2) When did embryo attachment evolve? Is it also a feature of marsupial pregnancy with its different forms of fetal-maternal relationships (see Chapter 3)?

With respect to the question of interspecific variation, or lack thereof, of embryo attachment, the case of hoofed animals is particularly interesting. Remember that, in the mouse, a consequence of embryo attachment is epithelial apoptosis. In epitheliochorial placentation, the luminal epithelium survives and becomes part of the definitive fetal-maternal interface, or some of the epithelial cells fuse with the trophoblast, as in the sheep. Does this mean that there is no embryo attachment, or at least not one that is based on integrin-ECM interaction? Or is the signaling downstream of integrins different in pigs, cattle, and sheep, compared to mice and humans?

In fact, proper integrin/OPN-based embryo attachment is well-documented in pigs (reviewed in Johnson et al. 2021, Johnson et al. 2023) and ruminants (reviewed in Green et al. 2021). Hence, it is likely that integrin-based embryo attachment was also present in the common ancestor of Boreoeutheria (Figure 2.3C). The fact that there is integrin but not cell death in all eutherians implies that it is the downstream effects of integrin signaling on LE cells that must differ between eutherian species, i.e., cell death is not an inevitable consequence of attachment via integrins. But

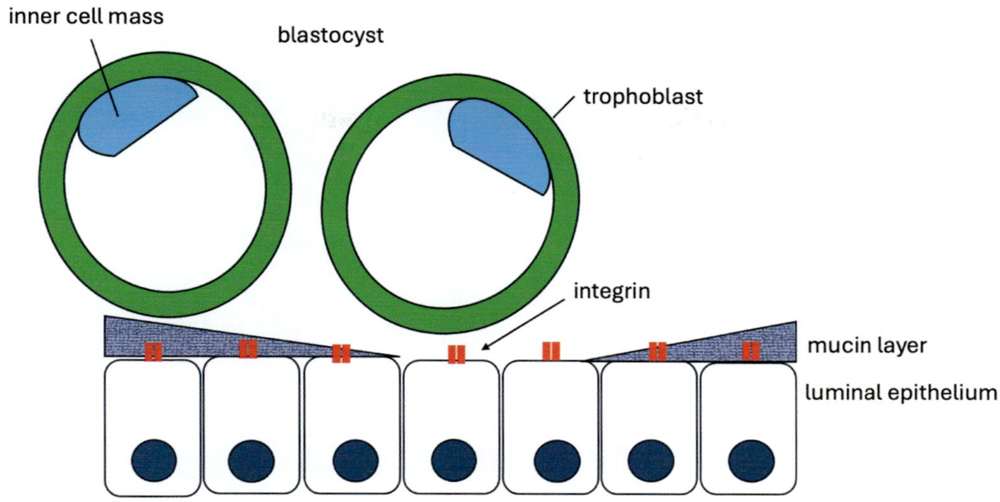

FIGURE 4.2 For an early embryo, called a blastocyst, to attach to the luminal epithelium of the endometrium, the epithelial cells have to shed their mucin cover (refer to Figure 4.1) in order to gain access to integrin receptors to form a firm attachment. In other words, embryo attachment requires that the luminal epithelium lose some of its epithelial polarity. (Image by GPW, CC BY-NC.)

what is known about Afrotheria and Xenarthra, i.e., the even more basally branching eutherian lineages?

Among afrotherians, the placentation of the African elephant (*Loxodonta africana*) has been investigated, but to our knowledge, detailed molecular studies of the attachment process have not been published.[8] Nevertheless, it is interesting to note that apparent attachment does not lead to apoptosis of the LE cells. Instead, the elimination of the LE is due to protrusions from the trophoblast that lift the LE cells off their basal membrane (Allen and Stansfield 2021). This mode of epithelial erosion is also found in a lizard, *Trachylepis ivensi* (Blackburn and Flemming 2012), which represents a rare form of reptilian invasive placentation and is phylogenetically independent from what is happening in elephants. It is thus likely that the attachment-dependent apoptosis of LE cells is a derived condition within the Euarchontoglires (see Figure 2.4 for phylogenetic orientation).

But what about marsupials, the sister clade of eutherians? These are characterized by relatively short gestation and very brief fetal-maternal contact (see Chapter 3). To our knowledge, integrins and their ligands have not been investigated, but there is some data on mucin expression and the histology of the FMI, in particular in the polyovular and ancestrally representative gray short-tailed opossum (*Monodelphis domestica*), as well as in the more derived Tamar wallaby, with an extended gestation compared to other marsupials (see Chapter 3). In *Monodelphis,* mucin was found in the endometrial transcriptome and has been immunohistochemically localized, as expected, on the luminal epithelium in non-cycling females, as well as in late gestation (Griffith et al. 2017), after the fetus "hatched" from its shell coat.[9] It is unlikely that the opossum forms any real epithelial attachment, not the least because during late gestation, the luminal epithelial cells are blebbing, i.e., budding off large cytoplasmic vesicles, akin to apocrine secretion, which seems to make attachment impossible (Figure 4.3). The same phenomenon also occurs in the late estrus cycle when ovulation happens, but no embryo develops and is thus a tissue-autonomous phenomenon (Griffith et al. 2019). In the epitheliochorial placentation of the Tamar wallaby, a firm embryo attachment is also unlikely, in contrast to the epitheliochorial placentation of pigs and ruminants (see above). This can be inferred from the fact that the late gestation fetus of a wallaby is easily separated from the uterine wall (see caption of Figure 2 in (Renfree and Shaw 2002) as well as (Dudley et al. 2024)).

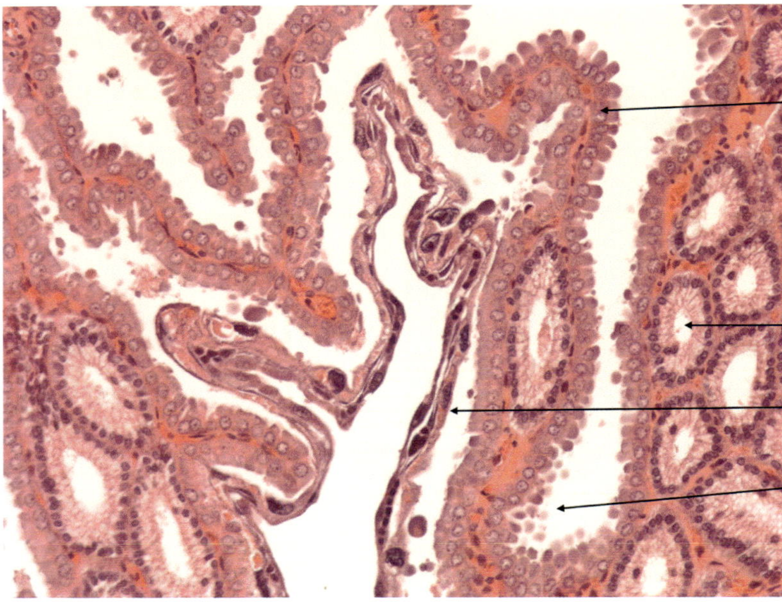

FIGURE 4.3 Fetal-maternal interface of a late pregnant opossum, *Monodelphis domestica*. There is no direct attachment between the fetal trophoblast (placenta) and the maternal luminal epithelium of the uterine endometrium. Instead, the maternal epithelial cells are blebbing, giving off large vesicles from their apical surface, a reaction that also occurs in the non-pregnant cycle and is thus internally regulated. (Image by Dan Stadtmauer and GPW, CC BY-NC.)

Nevertheless, during fetal contact, there are signs of partial EMT in marsupials, despite a lack of proper attachment. For instance, Kin and collaborators have identified smooth-muscle actin immunoreactivity in late gestation LE cells in opossum (Figure 5.3 in Kin et al. 2014), a sign of loss of epithelial polarity. In eutherians with invasive placentation, the cell adhesion molecule Desmoglein-2, a molecule necessary for epithelial integrity (Singh and Aplin 2015), is redistributed, apparently in preparation for trophoblast invasion (Preston et al. 2004, 2006). Interestingly, similar re-distribution has been reported in the LE of the dunnart, *Sminthopsis crassicaudata* (Dudley et al. 2015), the brush-tailed possum, *Trichosurus vulpecula*, and the Tammar wallaby, *Macropus eugenii* (Laird et al. 2018). This collection of species includes species with invasive trophoblast as well as those without trophoblast invasion, and thus these changes are unlikely to be related to the invasiveness of the embryo per se. These intriguing results are reminiscent of inflammation-related loss of epithelial polarity, suggesting that the attenuation of LE polarity might be ancestrally a cell-biological consequence of epithelial stress due to embryo contact, rather than an adaptation to support embryo attachment and implantation, as it seems to be in eutherians. This conclusion is consistent with the observation that epithelial remodeling is more related to phylogeny in marsupials than to the mode of fetal-maternal interaction (Laird et al. 2017).

Given the material reviewed above, the most likely scenario for the evolution of embryo attachment is that it evolved in the course of the origin of hemochorial placentation in the stem lineage of eutherians or within the eutherians before the ancestor of Laurasiatheria, i.e., the common ancestor of humans, mice, and hoofed animals. Furthermore, a cell-biological "seed" for the evolution of embryo attachment was the partial loss of epithelial polarity, due to unknown factors probably related to stress or an inflammatory reaction due to the presence of the blastocyst. This "seed" is present in marsupials without proper embryo attachment and thus is a feature shared between marsupials and eutherians. Loss of epithelial polarity of the LE is likely older than embryo attachment, as such, and more likely an enabling factor for the evolution of proper embryo attachment, rather than its consequence.

INTERLUDE: WHEN DO WE TALK OF IMPLANTATION?

In comparative reproductive biology, the term "embryo implantation" is often used in a rather loose way. In the broadest sense, any establishment of a fetal-maternal contact is sometimes called "implantation". This includes cases like the pig, where the fetus only attaches firmly to the luminal epithelium of the endometrium,[10] even though experts clearly state that implantation is an inappropriate term for the situation in pigs (Johnson et al. 2021). There is also confusion when it comes to distinguishing interstitial and "superficial" implantation. Interstitial implantation is clearly delineated as the case where the embryo is fully embedded in the endometrial stroma, as is the case in humans. But superficial implantation is sometimes loosely used to include mouse and rabbit implantation as well as pigs and cattle (for instance McGowen et al. 2014). The reason is that in the mouse and rabbit, the embryo implantation is "superficial" in the sense that the blastocyst is trapped in a swollen, tube-shaped uterus, rather than sinking into the endometrium, after which it is overgrown by the endometrium. This is certainly a different kind of implantation in terms of the process than the one in humans, but not in terms of the outcome. It still includes the erosion of the luminal endometrium, the transformation of the stroma into the decidua, and the establishment of a hemochorial placenta. To lump this together with the pig fetal-maternal interface as "superficial" implantation (as inMcGowen et al. 2014) is clearly not meaningful. The pig attachment is a fundamentally different situation than that in the mouse and rabbit in terms of the cell biology of the fetal-maternal interface. What shall we call implantation then?

Maybe it is helpful to say that "*implantation is a kind of establishment of the fetal-maternal interface where at least part of the maternal tissue is replaced by fetal/placental tissue*" so that in its mature form of placentation, we have a hybrid tissue consisting of fetal and maternal components. That includes all forms of implantation leading to placentation types covered by the Otto Grosser classification (Grosser 1909), except epithelio-chorial placentation. After all, the term "implant" comes from the Latin "implantare" for putting a plant *into* the soil. Now, implantation colloquially means inserting an object into the body of a person or animal. This point is not merely semantic. It is relevant because of the cell biological consequences of implantation compared to apposition and attachment (see below).

FROM ATTACHMENT TO IMPLANTATION: THE INFLAMMATION PARADOX

What is inflammation, and why does it matter in mammalian reproduction? In eutherian mammals with an invasive placenta, embryo attachment leads, in one way or another (see above), to the erosion of part of the luminal epithelium. In all animals, the integrity of epithelia is closely monitored, and injuries inevitably lead to compensatory reactions to restore the integrity of the epithelium and the underlying stroma. This is easy to understand if one considers the fundamental importance epithelia have in defining compartments within the body, as well as in maintaining the boundary between the inside of the body and the outside environment.

Reactions to epithelial injury can be summarized under two perspectives: inflammation and wound healing. Inflammation is an immediate reaction to injury and engages the cells of the innate immune system (Medzhitov 2008). Wound healing is the long-term restoration of tissue integrity. Inflammation and wound healing are, of course, closely related, as the resolution of the inflammatory process usually leads to wound healing (Adler et al. 2020). Both inflammation and wound healing, or the lack thereof, present two paradoxa in the biology of eutherian placentation. In this section, we will deal with the role of inflammation as an obstacle to the evolution of embryo implantation. The paradox of wound healing will be discussed in the following section.

Inflammation is usually discussed in the context of infection, and in fact, is a necessary step in activating the adaptive immune system to combat germs and viruses. However, inflammation also plays a broader role than fighting infections (Medzhitov 2008, Kotas and Medzhitov 2015, Okabe and Medzhitov 2016). It is essential for the maintenance and restoration of tissue integrity. This can readily be seen in the case of so-called "sterile" inflammation, where tissue damage occurs without infection, as in the case of a sprained ankle or similar internal injuries. These injuries also lead to inflammation (for a recent review of sterile inflammation, see Zindel and Kubes 2020). Other forms of inflammation are caused by more subtle injuries, such as a consequence of lipid overload in adipocytes, causing cellular stress. Hence, inflammation is not only, and perhaps not primarily, a mechanism to fight infection but should be seen as a mechanism generally activated in response to compromised tissue integrity. It is activated when normal homeostatic mechanisms fail. Inflammation is thus a tissue-level stress reaction (Adler et al. 2020).

Inflammatory processes are triggered by signals from so-called sentinel cells, mostly tissue-resident macrophages, mast cells, dendritic cells, as well as non-immune cells such as fibroblasts and even epithelia. These cells get activated when certain generic signs of infection or tissue damage are recognized. In the case of infections, the cells recognize macromolecular patterns typical for pathogens, so-called PAMPs, standing for Pathogen-Associated Molecular Patterns. The most well-known of these are LPS (lipo-poly saccharides, a component of the cell wall of Gram-negative bacteria, a.k.a. endotoxin) and mannose, a carbohydrate found on bacterial cell walls. Tissue damage is similarly recognized through so-called DAMPs, standing for Damage-Associated Molecular Patterns, like extracellular ATP, DNA, and others. These molecules are not supposed to be found outside the cell. If these molecules are found in the extracellular space, something went wrong.

On a broad level, the inflammatory process has three branches: (1) vasodilation, leading to additional blood to the place of injury and causing the characteristic redness of sites of inflammation, (2) vascular leakage, allowing plasma to seep into the tissue and leading to swelling, and (3) leukocyte recruitment. IL1 and TNF secreted from activated macrophages act on local endothelial cells to capture blood-resident neutrophils, allowing them to leave the bloodstream and enter the affected tissue. The first wave of leukocytes recruited to the site of inflammation are neutrophils. Neutrophils are highly effective in clearing pathogens by phagocytosis and the release of toxic chemicals from their granules. In addition, and primarily in the case of sterile inflammation, neutrophils are also effective in removing necrotic tissue debris and are an important source of growth factors. Finally, neutrophils undergo programmed cell death (apoptosis), the products of which are then cleared by macrophages. The latter process plays a role in reprogramming macrophages to so-called M2 macrophages, which initiates wound healing by secreting TGFβ1 and IL-10. Whether the role of neutrophils in switching off the inflammatory process and initiating wound healing requires a direct interaction of neutrophils with macrophages is still unclear (discussed in Zindel and Kubes 2020). Nevertheless, neutrophils can also lead to tissue damage when the transition to neutrophil clearance is unsuccessful, leading to a sustained inflammatory environment.

The second wave of leukocytes entering the damaged tissue are monocytes, the precursors of macrophages. They enter the area of injury as pro-inflammatory M1 cells, characterized by CCR2 expression, enhancing the pro-inflammatory environment, and over time are switched to become M2 macrophages. In some cases, this reprogramming happens under the influence of the signals emanating from apoptotic neutrophils or due to the influence of innate natural killer T cells (iNKT cells), which secrete IL4 and IL10 in response to the presentation of self-antigens by CD1d.

All these processes are mediated by a canonical set of signaling molecules such as IL1, IL8, IL2, IL12, TNF, IFNγ, and others, as well as small molecule mediators, such as prostaglandin E2, PGE2, and histamine. Any process with substantial contribution from these and related molecules and the cellular actors, such as macrophages and neutrophils, is often loosely attributed to as "inflammatory processes." This is also the case with human embryo implantation, leading to the notion of "good inflammation" (Mor et al. 2011).

Inflammation in human implantation: There are several lines of evidence that point to the possibility that embryo implantation is an inflammatory process, or rather a *process evolutionarily derived from inflammation*. From the clinical point of view, the most interesting is the observation that small injuries to the endometrium, as caused by needle biopsies, can increase implantation success in IVF treatment for infertility (Goel et al. 2017).[11] The interpretation, supported by correlative evidence of expression of inflammatory mediators, is that the injury triggers the inflammatory potential of the tissue and thus "primes" the endometrium for the expression of implantation-related inflammatory signals. This line of reasoning is plausible because during the normal ovarian cycle, the window of implantation, in humans and mice, is associated with the expression of inflammatory mediators (Mor et al. 2011). At the very least, this line of work points to a mechanistic overlap between generic inflammation and the process of embryo implantation.

The inflammation paradox has two components: (1) an evolutionary paradox (Chavan et al. 2017) and (2) a clinical one (Mor et al. 2011). The evolutionary paradox arises when one considers the evolutionary scenario of how embryo implantation may have arisen in evolution. Among viviparous species, embryo implantation is relatively rare and is thus likely evolutionarily derived in eutherians (see Chapter 3). Hence, one has to imagine that, at some time in the history of mammals, a population existed in which most of the individuals were viviparous but had no embryo implantation. In some females, the embryo was hatching from the egg coat and started to invade the endometrium. The first layer of maternal tissue the embryo encounters is the luminal epithelium, and this would have to be breached while evolving embryo implantation. But above, we have argued that injuring an epithelium elicits an inflammatory process, since this is a generic mechanism that ensures the restoration of tissue integrity. Causing inflammation in the uterus at the location of an embryo can have positive as well as negative consequences for the embryo. One can imagine that vascularization and vascular leakage, the first two "arms" of the inflammatory process (see above), could be beneficial to the embryo as they make blood-borne nutrients more accessible to the embryo. Also, ECM remodeling, typically occurring at the site of inflammation, is enhancing the ability of the embryo to implant itself into the uterus. On the other hand, the third branch of the inflammatory process, the recruitment of leukocytes, in particular neutrophils, is likely to be problematic. Neutrophil recruitment would be expected to create an inhospitable environment for the embryo. How exactly that would have occurred is, of course, not directly assessable, but the recent advances of neutrophil biology suggest a scenario.

As mentioned in the brief summary of sterile inflammation above, neutrophils, under normal circumstances, pave the way to healing by removing necrotic tissue and secreting growth factors. They also trigger the restorative phenotype of macrophages, so-called M2 (Serhan and Savill 2005, Sugimoto et al. 2016). However, if this transition from inflammation to tissue repair is unsuccessful, neutrophils and macrophages can enter a positive feedback loop, which exacerbates the inflammatory state and causes neutrophils to release toxins, leading to extensive tissue damage (Nathan 2022).

In the case of the initial stages of embryo implantation, we are not dealing with a short, damaging event, like a burn injury that can be resolved to the prior state after the damage is done. The embryo, as long as it is in the uterus, will continue injuring the endometrium, making resolution of the inflammatory reaction using the mechanisms described above difficult, if not impossible. Continued expression of damage signals (DAMPs) prevents the transition to healing, and the collateral tissue damage of neutrophil hyperactivation will eventually also affect the embryo. The expanding inflammatory reaction will trigger expulsion of the embryo in a process mechanistically analogous to emptying the intestinal tract by vomiting or diarrhea. The scenario presented here is entirely based on what is known about the physiology of sterile inflammation, rather than direct evidence, as we have no access to extant species that fully represent this hypothesized stage in the evolution of eutherian placentation.

This hypothesized chain of events is expected to be independent of the immunological status of the embryo, meaning that it is independent of whether the mother recognizes the embryo as genetically foreign or not. Instead, it is expected to precipitate from the tissue damage caused by the nidatory injury itself. The *innate* immune system would be activated whether the embryo is immunologically different from the mother or not, and is thus different from the widely acknowledged so-called "immunological" paradox of mammalian pregnancy (Medawar 1953). The consequence of this model is that embryo implantation, as we know it from eutherian mammals, required an evolutionary innovation that suppressed or modulated the inflammatory cascade at the site of embryo implantation. More about this below.

The clinical paradox is different from the evolutionary but may be mechanistically related. The clinical paradox is that while inflammation-like processes are beneficial to the establishment of pregnancy, i.e., implantation, the continuation of pregnancy in humans is constantly under threat from inflammatory processes (Romero et al. 2014). These can lead to premature birth with fatal consequences for the fetus/newborn, in particular in the absence of medical interventions that push the gestational age of viability to 22 weeks of gestation. Without clinical support, a human fetus becomes viable only after the 32nd week. While many risk factors have been identified that can increase the likelihood of premature birth, the vast majority of them converge to a common pathway, and that is inflammation in some part of the female reproductive tract and/or in the extraembryonic tissues of the fetus (Romero et al. 2014). How is it then that inflammatory mediators and/or processes can be beneficial at the beginning of pregnancy but so dangerous for the continuation of pregnancy later? In brief, and expanded later, we think the connection between the evolutionary and the clinical paradox is this: *implantation is intrinsically an inflammatory process, whereas the continuation of pregnancy after implantation depends on the suppression or resolution of the nidatory inflammation.* For the longest part of gestation, pregnancy is possible as long as the support of these anti-inflammatory mechanisms lasts. Any factor, including inflammatory gum disease (Tsikouras et al. 2024), that undermines the anti-inflammatory support can then lead to a breakdown of the pro-gestational state and precipitate premature birth or spontaneous abortion.[12]

As already mentioned, the scenario of the evolutionary inflammation paradox implies that extended pregnancy, as typical for eutherian mammals, requires several evolutionary innovations that have the primary function of switching a pro-inflammatory environment during the implantation process into an anti-inflammatory state necessary for the continuation of pregnancy. But what is this evolutionary innovation? Here, we propose what one can call the "*Decidua Hypothesis*," that is, the hypothesis that the evolutionary origin of a novel tissue type was the answer to the inflammation paradox. A detailed discussion of the nature and evolution of the decidua goes beyond the scope of this chapter. We will return to this idea briefly below and in more detail in Chapters 5 and 6. Here, we will continue with a discussion of the comparative biology of inflammatory mechanisms at the fetal-maternal interface to provide a fuller picture of how the inflammation paradox plays out in various lineages.

Inflammation in marsupial pregnancy: By now we have repeatedly made the point that when one speaks casually of "mammalian pregnancy," one actually has in mind the eutherian pregnancy, i.e., reproduction in humans, rodents, farm animals, cats and dogs, and even elephants. Other mammals, however, are substantially different from eutherians, not only with respect to female reproductive biology but importantly so. In particular, marsupials, opossums, dunnarts, koalas, kangaroos, and wallabies played an important role in inspiring the twin hypotheses of the *inflammation paradox* and the *decidua hypothesis* (see above).

Female reproductive biology in marsupials can be divided into two broad modes, one exemplified by the opossum and other so-called "primitive" marsupials, the other exemplified by wallabies and kangaroos (Macropodidae). The opossum-like mode of female reproduction is characterized by multiple ovulations, large litter size,[13] no systemic recognition of pregnancy, and a short gestational period, in fact, even shorter than the non-pregnant ovarian cycle (Freyer et al. 2003, Chavan et al. 2017). In contrast, the derived mode of female reproduction in marsupials is characterized by (usually) only one ovulation, as in humans, recognition of pregnancy, and an extended gestational period (Renfree 1972, Renfree and Shaw 2002, Freyer et al. 2007, Renfree 2010, Dudley et al. 2024). The structure of the phylogenetic tree of marsupials makes clear that the opossum mode of reproduction is likely more similar to the ancestral situation and that the macropod form of reproduction is derived within the marsupials (Luckett 1994) (Figure 4.4). The latter is thus an independent evolutionary origination of extended pregnancy, independent of that in eutherians. Hence, comparisons between eutherians and opossums, as well as between macropods and opossums, should be particularly informative.

When we speak here of the opossum, we usually mean the "laboratory" opossum species from Brazil, the short-tailed gray opossum (*Monodelphis domestica*) (Vandeberg 1990, VandeBerg and Robinson 1997). *Monodelphis* is easy to keep and breed in the lab. It is a much easier study organism than the North American opossum, *Didelphis virginiana*, a species much larger and requiring a more involved environment than that of a convenient laboratory animal. Earlier work on the North American opossum was done, but the differences to *Monodelphis* are not great as to require a separate treatment (Harder et al. 1993).

Opossum pregnancy is relatively short, about two weeks, compared to the three weeks of mouse pregnancy. Remarkable about the opossum is the long pre-hatching period of gestation. The embryo is separated from the mother by an eggshell coat for 12.5 days of gestation, at which time the eggshell is degraded, and the first physical contact between mother and embryo occurs (Selwood 2000, Griffith et al. 2017). After this contact, the expression of classical inflammatory mediators at the fetal-maternal contact zone progressively increases, IL1, IL6, IL8, IL17, as well as the enzyme PTGS2 and its product PGE2, leading to parturition after about two days. During the time of fetal-maternal contact, some subtle changes in the endometrial histology occur, like the replacement of the sub-epithelial layer of endometrial fibroblasts by a network of blood capillaries, suggesting an increased supply of oxygen and nutrients to the embryo as well as the recruitment of neutrophils (Griffith et al. 2017). The uterine glands increase in size and number and have an open lumen, suggesting increased secretory activity compared to uterine glands during the non-pregnant cycle. At the end of gestation, at a few places one can observe that the luminal epithelium is slightly breached by trophoblast cells (Koryu Kin and GPW personal observation), showing that even the opossum trophoblast is invasive, similar to what was described for the four-eyed possum, *Philander opossum* (Enders and Enders 1969), although it never comes to the establishment of an invasive placenta.[14] At the same time, the epithelium seems to greatly expand in area, since it folds upon itself, forming extensive epithelial folds. The epithelial cells start to bud off large pieces of cytoplasm akin to apocrine secretion (see Figure 4.3). The latter transformation, though, is embryo-independent since it also occurs during pseudopregnancy (Griffith et al. 2019).[15]

The cause and the biological role of the inflammatory processes during fetal-maternal contact in the opossum are not clear. One possible trigger could be the secretion of proteases by the trophoblast, which starts before the removal of the shell coat, and they are thus likely "hatching enzymes." The trophoblast continues to express proteases (Griffith et al. 2017) and thus could be attacking the luminal epithelium of the uterus. However, the idea that, in the opossum, the inflammatory processes represent a generic sterile inflammation is challenged by the discovery that many of the most important initial inflammatory mediators, IL1, IL6,[16] and IL17, are not produced by maternal cells, as one would expect in the case of a generic inflammatory process of the maternal tissue (Chavan et al. 2021, Stadtmauer et al. 2025). Instead, these mediators are produced by trophoblast cells. This phenomenon has been called "cooperative inflammation" (Stadtmauer and Wagner 2020) since it indicates that the inflammatory process is one that occurs through the contribution of inflammatory mediators from both the mother and the fetus. The fact that inflammatory mediators high up in the hierarchy of the inflammatory process are produced by the fetus shows that the quasi-inflammatory processes in the opossum are also in the "evolutionary interest" of the fetus. Otherwise, it would not have evolved as a character expressed by the fetus.

For the biological role of these processes, there are at least two candidates. On the one hand, as has been mentioned above, part of the inflammatory processes can lead to enhanced nutrient transfer to the embryo, because of increased blood flow and vascular leakage. In fact, during the phase of

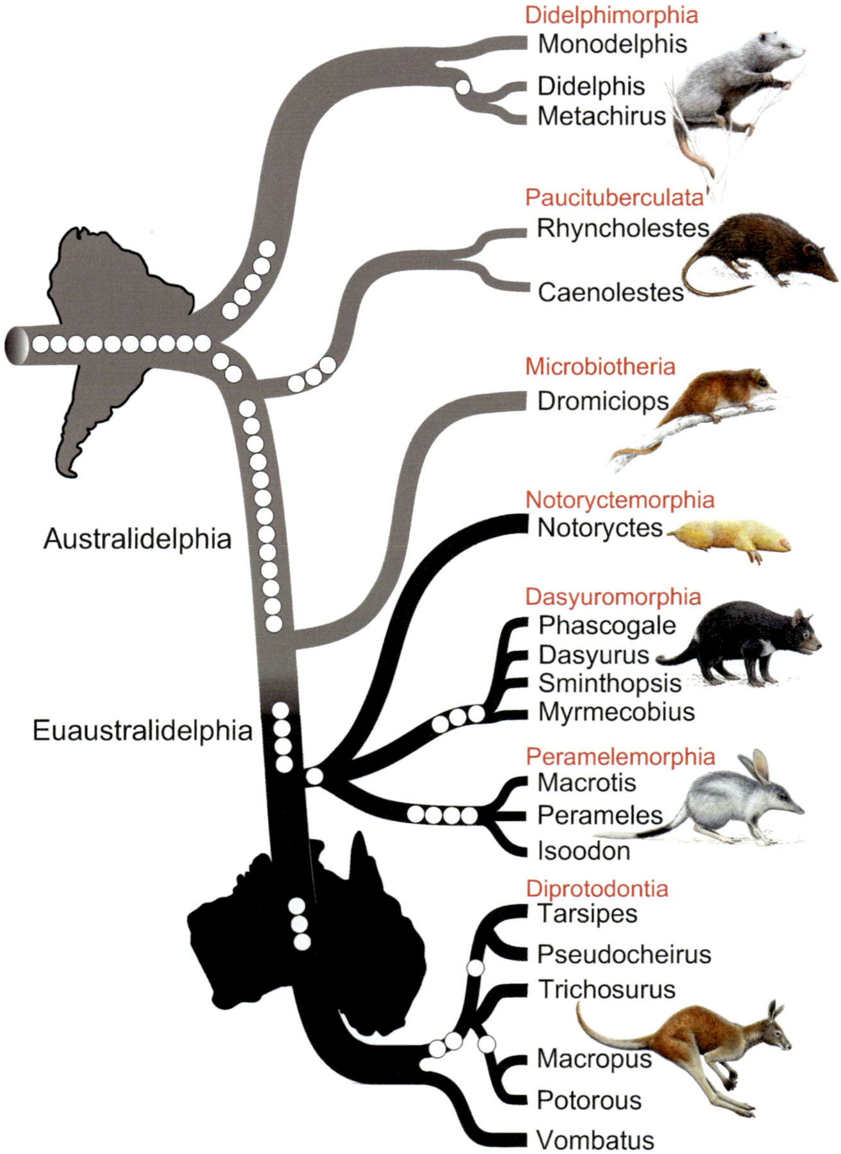

FIGURE 4.4 Phylogenetic relationships among major marsupial groups. This tree is based on the identity of transposable element insertions (Nilsson et al. 2010) (image is figure 2 in Nilsson et al. (2010) published under CC BY). Note the basal position of the lineage leading to modern-day opossums.

fetal-maternal contact, the vascularization of the endometrium is increasing, and most of the fetal prepartum growth is happening. However, attempts to test this hypothesis by blocking some of the inflammatory mediators and measuring the fetal biomass have not succeeded in demonstrating a nutritional role (Stadtmauer et al. 2026). The alternative hypothesis, although not really exclusive to the first, is the idea that the inflammatory mediators supplied by the fetus are a parturition signal (Hansen et al. 2017), i.e., a signal from the fetus to initiate the birth process. To our knowledge, this hypothesis has also not been tested experimentally.

Given that the age of the most recent common ancestor of therian mammals, i.e., the ancestor of eutherian and marsupial mammals, has been estimated to be between 200 and 250 Mio years in the past (Liu et al. 2017), it is not surprising that neither the opossum nor the eutherians would represent the situation hypothesized to have been present at the time when the first mammalian fetal-maternal contact occurred. The comparative evidence still suggests that the processes during eutherian implantation and opossum fetal-maternal contact are homologous to a generic inflammatory process but not identical to it, neither in eutherians nor in the opossum. The most likely scenario is that divergent evolution in marsupials and placentals led to different forms of biological "instrumentalization" (functionalization) of the ancestral sterile inflammation due to the embryonic or fetal contact with the endometrium. In eutherians, the evolutionary trajectory led to implantation, subsequent suppression of inflammation, and extended pregnancy. On the other hand, in at least some marsupial lineages like the opossum, the inflammatory process may have been co-opted to trigger parturition. It is thus interesting to ask what happened within marsupials when, in macropods, extended gestation evolved, independent of what happened in eutherians.

In one macropod, the tammar wallaby (*Notomacropus eugenii*), it has been shown that the rupture of the shell coat and the contact between the mother and the fetus lead to a rather muted and incomplete inflammatory reaction (Dudley et al. 2024). The wallaby fetus is also not invasive and does not cause a nidatory injury. This is thus an alternative strategy to effect longer gestation, namely, completely avoid a nidatory inflammation, rather than allow it and then turn it off, as is the case for eutherians with invasive placentation.

The decidua hypothesis: A corollary to the inflammation paradox is that, in eutherians, an evolutionary innovation arose that resolved the inflammation and allowed the evolution of extended fetal-maternal contact, i.e., extended placentation and pregnancy. The question thus is, what was this evolutionary innovation or innovations? – One answer is the *Decidua Hypothesis*, the idea that the resolution of the inflammation caused by implantation is effected by a novel cell type, the endometrial stromal fibroblast. The evolutionary and cell biology of the decidua is a complex story that will be discussed in a separate chapter (Chapter 6), and challenges to the nidatory inflammation and decidual hypotheses will be discussed toward the end of Chapter 5.

FROM IMPLANTATION TO PLACENTATION: THE TISSUE BIOLOGICAL PARADOX

Cells in multicellular organisms rarely act alone. With few exceptions, they are integrated into a tissue with multiple cell types[17] (Adler et al. 2023), or are migratory cells that often change tissue context like immune cells (Pavličev and Wagner 2024). Composite tissues, as one may call those consisting of multiple cell types, are configurations of cell types that mutually regulate each other's phenotype and abundance. A recent model suggests that composite tissues have at least four categories of cells (Adler et al. 2020): a parenchymatic cell type, endothelial cells, fibroblasts, and tissue resident macrophages. Parenchymatic cells are usually, but not always, of epithelial origin and perform the specialized functions of the tissue type. Endothelial cells form the vasculature that supplies nutrients and oxygen, and the fibroblasts provide much of the ECM for the tissue and are thus responsible for the mechanical integrity of the tissue. Macrophages are monitoring tissue integrity and removing cellular debris.

It is important to note that these *cell categories* are not *cell types*, but different cell types can take the role of a cell category in different tissues. For instance, it is well established that tissue-resident macrophages come in tissue-specific varieties that likely are different cell types in the evolutionary sense (Arendt et al. 2016). For instance, in the central nervous system, there is a cell type called microglia, which belongs to the macrophage cell type family and performs the role of macrophages in the brain; in (lamellar) bone the so-called osteoclasts, cells that remove bone substance, are also members of the macrophage family; in the liver the resident macrophage is called Kupffer cell, etc. The same is true for tissue-specific fibroblasts, like the stellate cells of the liver or the endometrial stromal fibroblasts of the uterus.

It is believed that the constellation of cell types in a composite tissue is a homeostatic unit, meaning that they mutually monitor and regulate each other's activities and abundance. Experimental evidence has been produced for feedback regulation between fibroblasts and macrophages (Zhou et al. 2018). An exemplary macroscopic phenomenon reflecting the self-stabilizing nature of tissues is wound healing, where tissue integrity is restored by growth and differentiation of additional cells. Of course, like every biological process, wound healing can go wrong, as in fibrosis, where parenchymatic cells are replaced by inert collagen instead of new parenchymatic cells, thus leading to progressive loss of tissue functionality.

And here is the tissue-biological paradox of eutherian placentation: the endometrium is a composite tissue just like many other tissues in the mammalian body, and can regenerate and heal, most impressively demonstrated in the human monthly regeneration of endometrial tissue after menstruation. We already argued that the implantation of the embryo into the uterus is an injury to the endometrium, the nidatory injury. Why then is the endometrium not healing after the initial inflammatory reaction has been resolved? If healing were to proceed, it would be incompatible with the continuation of hemochorial placentation!

Three reactions of the tissue to invasion by a foreign body are plausible. Encapsulation, as is the case with multicellular parasitoids, the suppression of healing and the establishment of a novel, alternative tissue homeostasis.

Encapsulation is a reaction of animals against the invasion by a foreign body that is too large to be phagocytosed. This mode of defense is best documented in insects, where it is also associated with melanization at the surface of the object (Streams 1971, Maramosch and Shope 1975). Encapsulation is also known in vertebrates, such as fish, to protect against parasites. For instance, eels encapsulate nematode parasites (Bracamonte et al. 2021). The character of encapsulation limits its applicability for dealing with blastocysts, since isolating the blastocyst from the rest of the tissue prevents provisioning of the embryo so that it can grow and develop. Hence, encapsulation is not an option for evolving a successful reproductive strategy. Nevertheless, encapsulation-derived processes could contribute a part to the implantation reactions, for instance, to regulate the degree of invasion.

Evidence for the second possibility, active suppression of the wound healing response, was discovered in the lab of Adrian Erlebacher and reported in two important papers (Nancy et al. 2018, Osokine et al. 2022). In Nancy et al. 2018 the authors showed that decidual cells in mice accumulate repressive chromatin markers (tri-methylation of lysine 27 on histone 3, H3K27me3) at a large number of genes, particularly genes known to be involved in fibroblast activation during wound healing, i.e., the transformation of fibroblasts into myofibroblasts. This chromatin methylation is mediated by a methyl transferase called EZH2, standing for "enhancer of zeste homolog 2" (which is not really a helpful name). In Osokine et al. (2022), the authors show that a knockout of EZH2 leads to pregnancy failure in mid-pregnancy. The decidual cells around the implantation site assume the phenotype of a myofibroblast, i.e., expression of alpha smooth muscle actin (aSMA, *ACTA2*), while still undergoing polyploidization, as decidual cells usually do in mice. This experiment shows that the elimination of EZH2 allowed the fibroblast activation pathway to be triggered at the implantation site and that the activation of the wound healing cascade is incompatible with the continuation of pregnancy. This is direct experimental evidence that endometrial tissue homeostasis had to be suppressed in order to allow sustained invasive placentation to arise.

The discovery of suppressed wound healing and the associated fibroblast activation at the site of implantation raises another important question. At the implantation site, some cells of the endometrium are eliminated, or breached, like the luminal epithelium, new cell types differentiate, like the decidual cells, and other cell types are added from the embryo: the chorion that separates the embryo from the maternal tissue, and some trophoblast cells invade the endometrium. The invasive cells are, for example, the extravillous trophoblast cells that replace the endothelial cells of the spiral arteries in humans, or other extra-placental trophoblast cells in other species (like rats, and also mice; Stadtmauer et al. 2025). How is it that this tissue, the decidua, can be maintained until the end of pregnancy, which in humans means for several months? Is it that the decidua is a metastable configuration that happens to not collapse for a limited amount of time? Or is the decidua an alternative tissue type with intrinsic homeostatic capabilities?

The questions raised at the end of the last paragraph do not have an experimentally grounded answer yet. They are, nevertheless, a logical consequence of current thinking about the nature of tissues (Adler et al. 2020, DiFrisco et al. 2020, Pavličev et al. 2024) and the discovery of the suppression of generic wound healing reactions in the fibroblast population of the endometrium after implantation. The answers to the above questions will likely be species-specific, with different degrees of integration between fetal and maternal cells into a fetal-maternal unit. An interesting example in this case is the fetal-maternal interface of the Armadillo.

The Armadillo is an interesting species to study because it belongs to the clade of Xenarthra, which, together with the Afrotheria (elephants, hyrax, tenrecs, etc.), forms a clade Atlantogenata, that splits off from the other eutherian lineages right at the root of Eutheria. Comparing animals from these groups with those of the rest of the placentals is thus particularly informative about the very origin of the eutherian condition. Technically, the placenta of armadillos is hemochorial, at least that of the nine-banded armadillo, *Dasypus novemcinctus*, found in North America (Enders 1960, Enders and Welsh 1993). That means that the trophoblast is in direct contact with maternal blood, but the anatomical relationship is quite different from that in humans and mice. The difference to humans is that the armadillo endometrium has a system of pre-formed blood lacunae (also called "sinuses") into which individual placental villi grow, each transversing the endometrium in a narrow canal (Figure 4.5) (Chavan and Wagner 2016). This situation can be thought of as a form of hemochorial placentation with minimal injury to the endometrium. In contrast, the placental bed of humans is a broad, open wound covered by the placenta. It is also not entirely clear whether and what kind of decidual cells the armadillo has, and whether they have also been modified to prevent fibroblast activation. In any case, this is an example of an effective hemochorial placentation with minimal injury to the maternal tissue, maybe related to a limited ability to resolve the inflammation and tissue-biological paradoxa. In contrast, sustained large injuries to the endometrium, as in humans, likely required additional innovations that either suppressed endometrial tissue homeostasis or replaced it with an alternative homeostatic tissue, the *decidua vera*.

FROM PLACENTATION TO IMMUNE TOLERANCE: THE IMMUNOLOGICAL PARADOX

While the so-called immunological paradox of mammalian pregnancy was first recognized in 1953 by Medawar, we present it here as the last of four pregnancy-related paradoxa. The reason is that the term "immunological paradox" is misleading, since it only refers to the problem of how to protect the fetus from the *adaptive immune system*, while the inflammation paradox discussed above is also related to the immune system, specifically the innate immune system. The other reason is that it takes time to mount an adaptive immune response, while the other issues, like the nidatory inflammation, play out over shorter timescales. The time required for allograft rejection is highly variable and can range from days to months after solid organ transplantation (Colvin and Smith 2005). In addition, the initiation of an adaptive immune response is downstream of the inflammatory reaction of the innate immune system, which is necessary to activate the adaptive immune system. In fact, if the attachment and implantation-related inflammation could be completely avoided, the adaptive immune response would also be less of a worry. The longer timescale of the adaptive immune reaction also means that the evolutionary drive to modify or avoid adaptive immune reactions would become necessary only after the gestational length evolved to be long enough for adaptive immune responses to arise. Nevertheless, most if not all eutherian mammals have evolved gestational lengths long enough that adaptive immune responses are a concern. It is thus not surprising that reproductive immunology, as a medical discipline, is mostly (but not exclusively) concerned with the

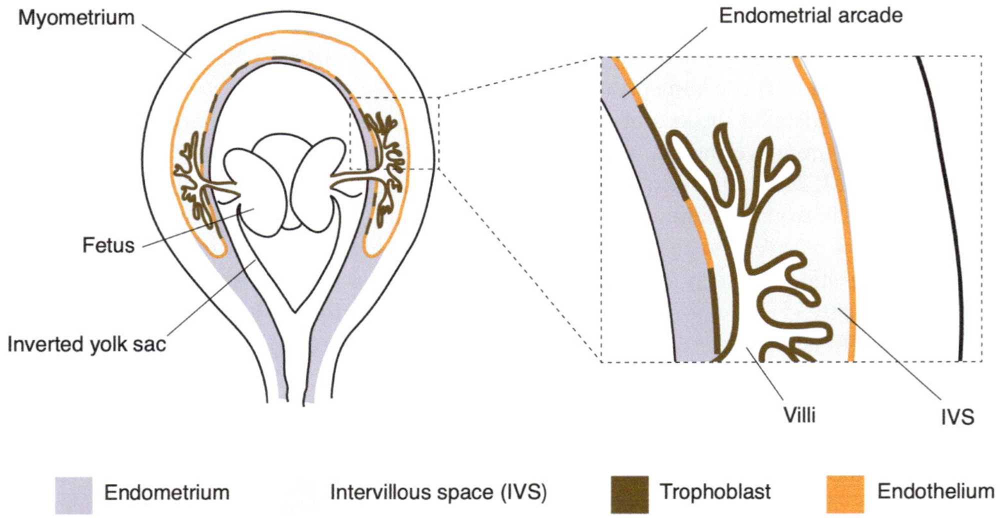

FIGURE 4.5 Schematic representation of the fetal-maternal interface of the nine-banded armadillo, *Dasypus novemcinctus*. The villi from the embryo are growing into the maternal endometrium and enter a pre-formed blood space in which they ramify. IVS = inter-villus space. (Figure 6 from A. R. Chavan and G. P. Wagner (2016), published open access under CC license.)

regulation of the adaptive immune system at the fetal-maternal interface. In order to appreciate how the fetus can be protected against allorecognition and rejection by the adaptive immune system, we may first have a look at how transplants are recognized and rejected.

In general, the adaptive immune system is activated and directed toward specific pathogens through the presentation of antigenic peptides by so-called major histocompatibility complex molecules (MHC). The name of MHC already betrays its role in allograft rejection, but its main function is to alert the adaptive immune system about the presence of pathogens. There are two types of MHC molecules with distinct roles in adaptive immunity. MHC class I (MHC-I) molecules are expressed on almost all cells of the body and "report" about the proteome composition inside the cells. This is important to identify virus-infected cells and ensure their elimination by cytotoxic lymphocytes (CTL), which recognize non-self peptides presented by MHC-I molecules. On the other hand, MHC class II (MHC-II) is expressed by professional antigen-presenting cells (APC), which take up proteins from the extracellular space and process them to be presented on their cell surface with MHC-II molecules. The APC migrates from the location of the infection/inflammation to the next draining lymph nodes and "educates" naïve T cells about the presence of allo-antigens.

The most logical way that an allograft becomes subject to an adaptive immune attack seems to be the presentation of graft-specific peptides to T cells and/or APC, either on MHC-I receptors on graft cells directly or by uptake of graft proteins by APCs and presentation by MHC-II in lymph nodes. In fact, some amount of allograft rejection is due to these pathways, but in transplant biology, this is called the "minor" pathway. In contrast, the "major" pathway of allograft rejection is due to the recognition of non-self MHC molecules themselves, rather than the peptides that they carry. MHC is called a "complex" because different genes belonging to the family of MHC genes are clustered on the same chromosome. Among them, some family members are highly polymorphic, i.e., there are many different alleles in the population such that many individuals have different alleles of an MHC gene. In particular, the so-called HLA-A genes, coding for part of the MHC-I molecular complex, are highly polymorphic in the human population. By 2022, over 7,000 alleles have been identified, and it is thus unlikely that any two individuals have exactly the same HLA-A alleles. The major allograft rejection pathway is based on the recognition of non-self HLA-A proteins in two ways: a direct and an indirect pathway.

In the direct pathway, the non-self HLA-A molecule is recognized by a CD8+ T cell, examining the MHC-I molecule on a graft cell. The indirect pathway is based on the uptake of some HLA-A proteins by host APCs and presentation of their peptides in the same way as other antigens are presented by APCs.

From these considerations, it follows that one way for the conceptus to protect itself from adaptive immune detection and destruction is to reduce the presentation of MHC molecules on those cells that are most directly in contact with maternal blood. These are, of course, the trophoblast cells that constitute the placental surface. In fact, MHC-II molecules are completely absent on syncytiotrophoblasts of mice and humans, which is not surprising because trophoblast cells are not APCs. Also, the expression of MHC-I molecules is much reduced on trophoblast cells, in particular the HLA-A protein, which is the most polymorphic and thus most likely to elicit a T cell reaction. However, not all HLA genes are suppressed in trophoblast cells. This is surprising, since at least the HLA-C locus is moderately polymorphic and thus prone to elicit a T cell-based rejection. In fact, the reduction of MHC-I molecules presents another problem for the maternal immune system.

What keeps the placenta to still present a subset of HLA proteins? The presentation of peptides of a cell's HMC-I not only allows T cells to identify cells that are either infected by a virus or are otherwise stressed. MHC-I is like an ID card for the cell that ensures that the cell is a member of the host body. A cell that does not express any HMC-I molecules and the associated intracellular peptides on its surface is suspicious, as it could either be a parasite or a tumor cell not playing by the rules. Hence, the body has to ensure that all cells express their HMC-I to reveal their identity. If they do not, they will be attacked by natural killer cells (NK). That would also apply to trophoblast cells if no MHC-I proteins are presented, with catastrophic consequences for the embryo. That is likely the reason that trophoblast cells in humans still express HLA-C proteins, even though that can lead to some degree of genetic incompatibility among couples.

While the reduced expression of HMC molecules is the main protection for the embryo against immune attack, the activity of APCs and T cells needs to be further reduced, because there is a chance that fetal cells, other than trophoblasts, can enter the maternal compartment in spite of the protective trophoblast layer. The reason is that the trophoblast layer can suffer slight injuries that allow fetal cells to cross the trophoblast-decidual border. To prevent immune detection of fetal cells in the placental bed, the trafficking of T cells and APCs is severely restricted in the endometrium. In fact, both the human and the mouse decidua are either completely (mouse) or largely (human) devoid of lymph vessels (Nancy et al. 2012). In the mouse decidua, there is a population of dendritic cells (DC), the main form of APC, but they are entrapped there and cannot travel to the draining lymph nodes of the uterus. T cells that can be found in the decidua of humans and mice are unlikely to be specific to fetal antigens and thus likely do not play a role in immune surveillance during pregnancy (Erlebacher 2013a, 2013b).

The summary above is the most basic outline of what is known about the reproductive immunology of humans and mice, raising the question of what is known about other animals. In particular, it is interesting to ask what the situation is with the trophoblast of epithelio-chorial species such as the pig, the cow, and the horse. In the pig, there does not seem to be an expression of both MHC-I and II genes in the peri-attachment and term trophoblast (Ramsoondar et al. 1993, Ramsoondar et al. 1999). In contrast, in the cow MHC-I gene expression has been detected in trophoblast cells (Davies et al. 2006), which might be related to the observation that MHC-I recognition at birth may contribute to placental release, i.e., MHC-I compatible pregnancies see a higher incidence of placental retention after birth (Davies et al. 2004). In the horse, MCH-I is expressed on the extra-placental trophoblast cells that form the endometrial cup, a transient endocrine structure made up of trophoblast cells clustered in tightly packed patches in the endometrium. Endometrial cups elicit a vigorous CTL response and eventually get eliminated after day 120 of pregnancy (Antczak and Allen 2021).

No information could be found for species from more ancestrally diverging lineages such as elephant, tenrec, hyrax, or armadillos. It is thus unclear whether the situation we see in humans and mice is an ancestral (synapomorphic) feature of hemochorial placentation.

MAMMALIAN PLACENTATION: PULLING TOGETHER A STRING OF EVOLUTIONARY INNOVATIONS

Hemochorial placentation, as we find it represented in human pregnancy, was likely the ancestral form of placentation in eutherians (Chapter 3). It is the result of overcoming a number of cell-biological constraints, which necessitated a corresponding number of evolutionary innovations that, in aggregate, are not seen in any other group of animals. This assessment implies that the evolution of eutherian placentation was the result of a long and complicated evolutionary history about which we know very little, except for the outcome. It likely played out over about 170 Mio years of Earth's history, of which no side branches survived to our time. That means we have no extant species that could represent intermediate stages in the evolution from the therian to the eutherian ancestor, revealing the order of steps leading to eutherian hemochorial placentation. The only way we can gain some limited understanding is to analyze the functional and cell biological processes involved and maybe eventually reconstruct a plausible scenario based on inferred functional interdependencies. A major obstacle to achieving this is the lack of mechanistic evidence about the fetal-maternal relationship in non-model organisms, in particular those diverging from the base of therian and eutherian clades, other than the lineages leading to model organisms. Yet another question, raised by the implied history of placentation, is "What was driving the origin of this extraordinary string of evolutionary innovations?" Citing the obvious advantages of intra-uterine development is not sufficient, given that there are many vertebrates and even invertebrates that have some form of viviparity (see Chapter 3) and thus would potentially be able to benefit from eutherian-like placentation. There are two avenues of reasoning we can employ to reflect on this question.

One interesting observation is that all marsupial neonates are altricial, while truly precocial neonates are limited to eutherian lineages. Moreover, even the members of the most basally diverging lineages have an abundance of species with precocial neonates, such as elephants, which belong to Afrotheria (Figure 4.6). Could the evolution of extended gestation ultimately be driven by a selective advantage of giving birth to relatively capable newborns? Clearly, the trend toward precocial neonates can be reversed, not least given the relative altricial nature of human newborns, compared to that of our primate relatives.[18]

Another group of factors to consider is less related to the adaptive forces shaping evolutionary outcomes. These are genomic features that enable fast gene regulatory network evolution, namely, transposable elements. It has been widely acknowledged and documented that transposable elements can contribute "pre-fabricated" genetic elements that make the likelihood of adaptive, or at least non-destructive, mutational events higher than expected from simple nucleotide substitutions (Marino-Ramirez et al. 2005, Feschotte 2008, Oliver and Greene 2009, Rebollo et al. 2012). This is the case both with the evolutionary origin of protein domains, such as the PAX domain, or cis-regulatory elements like alternative promoters and enhancers. Transposable element invasions and gene regulatory network innovations are associated with the evolution of mammalian female reproduction, e.g., with respect to decidual cell evolution (Kunarso et al. 2010, Lynch et al. 2011, Emera and Wagner 2012, Lynch et al. 2015).

In any case, the evolution along the stem lineage of eutherian mammals represents a period of extraordinary evolutionary innovation that challenges a basic assumption of classical neo-Darwinian evolutionary theory, i.e., the assumption of uniformitarianism that Darwin acquired from Charles Lyell's theory of earth history. Uniformitarianism assumes that processes in the past are essentially the same as the ones we can observe today. For geology, this means that the Earth's surface in the past was shaped by processes of volcanic activity, tectonic folding, and erosion, i.e.,

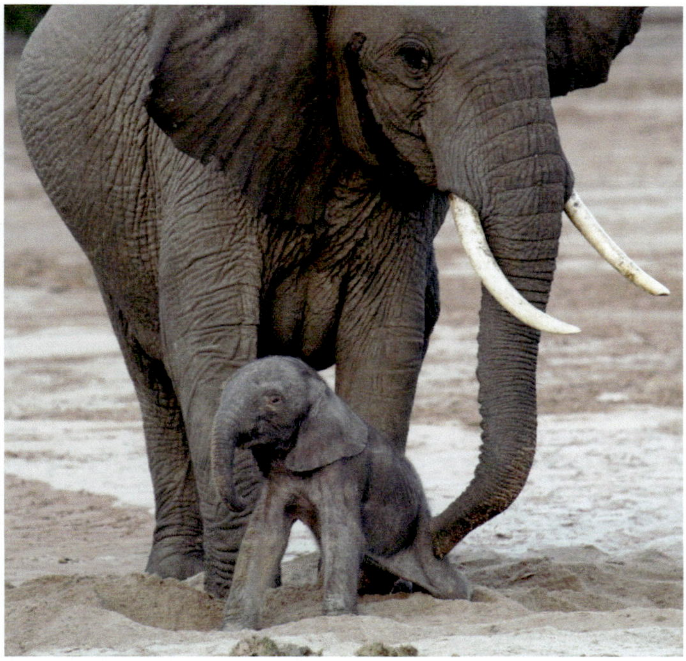

FIGURE 4.6 Newborn African elephant calf showing its precocial nature, i.e., open eyes and able to stand and walk soon after being born. (Image credit: Monica Bond, The Wild Nature Institute, NH, permission received 12/5/25.)

all processes that can still occur and can be studied today. For biology, this means that processes like mutation, recombination, and natural selection observable in populations today are the same as those that shaped evolution in the past. While this is still defensible as a broad principle, it does not mean that the genomic mechanisms of innovation and their likelihood cannot differ between lineages and periods of Earth's history. Transposable element invasion into one lineage but not another at a certain period in Earth's history can change the parameters and dynamics of evolutionary change in one lineage compared to another. Historicity has a deeper impact on natural history than just a string of the same kind of random events.

NOTES

1. Quoted from R. Moore, *Niels Bohr: the Man and the Scientist* (1967), p. 140.
2. This notion does not cover the technical meaning of paradoxa in logic and mathematics, where it refers to self-contradicting statements such as "This sentence is false." But these ideas are not helpful in the current context.
3. For that reason, the "common wisdom" that "you can not be 'half pregnant' " is really not true, as many of "common wisdoms" are. A female can carry a fertilized egg but not have a fully developed placenta in her body, which means that the pregnant state has not been fully established and she is thus partially pregnant. Pregnancy is the stepwise development toward birth.
4. In the literature, the basal membrane is often called the "basement" membrane, which I guess is a bastardization of the original term "basal" membrane, which is named after the basal, rather than the apical, side of the epithelial cells. There is also a distinction between "basal lamina" and "basal membrane", where the former is a thin layer directly produced by the epithelial cells consisting of Collagen 4 and Laminin, while the latter includes also fibrillar collagen from the mesenchymal extracellular matrix.

5. There is an unfortunate incongruence in anatomical terminology, where strictly speaking the "epi-thelia are covering the organism toward the outside of the body, but "epithelially" organized cell layers within the body" have various names like endothelium (the lining of blood and lymph vessels) or mesothelium, the lining of the celomatic body cavity. When we are writing here about epithelia, we mean any tissue of epithelial-like organization not just the body cover.
6. Many more molecular details of the attachment and implantation process have been discovered since 1993, but in terms of the cell biological concepts involved, the cited paper is still one of the best available.
7. Also known as TACE for TNF alpha converting enzyme.
8. This assessment is based on PubMed searches with the query on 08/11/2023: (embryo attachment AND "X"), "X" being "elephant," "Loxodonta," "Elephas," "hyrax," "Afrotheria," "armadillo," "Xenarthra."
9. Curiously, in pre-hatching, mid-gestation, endometrium, no mucin reactivity was reported. This is strange because at that stage the embryo would not be able to attach, because it is separated from the maternal tissue by a shell coat. Whether this is a false negative finding requires further investigation.
10. It should be noted for fairness that one of us, GPW, when working on pig reproduction do often call embryo attachment "implantation" in everyday lab-conversations and notetaking!
11. The question whether scratch injuries to the endometrium is an effective treatment to increase implantation success is still controversial (Lensen, S., C. Venetis, E. H. Y. Ng, S. L. Young, A. Vitagliano, N. S. Macklon and C. Farquhar (2019). "Should we stop offering endometrial scratching prior to in vitro fertilization?" *Fertil Steril* **111**(6): 1094–1101), although there are also questions about the design of studies contradicting the original findings (G. Mor, personal communication).
12. The distinction between premature birth and spontaneous abortion is based on gestational age and is entirely conventional.
13. For the Tasmanian devil, *Sarcophilus harrisii*, for which litters of up to 30 neonates have been documented, most of which of course perish because the mother does not have that many nipples to nourish them.
14. This observation is important to show that the classification of the opossum placenta and that of say hoofed eutherians as "epithelia-chorial" is problematic, since the non-invasive character of the opossum placenta is due to the short post-contact period of placentation, which does not give enough time to establish a hemochorial placenta, besides the likely fact that the opossum would not be able to sustain such an arrangement at the FMI.
15. In the opossum, pseudopregnancy is caused by exposure of a female to the pheromones of a male, which induce ovulation. If no fertilization occurs, the female reproductive tract undergoes many of the changes described here.
16. The interpretation of IL6 expression is complicated because of the highly pleiotropic nature of this signal, including a role in nutrient mobilization as for instance during physical activity (Kistner, T. M., B. K. Pedersen and D. E. Lieberman (2022). "Interleukin 6 as an energy allocator in muscle tissue." *Nat Metab* **4**(2): 170–179).
17. An interesting vertebrate tissue consisting of only one cell type is cartilage, which consists only of chondrocytes and ECM.
18. Human "altriciality" is due to delayed maturation, with pregnancy length comparable to other great apes.

REFERENCES

Adler, M., A. R. Chavan and R. Medzhitov (2023). "Tissue biology: in search of a new paradigm." *Annu Rev Cell Dev Biol* **39**: 67–89.

Adler, M., A. Mayo, X. Zhou, R. A. Franklin, M. L. Meizlish, R. Medzhitov, S. M. Kallenberger and U. Alon (2020). "Principles of cell circuits for tissue repair and fibrosis." *iScience* **23**(2): 100841.

Allen, W. R. T. and F. J. Stansfield (2021). "Placentation in the African elephant (*Loxodonta africana*)." *Adv Anat Embryol Cell Biol* **234**: 181–204.

Antczak, D. F. and W. R. T. Allen (2021). "Placentation in equids." *Adv Anat Embryol Cell Biol* **234**: 91–128.

Aplin, J. D. and P. T. Ruane (2017). "Embryo-epithelium interactions during implantation at a glance." *J Cell Sci* **130**(1): 15–22.

Arendt, D., J. M. Musser, C. V. H. Baker, A. Bergman, C. Cepko, D. H. Erwin, M. Pavlicev, G. Schlosser, S. Widder, M. D. Laubichler and G. P. Wagner (2016). "The origin and evolution of cell types." *Nat Rev Genet* **17**(12): 744–757.

Blackburn, D. G. and A. F. Flemming (2012). "Invasive implantation and intimate placental associations in a placentotrophic African lizard, *Trachylepis ivensi* (scincidae)." *J Morphol* **273**(2): 137–159.

Bracamonte, S. E., K. Knopf and M. T. Monaghan (2021). "Encapsulation of Anguillicola carassus reduces the abundance of adult parasite stages in the European eel (*Anguilla anguilla*)." *J Fish Dis* **44**: 771–782.

Brosens, J. J., M. S. Salker, G. Teklenburg, J. Nautiyal, S. Salter, E. S. Lucas, J. H. Steel, M. Christian, Y. W. Chan, C. M. Boomsma, J. D. Moore, G. M. Hartshorne, S. Sucurovic, B. Mulac-Jericevic, C. J. Heijnen, S. Quenby, M. J. Koerkamp, F. C. Holstege, A. Shmygol and N. S. Macklon (2014). "Uterine selection of human embryos at implantation." *Sci Rep* **4**: 3894.

Cha, J., X. Sun and S. K. Dey (2012). "Mechanisms of implantation: strategies for successful pregnancy." *Nat Med* **18**(12): 1754–1767.

Chavan, A. R., O. W. Griffith, D. J. Stadtmauer, J. Maziarz, M. Pavlicev, R. Fishman, L. Koren, R. Romero and G. P. Wagner (2021). "Evolution of embryo implantation was enabled by the origin of decidual stromal cells in eutherian mammals." *Mol Biol Evol* **38**(3): 1060–1074.

Chavan, A. R., O. W. Griffith and G. P. Wagner (2017). "The inflammation paradox in the evolution of mammalian pregnancy: turning a foe into a friend." *Curr Opin Genet Dev* **47**: 24–32.

Chavan, A. R. and G. P. Wagner (2016). "The fetal-maternal interface of the nine-banded armadillo: endothelial cells of maternal sinus are partially replaced by trophoblast." *Zoological Lett* **2**: 11.

Colvin, R. B. and R. N. Smith (2005). "Antibody-mediated organ-allograft rejection." *Nat Rev Immunol* **5**(10): 807–817.

Davies, C. J., J. A. Eldridge, P. J. Fisher and D. H. Schlafer (2006). "Evidence for expression of both classical and non-classical major histocompatibility complex class I genes in bovine trophoblast cells." *Am J Reprod Immunol* **55**(3): 188–200.

Davies, C. J., J. R. Hill, J. L. Edwards, F. N. Schrick, P. J. Fisher, J. A. Eldridge and D. H. Schlafer (2004). "Major histocompatibility antigen expression on the bovine placenta: its relationship to abnormal pregnancies and retained placenta." *Anim Reprod Sci* **82–83**: 267–280.

Denker, H. W. (1993). "Implantation: a cell biological paradox." *J Exp Zool* **266**(6): 541–558.

Dey, S. K., H. Lim, S. K. Das, K. Reese, B. C. Paria, T. Daikoku and H. Wang (2004). "Molecular cues to implantation." *Endocrine Rev* **25**: 341–373.

DiFrisco, J., A. C. Love and G. P. Wagner (2020). "Character identity mechanisms: a conceptual model for comparative-mechanistic biology." *Biol Philos* **35**: 43–44.

Dudley, J. S., C. R. Murphy, M. B. Thompson and B. M. McAllan (2015). "Desmoglein-2 during pregnancy and its role in the evolution of viviparity in a marsupial (*Sminthopsis crassicaudata*; Dasyuridae)." *J Morphol* **276**(3): 261–272.

Dudley, J. S., M. B. Renfree, G. P. Wagner and O. W. Griffith (2024). "The extension of mammalian pregnancy required taming inflammation: independent evolution of extended placentation in the tammar wallaby." *Proc Natl Acad Sci U S A* **121**(42): e2310047121.

Emera, D. and G. P. Wagner (2012). "Transformation of a transposon into a derived prolactin promoter with function during human pregnancy." *Proc Natl Acad Sci U S A* **109**(28): 11246–11251.

Enders, A. C. (1960). "Development and structure of the villous haemochorial placenta of the nine-banded armadillo (*Dasypus novemcinctus*)." *J Anat* **94**: 34–45.

Enders, A. C. and R. K. Enders (1969). "The placenta of the four-eye opossum (Philander opossum)." *Anat Rec* **165**(3): 431–449.

Enders, A. C. and A. O. Welsh (1993). "Structural interactions of trophoblast and uterus during hemochorial placenta formation." *J Exp Zool* **266**(6): 578–587.

Erlebacher, A. (2013a). "Immunology of the maternal-fetal interface." *Annu Rev Immunol* **31**: 387–411.

Erlebacher, A. (2013b). "Mechanisms of T cell tolerance towards the allogeneic fetus." *Nat Rev Immunol* **13**(1): 23–33.

Feschotte, C. (2008). "Transposable elements and the evolution of regulatory networks." *Nat Rev Genet* **9**: 397–405.

Freyer, C., U. Zeller and M. B. Renfree (2003). "The marsupial placenta: a phylogenetic analysis." *J Exp Zool A Comp Exp Biol* **299A**(1): 59–77.

Freyer, C., U. Zeller and M. B. Renfree (2007). "Placental function in two distantly related marsupials." *Placenta* **28**(2–3): 249–257.

Goel, T., R. Mahey, N. Bhatla, M. Kalaivani, S. Pant and A. Kriplani (2017). "Pregnancy after endometrial scratching in infertile couples undergoing ovulation induction and intrauterine insemination cycles-a randomized controlled trial." *J Assist Reprod Genet* **34**(8): 1051–1058.

Green, J. A., R. D. Geisert, G. A. Johnson and T. E. Spencer (2021). "Implantation and placentation in ruminants." *Adv Anat Embryol Cell Biol* **234**: 129–154.

Griffith, O. W., A. R. Chavan, M. Pavlicev, S. Protopapas, R. Callahan, J. Maziarz and G. P. Wagner (2019). "Endometrial recognition of pregnancy occurs in the grey short-tailed opossum (*Monodelphis domestica*)." *Proc Biol Sci* **286**(1905): 20190691.

Griffith, O. W., A. R. Chavan, S. Protopapas, J. Maziarz, R. Romero and G. P. Wagner (2017). "Embryo implantation evolved from an ancestral inflammatory attachment reaction." *Proc Natl Acad Sci U S A* **114**(32): E6566–E6575.

Grosser, O. (1909). *Vergleichende Anatomie und Entwicklungsgeschichte der Eihäute und der Placenta*. Vienna, W. Braumüller.

Haig, D. (1993). "Genetic conflicts in human pregnancy." *Q Rev Biol* **68**(4): 495–532.

Hansen, V. L., L. S. Faber, A. A. Salehpoor and R. D. Miller (2017). "A pronounced uterine pro-inflammatory response at parturition is an ancient feature in mammals." *Proc Biol Sci* **284**(1865).

Harder, J. D., M. J. Stonerook and J. Pondy (1993). "Gestation and placentation in two New World opossums: *Didelphis virginiana* and *Monodelphis domestica*." *J Exp Zool* **266**(5): 463–479.

Johnson, G. A., F. W. Bazer and H. Seo (2021). "The early stages of implantation and placentation in the pig." *Adv Anat Embryol Cell Biol* **234**: 61–89.

Johnson, G. A., R. C. Burghardt, F. W. Bazer, H. Seo and J. W. Cain (2023). "Integrins and their potential roles in mammalian pregnancy." *J Anim Sci Biotechnol* **14**(1): 115.

Kin, K., J. Maziarz and G. P. Wagner (2014). "Immunohistological study of the endometrial stromal fibroblasts in the opossum, *Monodelphis domestica*: evidence for homology with eutherian stromal fibroblasts." *Biol Reprod* **90**(5): 111.

Kistner, T. M., B. K. Pedersen and D. E. Lieberman (2022). "Interleukin 6 as an energy allocator in muscle tissue." *Nat Metab* **4**(2): 170–179.

Kotas, M. E. and R. Medzhitov (2015). "Homeostasis, inflammation, and disease susceptibility." *Cell* **160**(5): 816–827.

Kunarso, G., N. Y. Chia, J. Jeyakani, C. Hwang, X. Lu, Y. S. Chan, H. H. Ng and G. Bourque (2010). "Transposable elements have rewired the core regulatory network of human embryonic stem cells." *Nat Genet* **42**(7): 631–634.

Laird, M. K., H. McShea, B. M. McAllan, C. R. Murphy and M. B. Thompson (2017). "Uterine remodelling during pregnancy and pseudopregnancy in the brushtail possum (*Trichosurus vulpecula*; Phalangeridae)." *J Anat* **231**(1): 84–94.

Laird, M. K., H. McShea, C. R. Murphy, B. M. McAllan, G. Shaw, M. B. Renfree and M. B. Thompson (2018). "Non-invasive placentation in the marsupials *Macropus eugenii* (Macropodidae) and *Trichosurus vulpecula* (Phalangeridae) involves redistribution of uterine Desmoglein-2." *Mol Reprod Dev* **85**(1): 72–82.

Lensen, S., C. Venetis, E. H. Y. Ng, S. L. Young, A. Vitagliano, N. S. Macklon and C. Farquhar (2019). "Should we stop offering endometrial scratching prior to in vitro fertilization?" *Fertil Steril* **111**(6): 1094–1101.

Liu, L., J. Zhang, F. E. Rheindt, F. Lei, Y. Qu, Y. Wang, Y. Zhang, C. Sullivan, W. Nie, J. Wang, F. Yang, J. Chen, S. V. Edwards, J. Meng and S. Wu (2017). "Genomic evidence reveals a radiation of placental mammals uninterrupted by the KPg boundary." *Proc Natl Acad Sci U S A* **114**(35): E7282–E7290.

Luckett, W. P. (1994). "Suprafamiliar relationships within Marsupialia: resolution and discordance from multidisciplinary data." *J Mammal Evol* **2**: 255–283.

Lynch, V. J., R. D. Leclerc, G. May and G. P. Wagner (2011). "Transposon-mediated rewiring of gene regulatory networks contributed to the evolution of pregnancy in mammals." *Nat Genet* **43**(11): 1154–1159.

Lynch, V. J., M. C. Nnamani, A. Kapusta, K. Brayer, S. L. Plaza, E. C. Mazur, D. Emera, S. Z. Sheikh, F. Grutzner, S. Bauersachs, A. Graf, S. L. Young, J. D. Lieb, F. J. DeMayo, C. Feschotte and G. P. Wagner (2015). "Ancient transposable elements transformed the uterine regulatory landscape and transcriptome during the evolution of mammalian pregnancy." *Cell Rep* **10**(4): 551–561.

Maramosch, K. and R. E. Shope (1975). *Invertebrate Immunity: Mechanisms of Invertebrate Vector-parasite Relations*. New York, San Francisco, London, Academic Press.

Marino-Ramirez, L., K. C. Lewis, D. Landsman and I. K. Jordan (2005). "Transposable elements donate lineage-specific regulatory sequences to host genomes." *Cytogenet Genome Res* **110**(1-4): 333–341.

McGowen, M. R., O. Erez, R. Romero and D. E. Wildman (2014). "The evolution of embryo implanatation." *Int J Dev Biol* **58**: 155–161.

Medawar, P. B. (1953). Some immunological and endocrinological problems raised by the evolution of viviparity in vertebratges. *Evolution*. R. Brown and J. F. Danielli. New York, NY, Academic Press: 320–338.

Medzhitov, R. (2008). "Origin and physiological roles of inflammation." *Nature* **454**(7203): 428–435.

Mor, G., I. Cardenas, V. Abrahams and S. Guller (2011). "Inflammation and pregnancy: the role of the immune system at the implantation site." *Ann N Y Acad Sci* **1221**: 80–87.

Nancy, P., J. Siewiera, G. Rizzuto, E. Tagliani, I. Osokine, P. Manandhar, I. Dolgalev, C. Clementi, A. Tsirigos and A. Erlebacher (2018). "H3K27me3 dynamics dictate evolving uterine states in pregnancy and parturition." *J Clin Invest* **128**(1): 233–247.

Nancy, P., E. Tagliani, C. S. Tay, P. Asp, D. E. Levy and A. Erlebacher (2012). "Chemokine gene silencing in decidual stromal cells limits T cell access to the maternal-fetal interface." *Science* **336**(6086): 1317–1321.

Nathan, C. (2022). "Nonresolving inflammation redux." *Immunity* **55**(4): 592–605.

Nilsson, M. A., G. Churakov, M. Sommer, N. V. Tran, A. Zemann, J. Brosius and J. Schmitz (2010). "Tracking marsupial evolution using archaic genomic retroposon insertions." *PLoS Biol* **8**(7): e1000436.

Okabe, Y. and R. Medzhitov (2016). "Tissue biology perspective on macrophages." *Nat Immunol* **17**(1): 9–17.

Oliver, K. R. and W. K. Greene (2009). "Transposable elements: powerful facilitators of evolution." *BioEssays* **31**: 703–714.

Osokine, I., J. Siewiera, D. Rideaux, S. Ma, T. Tsukui and A. Erlebacher (2022). "Gene silencing by EZH2 suppresses TGF-beta activity within the decidua to avert pregnancy-adverse wound healing at the maternal-fetal interface." *Cell Rep* **38**(5): 110329.

Pavlicev, M., J. DiFrisco, A. C. Love and G. P. Wagner (2024). "Metabolic complementation between cells drives the evolution of tissues and organs." *Biol Lett* **20**(11): 20240490.

Pavlicev, M. and G. P. Wagner (2024). "Reading the palimpsest of cell interactions: what questions may we ask of the data?" *iScience* **27**(5): 109670.

Preston, A. M., L. A. Lindsay and C. R. Murphy (2004). "Progesterone treatment and the progress of early pregnancy reduce desmoglein 1&2 staining along the lateral plasma membrane in rat uterine epithelial cells." *Acta Histochem* **106**(5): 345–351.

Preston, A. M., L. A. Lindsay and C. R. Murphy (2006). "Desmosomes in uterine epithelial cells decrease at the time of implantation: an ultrastructural and morphometric study." *J Morphol* **267**(1): 103–108.

Ramsoondar, J., R. J. Christopherson, L. J. Guilbert and T. G. Wegmann (1993). "A porcine trophoblast cell line that secretes growth factors which stimulate porcine macrophages." *Biol Reprod* **49**(4): 681–694.

Ramsoondar, J. J., R. J. Christopherson, L. J. Guilbert, W. T. Dixon, A. Ghahary, S. Ellis, T. G. Wegmann and J. A. Piedrahita (1999). "Lack of class I major histocompatibility antigens on trophoblast of periimplantation blastocysts and term placenta in the pig." *Biol Reprod* **60**(2): 387–397.

Rebollo, R., M. T. Romanish and D. L. Mager (2012). "Transposable elements: an abundant and natural source of regulatory sequences for host genes." *Annu Rev Genet* **46**: 21–42.

Renfree, M. and G. Shaw (2002). Reproduction in monotremes and marsupials. *Encyclopedia of Life Sciences*. New York, Wiley and Sons: 1–5.

Renfree, M. B. (1972). "Influence of the embryo on the marsupial uterus." *Nature* **240**(5382): 475–477.

Renfree, M. B. (2010). "Marsupials: placental mammals with a difference." *Placenta* **31**: S21–S26.

Romero, R., S. K. Dey and S. J. Fisher (2014). "Preterm labor: one syndrome, many causes." *Science* **345**(6198): 760–765.

Selwood, L. (2000). "Marsupial egg and embryo coats." *Cells Tissues Organs* **166**(2): 208–219.

Serhan, C. N. and J. Savill (2005). "Resolution of inflammation: the beginning programs the end." *Nat Immunol* **6**(12): 1191–1197.

Singh, H. and J. D. Aplin (2015). "Endometrial apical glycoproteomic analysis reveals roles for cadherin 6, desmoglein-2 and plexin b2 in epithelial integrity." *Mol Hum Reprod* **21**(1): 81–94.

Stadtmauer, D. J., S. Basanta, J. D. Maziarz, A. G. Cole, G. Dagdas, G. R. Smith, F. van Breukelen, M. Pavlicev and G. P. Wagner (2025). "Cell type and cell signalling innovations underlying mammalian pregnancy." *Nat Ecol Evol* **9**: 1469–1486.

Stadtmauer, D. J., J. D. Maziarz, O. W. Griffith and G. P. Wagner (2026). "Fetal inflammatory signals regulate maternal investment in a pregnant marsupial." PLoS Biol 24(2): e3003670. https://doi.org/10.1371/journal. pbio.3003670.

Stadtmauer, D. J. and G. P. Wagner (2020). "Cooperative inflammation: the recruitment of inflammatory signaling in marsupial and eutherian pregnancy." *J Reprod Immunol* **137**: 102626.

Streams, F. A. (1971). "Encapsulation of insect parasites in superparasitized hosts." *Entomologia Experimentalis et Applicata*. 14: 484-490.

Sugimoto, M. A., L. P. Sousa, V. Pinho, M. Perretti and M. M. Teixeira (2016). "Resolution of inflammation: what controls its onset?" *Front Immunol* **7**: 160.

Sun, X., L. Zhang, H. Xie, H. Wan, B. Magella, J. A. Whitsett and S. K. Dey (2012). "Kruppel-like factor 5 (KLF5) is critical for conferring uterine receptivity to implantation." *Proc Natl Acad Sci U S A* **109**(4): 1145–1150.

Thathiah, A., C. P. Blobel and D. D. Carson (2003). "Tumor necrosis factor-alpha converting enzyme/ADAM 17 mediates MUC1 shedding." *J Biol Chem* **278**(5): 3386–3394.

Thathiah, A. and D. D. Carson (2004). "MT1-MMP mediates MUC1 shedding independent of TACE/ADAM17." *Biochem J* **382**(Pt 1): 363–373.

Tsikouras, P., E. Oikonomou, K. Nikolettos, S. Andreou, D. Kyriakou, C. Damaskos, N. Garmpis, V. Monastiridou, T. Nalmpanti, A. Bothou, G. Iatrakis and N. Nikolettos (2024). "The impact of periodontal disease on preterm birth and preeclampsia." *J Pers Med* **14**(4): 345. https://doi.org/10.3390/jpm14040345

Vandeberg, J. L. (1990). "The Gray Short-Tailed Opossum (*Monodelphis domestica*) as a model didelphid species for genetic research." *Australian J Zool* **37**(3): 235–247.

VandeBerg, J. L. and E. S. Robinson (1997). "The laboratory opossum (*Monodelphis domestica*) in laboratory research." *ILAR J* **38**(1): 4–12.

Wagner, G. P. and G. B. Müller (2002). "Evolutionary innovations overcome ancestral constraints: a re-examination of character evolution in male sepsid flies (Diptera: Sepsidae)." *Evol Dev* **4**(1): 1–6; discussion 7-8.

Zhou, X., R. A. Franklin, M. Adler, J. B. Jacox, W. Bailis, J. A. Shyer, R. A. Flavell, A. Mayo, U. Alon and R. Medzhitov (2018). "Circuit design features of a stable two-cell system." *Cell* **172**(4): 744–757.e717.

Zindel, J. and P. Kubes (2020). "DAMPs, PAMPs, and LAMPs in immunity and sterile inflammation." *Annu Rev Pathol* **15**: 493–518.

5 The Natural History of Decidua

In the previous chapter, we made the argument that some of the paradoxical features of the mammalian FMI were able to evolve because of a novel tissue and the associated cell types, i.e., the decidua. Specifically, we argued that the switch from "attachment & nidatory inflammation" to an anti-inflammatory state became possible due to the evolution of the decidua, which, according to the present model, exerts an anti-inflammatory influence at the implantation site. In addition, for the tissue-biological and the immunological paradox, a role of the decidua has been identified. Adrian Erlebacher and colleagues, for instance, have shown that decidual stromal cells suppress the expression of wound healing-related genes, thereby resolving the tissue-biological paradox (Nancy et al. 2018, Osokine et al. 2022). They have also shown that during placentation, the endometrium of mice prevents the immigration of T cells and the emigration of antigen-presenting cells to lymph nodes, thereby contributing to immune tolerance toward the embryo (see Chapter 4). Hence, the theory is that the fetal-maternal interface is the locus of a number of cell-biological innovations that make eutherian pregnancy possible. In this and the following chapters, we trace the outlines of the evolution of the eutherian decidua, in particular its cellular components. The title of this chapter points to the fact that here we will focus on the phylogenetic distribution of decidua and its overt function. More molecular and mechanistic aspects of decidua and their evolution will be the focus of the next chapter.

Since the availability of single-cell (SC) technologies, SC transcriptomics, and SC epigenetics, the cell biology of decidua and decidual cells has been the subject of intense study (Vento-Tormo et al. 2018, Wang et al. 2020, Garcia-Alonso et al. 2021, Stadtmauer and Wagner 2021, Arutyunyan et al. 2023, Yang et al. 2023, Stadtmauer et al. 2025). The results of these studies reopened many conceptual issues that were beyond the reach of the classical comparative research tradition based on histological methods and careful observation, including "neo-classical" work in the image of the molecular biology of the late 20th and early 21st century. An example is the question "What is the relationship, in humans and other apes, between decidual cells of pregnancy and the decidualization during the luteal phase of the menstrual cycle?" Nevertheless, we want to introduce the "natural history" of decidual cells and decidualization before reflecting upon the implications of the more recent single-cell research, since the former will set the stage for what we expect of the latter to achieve, i.e., what we learn from the SC work depends on the context provided by the older literature. Much of current SC research of the fetal-maternal interface is focused on getting the demanding experimental and data-analytical challenges right. This is, of course, important, but cannot be an end in itself. Understanding the broad landscape of decidual biology first, even though some of it might require eventual revision in the light of newer research, is the background against which the newer work attains its meaning.

The decidual stromal cell is a cell type that develops, in most eutherian mammals that have decidualization, during the implantation process and persists for either the whole pregnancy or the initial parts of it, depending on the species (see below). In a minority of eutherian species, in particular the ones that menstruate, decidual cells become apparent even in the absence of a blastocyst, as is the case with humans.[1] This is called "spontaneous decidualization" and is clearly a derived character that does not need to be discussed here (but see Chapter 9). The product of spontaneous decidualization has been called "pre-decidual" cells in the classical gynecological and pathological literature (Kurman et al. 2019). Here, we first examine the evidence about the phylogenetic distribution of decidual cells. Then we look at the pattern of decidual phenotypes to infer shifting functional roles of the decidua.

DOI: 10.1201/9781032717777-5

PHYLOGENETIC DISTRIBUTION OF DECIDUAL CELLS

Although it is still difficult to identify decidual cells in a way that is operational and applicable to different species, some phylogenetic analyses have been conducted based on data from classical histological observations, most often the data assembled in (Mossman 1987). In histology, decidual cells are identified as endometrial stromal cells that are larger and more rounded than endometrial stromal fibroblasts with a large, round, pale nucleus, sometimes with glycogen and lipid inclusions in the cytoplasm. Based on this characterization, decidua were found only in eutherian species with one possible exception (see below). Mess and Carter thus concluded that decidual cells evolved in the stem lineage of eutherian mammals (Mess and Carter 2006). Needless to say, some questions remain that might be worth examining more closely.

First, we want to ask whether the absence of decidual cells in marsupials is correct. Most phylogenetic mapping studies of the fetal-maternal interface focus their taxon sampling on eutherians, for obvious reasons, and only one or a small handful of marsupials are included as outgroups (Mess and Carter 2006, Wildman et al. 2006, Elliot and Crespi 2009). Given that in eutherians the evolution of invasive placentation and the origin of decidua coincide, up to the resolution of the phylogenetic reconstruction, the question is whether, in cases of invasive marsupial placentation, there is evidence for a decidual reaction. While invasive trophoblasts have been reported from several marsupial taxa, such as Dunnarts (*Sminthopsis carassicaudata*), the quoll (*Dasyurus*), and others, in only one case, we found mention of a putative decidual reaction. That is the study about the gray four-eyed opossum, *Philander opossum* (Enders and Enders 1969). *Philander* is a member of the opossum clade from South America, and Enders and Enders report that near the *sinus terminalis*, which is a large blood vessel at the border between the bilaminar and trilaminar yolk sack placenta, the trophoblasts of the trilaminar placenta are penetrating the luminal epithelium at the tip of endometrial epithelial folds. At these sites of epithelial penetration, the nearby stromal cells assume a morphology similar to the histological characteristics of decidual cells. The authors write: "[...], at the tip of the fold [of the luminal epithelium] where the epithelium is penetrated, are several slightly enlarged fibroblasts which may constitute a primitive decidual reaction" (Enders and Enders 1969, p. 435).

How shall we assess this report? Is this evidence that the decidual cell type is older than the eutherian stem lineage? First, we need to note that, in marsupials, invasive placentation, when it occurs, is always very short-lived. If the ideas developed in Chapter 4 about the role of decidual cells are correct, one would not expect the functional need for a decidual cell type in marsupials, given the short placental phase of gestation in marsupials. But this inference is, of course, dependent on whether the inferred ancestral role of decidua is correct. More importantly, the penetration of the luminal epithelium is an injury, which should lead to the activation of the sub-epithelial fibroblasts. In contrast to inactive fibroblasts, which are usually thin, spindle-shaped with dense elongated nuclei, activated fibroblasts are more "plumb spindle-shaped" or dendritic with pale oval or round nuclei and abundant rough endoplasmic reticulum (Younesi et al. 2024). After epithelial injury, some of the associated fibroblasts express smooth muscle actin and become contractile and are called myo-fibroblasts. Hence, activated fibroblasts do look to some degree like decidual cells, with round pale nuclei and a more rounded cell shape. In addition, during differentiation, human endometrial fibroblasts go through a stage in which they are similar to activated myofibroblasts (Kim et al. 1999, Vento-Tormo et al. 2018, Stadtmauer and Wagner 2021, Chen et al. 2023), likely a remnant from their evolutionary origin from activated fibroblasts (see also Chapter 6). Hence, the important observation by Enders and Enders is likely a case of fibroblast activation as expected in the presence of an epithelial injury. This observation is also consistent with the hypothesis that invasive placentation in marsupials leads to a wound healing reaction that may be the starting point for the evolution of the decidual cell type (more about this scenario below and in Chapter 6). Even so, the situation in *Philander* should be empirically re-evaluated, for instance by immune-staining for smooth muscle actin.

In contrast to the decidual cells, which most likely are absent in marsupials, the developmental precursor cell type, the endometrial stromal fibroblast (ESF), has been identified in the opossum (Kin et al. 2014, Stadtmauer et al. 2025). Fibroblasts with protein expression profile consistent with ESF identity are found in a relatively (compared to, say, mouse) thin sub-epithelial layer. These cells exhibit expression of the mesenchymal marker vimentin, VIM, smooth muscle actin, SMA, and the transcription factors HoxA11, CEBPb, and PGR. During pregnancy, the sub-epithelial layer is reduced in size, replaced by a layer of blood capillaries (Griffith et al. 2017). It is not clear whether the ESF gets lost or is just diluted in the expanding uterine tissue during pregnancy. During the non-pregnant estrus cycle, the subepithelial layer is retained (Griffith et al. 2019). These observations show two things: (1) precursor cell types to decidual cells are present in a marsupial and are likely homologous to the decidual cells in eutherians; and (2) stromal cells play a minor role in regulating the fetal-maternal interface during the short period the fetus is in direct physical contact with the maternal tissue. In addition, decidual cells have not been identified in pregnant opossum endometrium with single-cell techniques (Stadtmauer et al. 2025).

Within the Eutheria, decidual cells have been reported in most clades, and in particular the early branching lineages of Afrotheria, Xenarthra, Euarchonoglires, and Laurasiatheria, which led Mess and Carter to conclude that "the presence of decidual cells is a plesiomorphic state for Eutheria" (Mess and Carter 2006), although this characterization is not very accurate. What the phylogenetic analysis is showing is that decidual cells are *apomorphic* (shared derived) for Eutheria, and plesiomorphic for each of the subclades of Eutheria, like Boreoeutheria, for instance. According to the data analyzed by Mess and Carter, the absence of decidua has been reported from Ferungulata (if that is still a clade), *Galago* (bushbabies), *Scalopus* (the eastern mole), *Echinops telfairi* (lesser hedgehog tenrec), and *Orycteropus afer* (aardvark).

Before we go on to discuss these possible cases of decidual cell loss, we want to mention another line of evidence that supports the notion that decidual cells evolved in the stem lineage of eutherians. This approach utilizes mechanistic knowledge about the differentiation of decidual cells. It has been shown that specific protein interactions are necessary for the differentiation of human decidual cells. One is a physical interaction between the transcription factors HoxA11 and FOXO1, which, together with post-translational modifications such as phosphorylation, turns the HoxA11 protein into a transcriptional activator (Lynch et al. 2009). If tested alone, HoxA11 is a transcriptional inhibitor (Roth et al. 2005). That ability to assume the role of a transcriptional activator in decidual stromal cells is limited to HoxA11 proteins from eutherian species, including the ancestrally reconstituted protein of the eutherian ancestor, and absent in opossum and the HoxA11 protein from the common ancestor of therian mammals (Lynch et al. 2008). This ability of eutherian Hoxa11 proteins depends on evolved changes in their reaction to phosphorylation at key amino acid residues (Nnamani et al. 2016). The phylogenetic distribution of Hoxa11 proteins that can substitute for the human protein in human endometrial stromal cells shows that some of the transcriptional machinery responsible for decidual cell differentiation in humans is limited to eutherians and absent in marsupials and more distantly related species like the chicken and monotremes, which implies that the decidual cell likely evolved in the stem lineage of eutherian mammals.

Another functionally important molecular feature is the activation of the transcription factor protein CEBPB. The eutherian version of this protein gets phosphorylated by GSK3, leading to the exposure of the trans-regulatory activation domain (Lynch et al. 2011). The ancestral therian version of that protein, in response to the same kinase, assumes an inactive conformation. This difference could be traced to three amino acid substitutions, which led to a slightly different location of the phosphorylated serine residues, with dramatic effects on protein structure. Also, this change could be traced back to the stem lineage of eutherians, further consolidating the conclusion that decidual cells, or at least a version of them, originated in the stem lineage of eutherian mammals.

The largest group of mammals reportedly without decidualization is the hoofed animals and their relatives (Ferungulata, comprising Carnivora, Perissodactyla, and Artiodactyla). This is interesting because this group must have secondarily reverted from invasive placentation to epitheliochorial placentation (Wildman et al. 2006, Elliot and Crespi 2009). Given the absence of invasion and assuming that the primary role of the decidua is to enable and sustain implantation, the inferred loss of decidual cells makes sense. Absence of invasion is best exemplified in pigs, where the conceptus only attaches but does not otherwise modify the luminal epithelium in any obvious way. No decidual reaction has been reported in pigs. The situation, however, is considerably more complicated because among hoofed animals, the pig seems to be the exception rather than representing the "norm." While deeply invasive placentation is absent from hoofed animals, there are various degrees of modifications and regional differences found in hoofed animals, which makes the wholesale characterization of this clade as "epitheliochorial" an oversimplification. For instance, in the horse, there is a population of extra-placental trophoblast cells, which invade the endometrial stoma, forming transient clusters of cells called endometrial cups, which seem to perform endocrine functions (Antczak and Allen 2021). In the cow, the specialized placental structures, placentomes consisting of maternal caruncles and fetal cotyledons (see Chapter 3), undergo a dynamic change in which, at least temporarily, the luminal epithelium can be replaced by a layer of trophoblast cells (Seo et al. 2024). In the sheep, the trophoblast erodes the luminal epithelium to some extent and fuses with the remaining epithelial cells, creating so-called heterokaryons, i.e., cells with nuclei from different cell types and individuals (Green et al. 2021). These changes are accompanied by a transformation of the underlying stroma, where fibroblasts assume the shape of decidual cells, and express decidual marker genes, such as SSP1 (a.k.a. Osteopontin, OPN), Vimentin (a pan-mesenchymal gene rather than decidua-specific), and smooth muscle actin (Johnson et al. 2003). This paper gives support to earlier reports in the classical literature, which reported histological signs of decidualization in other artiodactyls as well. For instance, Kellas published a study on the antelope *Oureba ourebi* (vernacular "oribi") reporting histological observations suggesting a decidual reaction in the stroma (Kellas 1966). He cites a statement by Mossman from 1937, where the latter claims that in hoofed animals one finds "… a definite change in the sub-epithelial connective tissue which suggests the early stages of decidual cell formation […]." Hence, there seems to be a correlation between the degree of luminal epithelial erosion/modification and the presence of at least some degree of decidual reaction in the stroma, even in ruminants. These observations are consistent with the phylogenetic inferences that non- or minimally invasive placentation in eutherians evolved from a more invasive form originating in the eutherian stem lineage and that, in animals like the pig, the lack of decidua is secondary, likely due to the lack of epithelial injury[2]. It would be interesting to study, in pigs that do not have a natural epithelial injury during pregnancy, the effect of luminal epithelial injury during diestrus on the sub-epithelial fibroblasts. Is the epithelial injury sufficient to still elicit a decidual-like reaction, like in mice and rats, as well as naturally during sheep pregnancy? It would also be important to understand whether what is recognized by "early stages of decidual reaction" in hooved animals is more similar to decidualization than to fibroblast activation, as suggested above for the marsupial.

The reported absence of decidual cells in bushbabies (Galago) is also in need of additional investigation. Galago belongs to the Strepsirrhine clade of primates, diverging from the rest of the primate lineage at the very basal node of crown primates. It forms a clade together with lemurs. The question of the ancestral status of the placenta in the strepsirrhine primates is controversial and interesting. Following the insightful discussion by Robert Martin from 2008, it seems most likely to represent a moderately invasive placentation (Martin 2008). This suggestion is supported by the description of a transient invasive form of placentation in *Galago demidoff* (Butler 1964; cited after Martin 2008). Should the absence of decidua be confirmed by additional investigations, it would most likely be a secondary loss, as inferred by Mess and Carter (2006).

The case of the eastern mole (*Scalopus aquaticus*) is even more complicated, as the relevant paper's (Prasad et al. 1979) publication history is rather complex (Carter 2005). In brief, the placenta of the eastern mole has been described as epithelio-chorial with no decidualization, an assessment that, according to Carter (2005), is wrong due to the mistaken identification of a syncytial trophoblast layer for a syncytial luminal epithelium. In the closely related European moles (*Talpa europea* and *T. occidentalis*), the placentation is uncontroversially endotheliochorial with large multinucleated and vacuolated decidual cells (Siniza et al. 2012). While the presence or absence of decidual cells in *Scalopus* was not assessed by Carter (2005), it is at least unlikely that the eastern mole is a complete exception.

In addition to the exceptions noted by Mess and Carter (2006), the case of the nine-banded armadillo (*Dasypus novemcinctus*) deserves notice. In 1958, Enders described a small number of putative decidual cells associated with the invasive villi of the placenta (Enders et al. 1958). In contrast, Kurt Bernischke denied the existence of decidual cells in the endometrium of the pregnant armadillo (Bernischke 2015). This controversy is likely due to a rather muted decidual reaction, because the armadillo placenta, though technically hemochorial, is minimally invasive (see Chapter 4).

Tenrecs are a clade of afrotherian mammals endemic to Madagascar, which retained (or potentially reacquired) a cloaca, a characteristic mostly found in marsupials and reptiles, including birds (Riedelsheimer et al. 2007). The body shape of tenrecs is highly polymorphic due to extensive convergent evolution to different lifestyles. It includes four species of hedgehog tenrecs, so called for their spines similar to those of hedgehogs. There is some disagreement about the presence of decidual cells in these animals. An early histological study of a single individual of the tailless hedgehog tenrec (*Tenrec ecaudatus*) described a decidual cell layer under the central hemophagous region of the placenta (Goetz 1938). This conclusion was confirmed by single-cell sequencing of mid-gestation samples, which identified a population of cells with decidual characteristics, such as IL15 expression (Stadtmauer et al. 2025). These cells differentiate from a population of endometrial stromal cells, as indicated by RNA velocity analysis. In contrast, a study of the lesser hedgehog tenrec (*Echinops telfairi*) failed to find histological evidence of decidual cells (Carter et al. 2004a, 2005), even though the placentation is clearly hemochorial with a hemophagous region like in the tailless hedgehog tenrec, making the loss of decidual cells rather unexpected. This case requires additional investigation to assess the presence or absence of decidual cells. If the absence of decidual cells in *Echinops telfairi* is confirmed, the question will arise: how does this species maintain a hemochorial placentation without the aid of decidual cells?

Finally, the case of the aardvark (*Orycteropus afar*) is also rather unclear. The aardvark also belongs to the Afrotheria and is thus of high phylogenetic interest. It belongs to the same subclade as the tenrecs, the Afroinsectiphilia. There is very little published data on the aardvark placenta and endometrium (Carter et al. 2004b), and the reference to the 1937 compilation by Mossman is not helpful (Mossman 1937), as is the reference to the fetal-maternal interface of other Afrotheria. For instance, Mossman describes the elephant decidua as "atypical" without explaining in what way it is atypical. It thus seems most parsimonious to assess the status of the decidua of the aardvark as unknown.

Returning to the question of the evolution of decidual cell type(s), there is a strong consensus that some kind of decidual cell is a shared derived feature of eutherians. Single-cell transcriptomics added another dimension to it, showing a stepwise increase in the number of decidual cell types in eutherians (Stadtmauer et al. 2025). The scenario arising from that study is the following (Figure 5.1): all therian mammals, and probably all gnathostomes with a Müllerian duct, share a fibroblast population that in mammals is called endometrial fibroblast. It is different from typical tissue fibroblasts, which one, for instance, also finds in the myometrium of the uterus. In Eutherians, from this endometrial stromal fibroblast (ESF), the decidual cell types arise during pregnancy or the menstrual cycle, if the latter exists. In all eutherians examined, there is an ECM-modifying population of decidual cells present, which could be called "pre-decidual" cells, because of the similarity between them and the decidual cells differentiating during the menstrual cycle of humans. Tenrecs only possess this "pre-decidual" cell type at their mature placental-endometrial interface, characterized also by expression of IL15, a factor known to cause the recruitment of natural killer cells. Among the rodents and primates, another cell type is added, called the endocrine decidual cell, because of the expression of endocrine factors like prolactin or oxytocin. In primates, there is only

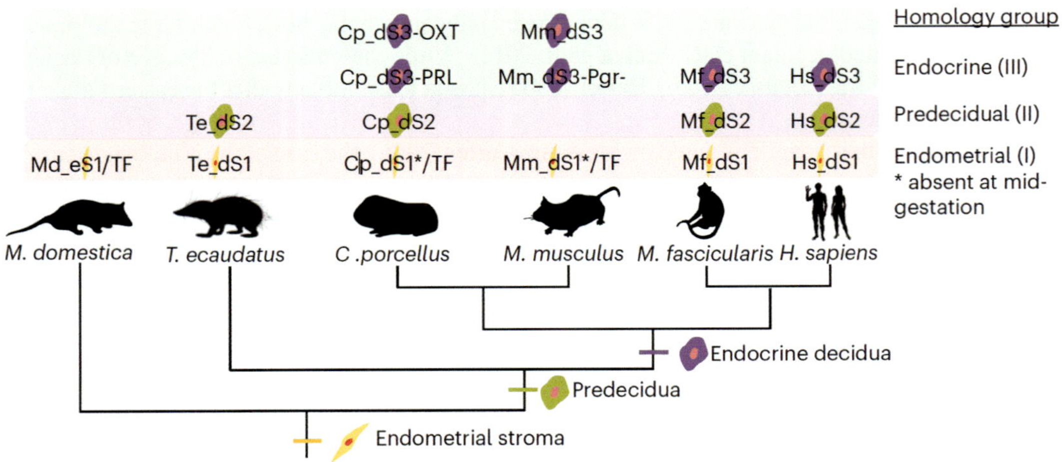

FIGURE 5.1 Hypothetical scenario of the complexification of the decidual cell inventory in therian evolution. All therians have endometrial stromal fibroblasts (ESF), likely inherited from at least the sarcopterygian Mullerian duct. In opossum and other marsupials, these cells are unable to differentiate into decidual cells. In the basally branching Afrotheria, here represented by tenrec, only one IL15-producing population of decidual cells is found. In primates and rodents, an additional type of DSC, an endocrine cell, evolved, with the greatest complexity of decidual cells found in rodents. (Image from figure 3 of Stadtmauer et al. (2005) published open access with MP and GPW as co-authors.)

one endocrine DSC, while in guinea pigs and mice, we find two endocrine DSC cell populations. Whether these are different cell types is not yet clear.

The question, where in the eutherian evolutionary history decidual cells were lost secondarily is still unclear, mostly due to the lack of detailed information about many non-model organisms. The strongest case for the loss of decidua is found for the ungulates. If claims of absence of decidua in other species are taken at face value, the loss of decidua would be rather sparsely distributed across the phylogenetic tree, i.e., a loss in one species and presence in relatively closely related species. An example could be the eastern mole (*Scalopus*) compared to the European moles (*Talpa*; see discussion above). However, given the low level of evidence in these cases, the pattern could easily be due to a small number of false negative reports. In the latter case, the reversion from invasive placenta and decidua to non-invasive and non-deciduate would be rare, limited to Ferungulata and perhaps *Galago* associated with loss of embryoimplantation which in itself is an interesting evolutionary pattern. Overall, the phylogenetic pattern is consistent with the hypothesis that decidual cells in eutherians originated once in the stem lineage of eutherian mammals, have diversified within the primates and even more so in rodents, and have been lost a few times when invasive decidualization was lost, in particular in hoofed animals and their relatives, and possibly in Galagos.

CHANGING FUNCTIONAL ROLES OF DECIDUA?

Here we want to briefly summarize the evidence and arguments presented in the paper by Arun Chavan and coauthors in 2016 (Chavan et al. 2016). Their main conclusion, relevant here, is that there seems to be a difference in the functional role of decidua in basally branching lineages of Eutheria, such as the Atlantogenata (comprising Xenarthra and Afrotheria), compared to Euarchontoglires. In mice, rats, and humans (representing Euarchontoglires), the decidua forms a continuous layer of tissue, separating the placenta from the deeper layers of the endometrium and the myometrium, which is retained until the end of pregnancy, even though reduced in depth. This layer of decidual tissue is essential for successful reproduction in humans. In the rare cases where the placenta erodes

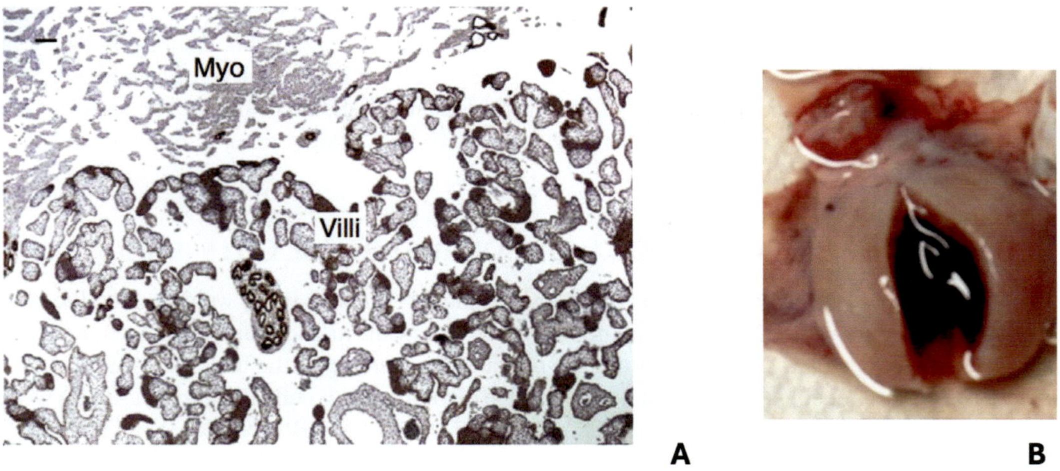

FIGURE 5.2 (A) Histological section of the fetal-maternal interface of the armadillo, *Dasypus novemcinctus*. To visualize the trophoblast cells, the section is stained with an antibody for cytokeratin, detected with HRP (brown precipitate). The fetal villi attach directly onto the maternal myometrium, thus representing a "physiological placenta accreta." (B) Postpartum armadillo uterus showing the blood clot in the uterine cavity. This finding shows that armadillo birth is associated with uterine bleeding even though the armadillo placentation is minimally invasive. (Image A is from figure 3, taken by Arun Chavan and published in Chavan et al. (2016), and image B was taken by GPW and published in Martin and Wagner (2019).)

the endometrium and comes into direct contact with the myometrium, the consequences can be catastrophic for the woman, a condition called "*placenta accreta*."[3] Normally, after birth, the *postpartum hemorrhage* is stopped by the contraction of the spiral arteries. With a *placenta accreta,* there are no spiral arteries between the placenta and the myometrium, and thus, they cannot stop the bleeding by arterial contraction. Without medical intervention, the consequence is maternal death. In contrast to this, species from the Atlantogenata have been shown, in later stages of gestation, to completely lack an endometrial separation between the placenta and the myometrium, a condition that can be called "*physiological placenta accreta*." That condition has been shown, for instance, for the nine-banded armadillo (Figure 5.2A) (Chavan and Wagner 2016). The post-partum armadillo uterus contains copious amounts of coagulated blood (Figure 5.2B) (Martin and Wagner 2019). Notably, putative decidual cells in armadillo do not form a compact layer as in human and mouse but are loosely associated with the invading placental villi (Enders et al. 1958). Other examples of a *physiological placenta accreta* are hyrax (*Procavia capensis*) and the lesser hedgehog tenrec (*Echinops telfairi*) (see Chavan et al., 2016 and the references therein) (Carter et al. 2004b). In Laurasiatherians, examples include the European mole (*Talpa europaea*) and two bats (the Indian false vampire bat, *Megaderma lyra,* and the neotropical disc-winged bat, *Thyroptera tricolor spix*). In these species, histological evidence suggests the presence of decidual cells at the beginning of pregnancy, but their absence later, in contrast to the situation in humans and mice.

The pattern summarized above suggests at least two functional types of deciduae. In the Atlantogenata, there is evidence for early decidualization probably necessary to regulate the inflammatory attachment and implantation reaction, whereas the decidua is dispensable in these animals[4] in later stages of pregnancy. In humans and mice, the pattern seems to be that there are different phases of decidual function. An early function is likewise probably related to inflammation, and a later function may be the regulation of the invasive phenotype of the placenta, a possible endocrine function, or the prevention of an adaptive immune response by the mother. These latter functions are necessary until the end of pregnancy. In fact, a major contributor to precipitate parturition in humans is decidual demise, a model called "decidual activation" (Casey and MacDonald 1988). The idea that the decidua has different functions in different eutherian lineages and in different phases of gestation matches well with the finding that *Tenrec ecaudatus* has only one major population of decidual cells, while humans have at least two, and the guinea pig has at least three (see Figure 5.2). We thus have to be open to the possibility that "the decidual cell" should be thought of as a cell type family rather than a unitary cell type, or a cell type with increasingly many physiological states accessible to them, as evolution proceeds.

CELLULAR ELEMENTS OF DECIDUA: DECIDUAL STROMAL CELLS (DSC)

Some histological characteristics of DCS have been mentioned above when we discussed the phylogenetic distribution of DSC across mammals. Here, we want to summarize what seems to be characteristic of decidual cells in order to get a better understanding of the biological role and evolutionary origin of decidual cells. Current knowledge about decidual cells is mostly based on work on the human endometrium during the menstrual cycle (Gellersen and Brosens 2014) and pregnancy (Suryawanshi et al. 2018), as well as from mice (Cha et al. 2012). To our knowledge, there is no broad-based characterization of decidual cells that is valid across eutherian species. Here we want to set the seed for such a characterization by summarizing what is known from humans and assessing, at this point largely through guesswork (which should be taken with a spoon of salt), what likely could be generalizable.

Condensing a large amount of literature, as summarized by Gellersen and Brosens in their magistral review of the field from 2014, the following features have been associated with decidual differentiation (Gellersen and Brosens 2014). At the tissue level, the differentiation of DSC is preceded by edema, i.e., the accumulation of fluid in the intercellular space, and the recruitment of leukocytes, in particular uterine natural killer cells (uNK) and macrophages (Mph). These features are not cell-intrinsic characteristics of DSC but are important with respect to models of decidual cell differentiation and their evolutionary origin.

In studies of human decidual cells, a small handful of "marker genes" are broadly used to recognize decidual cell differentiation. These are decidual prolactin (dPRL[5]), IGFBP1, and LEFTY2. All of them are secreted products, and their value for detecting decidual cells in other species is questionable, given that cell type identity is more based on transcription factor regulation rather than effector or signaling molecules (Arendt et al. 2016). Most clearly, that is the case for PRL, which is a signaling molecule that is expressed in human and mouse decidua (Soares 2004). This similarity is likely derived independently and does not represent a shared derived characteristic of decidual cells. While in apes there is only one *PRL* gene, in mice there are 26 PRL loci. Furthermore, their regulation is based on alternative promoters. In humans, extra-pituitary PRL expression depends on a primate-specific alternative promoter derived from the DNA transposon MER20 (Gerlo et al. 2006), which does not exist in mice. In rodents, one PRL paralog, Prl8a2, is expressed in decidual cells and is transcribed from an alternative promoter originating from the MER77 transposable element (Emera and Wagner 2012). Decidual PRL expression has probably evolved three to four times in Eutheria and is thus not a reliable character to identify decidual cells across wider phylogenetic distances (Emera et al. 2011). Even though, in the case of more closely related species, like rodents, PRL expression can be a useful criterion because the decidual expression of PRL has been established in one rodent species, *Mus musculus*, and is likely a shared derived character of rodents, as it is also expressed in some guinea pig decidual cells (Stadtmauer et al. 2025). Within rodents, and other clades with shared derived PRL expression, the phylogenetic evidence validates PRL expression as a criterion for the identification of DSC, as for instance in the spiny mouse (Bellofiore et al. 2017). To our knowledge, there is not enough data about IGFBP1 and LEFTY expression to assess their validity as DSC marker genes across species.

The analysis of decidual transcriptomes suggests three functional domains to be affected by DSC differentiation: ECM modification as noted above, secretion of cytokines and other signaling molecules, and changes to the cytoskeleton related to shape changes (Gellersen and Brosens

2014). Hence, broadly conceived, the biological role of DSC can be expected to be related to tissue re-organization, changing both the extracellular matrix as well as the cell type composition (dNK and dMph recruitment) via changes in the expression of signaling molecules and cell shape (cytoskeleton). Let us start with cell shape.

At the cell morphological level, decidualizing and decidualized cells differ from their precursors, the endometrial stromal fibroblasts (ESF), by signs of cellular activation and secretory activity: the nucleus transforms from a dense, elongated shape to a round, hematoxylin-pale-staining ball, suggesting a more open chromatin state and thus a more active transcriptional state. There is also an expansion of the cytoplasm, which gives the DSC a more rounded rather than spindle-shaped appearance. Within the cell, the transformation includes expansion of the rough endoplasmic reticulum and Golgi apparatus, also indicating a more active production of proteins (rough endoplasmic reticulum) and secretions (Golgi). Polyploidization has been found in mouse DSC but not in humans. Polyploidization could be seen as a device to increase the transcriptional output of the cell and is often encountered in secretory cells of glandular epithelia. Importantly, the cellular transformation is progesterone-dependent, consistent with the general reliance of eutherian pregnancy on active progesterone signaling.

Other changes associated with decidualization have to do with cell-cell contacts and communication as well as the extracellular matrix. There are signs of increased formation of gap-junctions as witnessed by increased expression of connexin 43 (CX43), ZO1, and cadherin 11. In mouse, CX43 is essential for decidualization and implantation (Okada et al. 2018). Decidual cells also express enzymes that remove some ECM components, a process that is also reflected in the formation of pseudopodia engulfing portions of the ECM. DSC add new elements to the ECM, most notable components of the basal membrane, Laminin and collagen IV. In fact, during decidualization in humans, the DSC become enclosed in a layer of basal membrane-like material.

Although the molecular mechanisms of decidual cell differentiation will be discussed in the next chapter, we want to briefly reflect on the use of transcription factor genes as markers of DSC identity. Based on first principles of molecular biology, the use of transcription factor genes is preferable for the identification of cell type identity across species to, say, signaling molecules (see Wagner 2014, and chapter 5). Yet, transcription factor markers can also impose problems. This can be illustrated with reference to the transcription factor Hoxa11. This transcription factor is known to be causally necessary for DSC differentiation in humans (Lynch et al. 2009, Nnamani et al. 2016), and even for the development of ESF in mice (Taylor et al. 1999, Chau et al. 2002, Milroy et al. 2005). However, Hoxa11 is also strongly expressed in myometrial cells (Figure 5.3) and thus seems to be more related to the regional identity of mesenchymal cells rather than ESF or DSC specifically. FOXO1, which is essential for DSC in humans does not seem to play the same role in mouse endometrium and is thus equally problematic, not to speak of the fact that FOXO1 is generally needed for regulating the oxidative stress response as well as carbohydrate metabolism, which appears to be of importance for DSC (Meng et al. 2023, Jia et al. 2024, Huang et al. 2025).

If a transcription factor-based generalizable profile of DSC exists, it will have to be a combination of expression features, rather than a specific transcription factor gene. From the limited amount of comparative data available, one can suggest a core profile of transcription factor genes that could be causal for the decidual cell identity. These are FOXO1, WT1, MEIS1, as well as HAND2 and FOS (Stadtmauer et al. 2025). Note that this list excludes many transcription factor genes experimentally verified to be essential for human decidualization, such as Hoxa11, Hoxa10, or CEBPB, for reasons discussed above.

One idea that is consistently associated with decidual differentiation is that the stromal cells assume an "epithelial" or at least an "epitheloid" phenotype. This idea relates to the observation that decidual cells are more polygonal than the spindle-shaped quiescent fibroblasts, as mentioned above, and has been related to the concept that decidualization includes an MET, i.e., a mesenchymal-to-epithelial transition. This in itself is an attractive idea, since it seems consistent with the "barrier" function against trophoblast invasion that the decidual cells play in human pregnancy (as

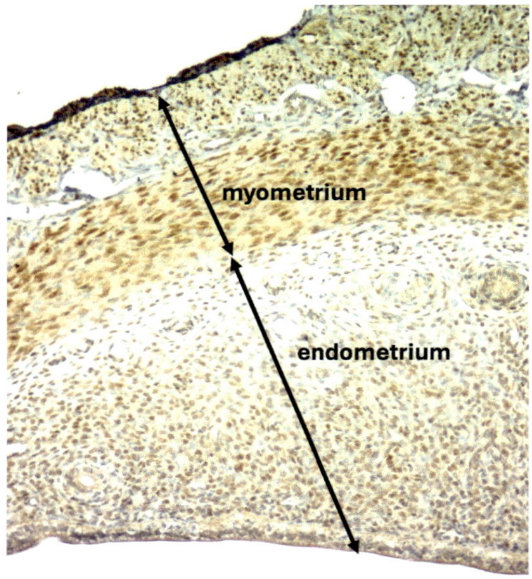

FIGURE 5.3 Cross section through the uterine wall of a gerbil, *Meriones unguiculatus*. The sections are stained with an antibody against the transcription factor Hoxa11 (brown precipitate). This image shows that both myometrial smooth muscle cells and stromal cells are positive for Hoxa11. (Image by GPW, CC BY-NC.)

discussed above). However, a critical review of the evidence for an MET during decidualization reveals that the concept is quite problematic. What is uncontroversial is that human decidual cells express some epithelial genes, such as collagen IV, laminin, as well as a higher level of cell-cell adhesion molecules, such as ZO1 (Zona Occludens 1) and Connexin 43 (Gellersen and Brosens 2014, Okada et al. 2018). However, it is a stretch to call these cells "epithelial" or even "epitheloid," as to our knowledge, nobody has demonstrated the key characteristic of epithelial cells, namely, an apical-basal polarity. With respect to the expression of transcription factors that are causally related to MET/EMT processes, that are *Snail, Slug,* and *Twist*, the evidence is rather unstable. Zhang and collaborators, in one of the pioneering papers that launched the idea that decidualization is an MET (Zhang et al. 2013, Okada et al. 2018), a slight reduction in Snail protein was reported in mouse and human cells (but without replication), although a 50% reduction in snail mRNA abundance is shown for mice via qPCR (it is unclear what the internal standard was). On the other hand, the rather extensive paper by Yu and colleagues, published in 2016, reports that expression of "neither Snail nor Slug was modulated" in their experiment (Yu et al. 2016). Re-examination of published bulk RNA seq results from in vitro decidualized human ESF (both immortalized and primary) consistently showed an increase in *Snail* RNA abundance (Longjun Wu and Günter Wagner, unpublished). Also, to our knowledge, none of the cytokeratin staining of human or mouse placentation sites shows cytokeratin in the stroma, while Zhang and collaborators reported cytokeratin in *in vitro* decidualization. Thus, while some epithelial genes are specifically expressed in human decidual cells, like Collagen IV, Laminin, and ZO1, the evidence for a proper MET during decidualization needs re-evaluation.

Of all the signs of decidual differentiation reported for humans, we want to take a guess at which of these signs could be part of a diagnostic profile projectable onto mammalian species other than humans. First are the signs of fibroblast activation, expansion of cytoplasm, round pale nuclei, which in fact have been used in classical comparative histological studies (see above). A likely general feature is also the progesterone dependence of DSC differentiation and maintenance, although this criterion is hard to implement in comparative studies. But nuclear progesterone receptor A expression could be used as a necessary criterion for DSC identity. Another likely projectable criterion is the association between decidualization and recruitment of cells of the innate immune system, in particular, uterine natural killer (uNK) cells and macrophages. ECM remodeling based on DSC-secreted MMPs is also a plausible candidate for a general decidual identity marker, given that embryo implantation and attachment are always associated with ECM remodeling. Intriguingly, the latter is also happening during pig embryo attachment, even though there is no implantation, enforcing a remodeling of the endometrium (Johnson et al. 2021). It is an interesting question whether DSC from all deciduate eutherian species secrete components of the basal membrane, laminin, and collagen IV. But the fact that, in Atlantogenata, the decidua does not form a protective layer, as in human and mouse, raises the possibility that this feature is limited to clades where the decidua is responsible for limiting the invasion of placental cells. This leaves morphological signs of cell activation, progesterone dependence, and hence PR expression, association with edema and leukocyte recruitment, and ECM remodeling as a preliminary list of potentially projectable criteria for identifying decidual stromal cells across mammals, in addition to a limited profile of transcription factor genes: FOXO1, WT1, MEIS1, as well as HAND2 and FOS. As said above, this summary should be understood more as a challenge to come up with a better list of criteria than a definite answer.

CELLULAR ELEMENTS OF DECIDUA: UTERINE NATURAL KILLER CELL (UNK)

As noted above, decidual stromal cells secrete signals such as IL15 that recruit innate lymphocytes to the endometrium, most notably uterine natural killer cells (uNK). In mice and related rodents (e.g., gerbil), uNK cells are easily recognizable in histological preparations because of their large (5 micro-meter) eosinophilic granules and are thus also known as large, granulated lymphocytes (LGL). Their other traditional name, granulated metrial gland cells, comes from their frequent localization in the metrial triangle of the mouse uterus, i.e., where the mesometrium meets the uterine tube. Immunologically, the uNK cells are characterized as CD56+ and CD16-, which is also important for their functional role, as will be explained below. In early pregnancy, these cells are the most abundant lymphoid cells and the second most abundant stromal cells besides decidual stromal fibroblasts. Their number decreases in later gestation, mostly due to cell death; thus, they seem to have their main function early in pregnancy. They are recruited from bone marrow cells and are attracted to the endometrium via IL15 expressed by DSC and decidual macrophages and differentiate there under the influence of IL15 and TGFB1.

The function of uNK cells is seen in two roles (Erlebacher 2013, Xie et al. 2022). On the one hand, they are involved in the remodeling of spiral arteries in collaboration with extra-placental trophoblast cells and uterine macrophages, a function important in early pregnancy stages. uNK cells are also involved in the production of a tolerogenic immunological environment for the placenta. In fact, uNK cells have a bipolar role, as they can assume both a tolerogenic and a cytotoxic phenotype. The latter is enabled by the content of the cytoplasmic granules, which contain, besides copious amounts of glycoproteins such as mucin 1, also lysosomal enzymes and perforin, the main cytotoxic molecule of lymphocytes. The cytotoxic form of uNK is induced by IL2, a major pro-inflammatory mediator, and blocked by interferon gamma (IFNG), which, in mice, they produce themselves. The role of a primarily tolerogenic rather than cytotoxic cell is also related to its immunological profile, i.e., being CD16 negative. CD16 is a cell surface receptor involved in degranulation and cytolysis, and thus its absence could be seen as a way to make uNK cells less cytotoxic. uNK cells also express a much larger repertoire of signaling ligands than NK cells in the peripheral blood. The tolerogenic role of uNK cells is likely related to their secretion of large amounts of IL-10, acting on decidual macrophages to assume an anti-inflammatory phenotype.

At this point, it is worth speculating about the importance of the bipolar nature of uNK cells, as both potentially pregnancy-enhancing and cytotoxic capabilities. Given this polarity, uNK cells could function as a switch for deciding about continuing pregnancy or aborting or resorbing an embryo. This model is also supported by evidence, in both mice and humans, which shows an involvement of uNK cell activation in pregnancy failure and embryo resorption (reviewed in Erlebacher 2013).

CELLULAR ELEMENTS OF DECIDUA: UTERINE MACROPHAGES

The decidua is also home to a uterus-specific macrophage population, called uterine or decidual macrophages (uMph or dMph). They constitute the second largest subpopulation of endometrial leukocytes and are characterized by the expression of an unusual surface antigen, CD209, a ligand of ICAM3 (intercellular adhesion molecule 3, a.k.a. CD50). CD209 is not found on peripheral blood macrophages except for the dermis and the lung stroma, in addition to the endometrium. The expression of CD209 is important to note because of its role in binding ICAM3, a cell surface molecule of uNK cells. During spiral artery remodeling uMph and uNK are seen to form cell dyads, suggesting a role of uMph in spiral artery remodeling, which could be mediated by CD209::ICAM3 binding. uMph are similar to anti-inflammatory IL10-expressing Mph, so-called M2 macrophages, as they are known from their role in the resolution of inflammation during wound healing. Finally, they also seem to play a role at the end of pregnancy when they become pro-inflammatory and are understood to play a role in decidual activation, as an initial step toward giving birth. uMph are a second example of a cell type family with generic functions in inflammation and wound healing, which plays a key role in the decidua of pregnancy. In the endometrium and, in particular, the decidual state of the endometrium, they assume anti-inflammatory and tissue-remodeling roles specific to the fetal-maternal interface.

CELLULAR ELEMENTS OF DECIDUA: TROPHOBLAST CELLS

Trophoblast cells constitute or originate from the outermost cell layer of the therian embryo and are not considered part of the endometrium. In the non-pregnant state, this is certainly true (besides the residual trophoblast cells that remain from previous pregnancies). But during pregnancy, most clearly in species with invasive placentation, trophoblast cells definitely become part of the decidual tissue. Many generic vertebrate tissues are composed of an epithelial part and a stromal part, as is the case with the endometrium. In hemochorial and endotheliochorial placentation, one can argue that the trophoblast layer of the placenta represents an additional epithelium or an epithelium that replaces the role of the luminal epithelium of the endometrium (Pavličev and Wagner 2024). The only odd thing about the trophoblast barrier layer as a substitute for the luminal epithelium is the polarity of the epithelium, since topologically the maternal stroma should be facing the basal, rather than the apical side of the trophoblast epithelium. While during implantation, loss of polarity of luminal epithelial cells has long been recognized, evidence for the trophoblast side is relatively recent. In fact, in the mouse, trophoblast development has been found to be associated with inversion of epithelial polarity (Ozguldez et al. 2023).[6]

In addition to the epithelial trophoblast barrier, often but not always syncytial, the trophoblast also gives rise to cells that leave the embryo and migrate into the stoma of the endometrium. In apes,[7] these cells are called extravillous trophoblast cells, referring to the villous morphology of the ape placenta. However, species with labyrinth placenta also have migratory trophoblast cells, such as mice and rats, which cannot be called extravillous, since there are no villi. To remove this ambiguity, it is better to speak of extra-placental trophoblast cells (EPT; Stadtmauer et al. 2025). Less radical then is the realization that the extraplacental trophoblast cells insert themselves into the decidual stroma, and even into the myometrium. For that reason, EPTs need to be considered as an element of the decidual tissue. In fact, some of these cells not only add to the cell inventory of the mesenchyme but actually replace another stromal cell element, the endothelial cells of the spiral arteries.

What about the trophoblasts of those (eutherian) species that have epitheliochorial placentation like the pig? In these species (with the important exception of the horse, which traditionally is called epitheliochorial), there is no physical mixing of maternal and embryonic cells.[8] It turns out that in these species the trophoblast is nevertheless engaged in an intense signaling exchange with the stroma, in particular during the early stages of pregnancy when attachment is happening. Most critically, in the pig during attachment, the trophoblast signals to maternal uterine macrophages via interferon gamma (IFNG), and they are the only source of IFNG in the uterus during this stage of gestation (McLendon et al. 2020, Johns et al. 2021, Cain et al. 2024). Hence, the integration of trophoblast cells into the cellular communication network of the endometrial stroma did not cease when the trophoblast cells were excluded from the endometrial tissue compartment.

CHALLENGES TO THE NIDATORY INFLAMMATION NARRATIVE AND THE DECIDUA HYPOTHESIS

Given the narrative that implantation includes inflammation-derived processes because the embryo causes a nidatory injury to the endometrium, the question arises: how broad is the explanatory scope of this idea? For instance, many, if not all, hoofed animals have a non-invasive, epitheliochorial placentation. Hence, there is technically no "implantation" into the endometrium, at most an attachment as discussed in the previous section ("implantation is a misnomer," p. 71 in Johnson et al. 2021). No overt injury to the endometrium can be detected in pig pregnancy, although limited invasive processes have recently been described in the sheep and cattle (Green et al. 2021). Does this mean that inflammation-derived processes do not play a role in pig pregnancy, for instance? Another part of the inflammation paradoxon is the idea that initially endometrial inflammation was caused by and may still be triggered by the hatching enzymes from the blastocyst. Intra-uterine hatching also happens in viviparous reptiles. Shouldn't we expect inflammation to proceed there and cause a "reptilian inflammation paradox"? Another challenge, specifically for the decidua hypothesis, is ectopic pregnancies, i.e., situations where the embryo establishes a placenta outside the uterus. How is this possible if we think the decidua is necessary for the establishment of pregnancy? Here, we want to discuss these three challenges to the inflammation/decidua narrative.

First, let us look at the initiation of pregnancy in epitheliochorial eutherian species. There are many non-hemochorial eutherian species, not the least because of the large number of artiodactyl species (e.g., antelopes). The best investigated among these in terms of their reproductive biology are farm animals, pig, cow, and sheep, for obvious reasons. The horse is a special case, not an artiodactyl, and has some invasive specializations (endometrial cups, i.e., transient clusters of trophoblast cells in the endometrial stroma) that make a comparison difficult (Antczak and Allen 2021).

Epitheliochorial placentation in eutherians evolved from a hemo- or endotheliochorial placentation (see Chapter 3). The ancestors of epitheliochorial eutherian species, such as the pig, likely had an invasive placenta with the associated inflammatory processes. Given this phylogenetic context, the question is whether inflammation-derived processes are still playing a role in the initiation of pregnancy, or whether they got lost with the loss of invasive implantation? The answer is that inflammation-related processes are still clearly detectable and likely play an important role, judging from the number of cells involved (see below).

In the pig, the blastocyst enters the uterus two days after fertilization (dpf) and then hatches from the zona pellucida and starts growing from <1 mm to 2 to 6 mm at day 10 pf. Then it undergoes additional growth and transformation, eventually assuming a filamentous shape of 800 to 1000 mm in length and a diameter of 1 mm by day 15 (reviewed in Johnson et al., 2021). The period of rapid elongation is critical for the development of the fetal-maternal relationship in the pig where the blastocyst is secreting copious amounts of signaling molecules such as estrogen, interleukin 1 beta (IL1b), interferon gamma (INFG) and interferon delta (IFND), prostaglandin E2 (PGE2) as well as transforming growth factors (TGFB1, 2, and 3). Most notable here are the secretion of pro-inflammatory signals, IL1b, and IFNG. At the same time, the blastocyst attaches to the luminal epithelium as described above. On the endometrial side, there is an accumulation of leukocytes at the sites of attachment, as well as extensive apoptosis in the endometrial stroma (McLendon et al. 2020), but which cells undergo cell death has not been determined. Among the leukocytes, a proliferating, activated population of T cells was detected, predominantly CD4+ T-helper cells and only a minority of CD8+ cytotoxic T cells. This composition suggests that both pro- and anti-inflammatory activities are in play during the attachment phase. This is also supported by the detection of T cell attracting chemokines (CXCL9, 10, and 11). At day 15 post fertilization (pf), an increase in macrophage and lymphocyte frequency was observed by single-cell analysis (Tian et al. 2022). The data from Tian and collaborators suggest that the lymphocytes were predominantly CD8+ cytotoxic T cells and a minority of CD4+ helper and regulatory T cells, contrary to the T cell quantification by McLendon et al. (2020). This discrepancy requires further attention. Maybe most significant is the observation that the porcine luminal epithelium is expressing large amounts of protease inhibitors, which might explain the lack of invasive nidation in the pig (Bazer and Johnson 2014).

The inflammatory processes in the pig endometrium depend on signals from the blastocyst. In particular, the role of IFNG has been documented by the production and insertion of IFNG -/- blastocysts into cycling females (Johns et al. 2021). At the macroscopic level, the result is paradoxical, as the uterus turns hyperemic and fibrotic, suggesting an upsurge of inflammatory processes. At the cell level, however, the lack of IFNG from the blastocyst leads to a loss of CD3+ T cells. Eventually, the blastocysts fragment and die by day 17pf.

A full understanding of the role of INFG and the other pro-inflammatory signals, as well as the role of the T cells, is still awaiting resolution. Nevertheless, it is clear that even in the epithelial placentation of the pig, certain inflammatory mechanisms are activated during the attachment phase of pregnancy, which decline substantially by day 20pf. McLendon and collaborators hypothesize that these attachment-associated inflammatory processes, as well as the inflammatory signals from the embryo, may be necessary for endometrial remodeling and increased vascularization for provisioning the embryos (McLendon et al. 2020). Hence, inflammation-derived mechanisms remain important even when no overt tissue injury to the endometrium is caused by the blastocyst. This suggests that inflammation-derived processes acquired essential roles for the establishment of pregnancy even when the putative primary trigger, tissue injury, is no longer present. Also notable is that important signals to initiate the inflammatory processes, in particular IFNG, emanate from the blastocyst rather than from the endometrium. In mice and humans (as well as guinea pigs; Stadtmauer et al. 2025), IFNG is primarily produced by uNK cells, while the pig is unique in expressing IFNG exclusively in the blastocyst during the attachment phase. This implies that the inflammation-related processes are in the "evolutionary interest" of the embryo.

Now, let us turn to the second question, the role of hatching enzymes in lizard placentation. Remember that the model suggests that uterine inflammation in mammals has its origin from hatching enzymes that the embryo expresses to either hatch from the zona pellucida (eutherians) or the shell coat (opossum), and which continue to be expressed during the embryo-maternal attachment and implantation. In viviparous reptiles, at least those that have a longer post-hatching residence time in the uterus, the same logic should apply, but there is no evidence that this is the case. Clearly, hatching enzymes of some kind need to be expressed to liberate the embryo from the eggshell.

Not a lot of work has been done on the problem outlined above, but the literature nevertheless suggests an explanation. In the case of therians, where we have some information, it seems that the hatching enzymes are exclusively produced by the trophoblast (Denker 1974, 1977, Brosens et al. 2014, Griffith et al. 2017). However, in lizards, proteolytic enzymes also seem to come from the luminal epithelium. In fact, a transcriptomic study of the pregnant and non-pregnant uterus of the skink *Chalcides ocellatus* shows that a highly upregulated gene ontology category in the pregnant uterus is proteases (Brandley et al. 2012). There are nine serine proteases and eight cathepsins, including secreted cathepsins, detected as upregulated in the pregnant *Chalcides ocellatus* uterus. It seems that intrauterine hatching in lizards is, in part, effected by maternal protease secretions, likely in addition to contributions from the embryo. If an epithelium, in this case the luminal epithelium, is actively secreting proteases, it will have to evolve resistance to its own secretions, as is the case in the digestive tract. In fact, the stomach and the gut are protected against their digestive enzymes through a mucus layer (Davenport 1971, Schmid-Schonbein 2008). It would be interesting to investigate the uterine mucus in viviparous lizards. Hence, it follows that the role of inflammatory processes during eutherian implantation could evolve only because the luminal epithelium does not contribute hatching enzymes for the breakdown of the embryo cover and is thus sensitive to the enzymes secreted by the embryo. Along these lines, the muted inflammatory response during early Wallaby pregnancy (Dudley et al. 2024) could be due to the involvement of the uterine epithelial protease secretions during fetal hatching (Denker and Tyndale-Biscoe 1986).

The third challenge we need to discuss is the question of how ectopic embryo implantation is possible without decidua. The decidua hypothesis claims that implantation and extended maintenance of the embryo depend on the presence and the actions of decidual stromal cells. A challenge to this hypothesis is the existence of ectopic pregnancies (Figure 5.4), i.e., pregnancies where the blastocyst implants outside the uterine lumen or endometrium.[9] In humans, ectopic pregnancies occur on average in 2% of pregnancies, but there are both environmental (risk factors) and genetic differences between populations. Ectopic implantation sites include the oviduct (all parts from fimbria to ampulla and isthmus, i.e., tubal pregnancy), the cervix, the ovary, or other places in the peritoneum (abdominal pregnancy). By far the most frequent ectopic implantation site is the oviduct (95%), where the ovum is fertilized and from where it should move to the uterus (Stock 1991). During a tubal pregnancy, the embryo usually does not survive, but exceptions are known when it has survived until the 14th week of pregnancy (Elmoheen et al. 2020). Abdominal pregnancies, in contrast, can proceed to full term. Of course, the baby needs to be delivered by surgery. Abdominal pregnancy can occur secondary to a burst uterus, where the baby is found in the abdominal cavity, but the placenta is still attached to uterine tissue. More problematic to explain are full-term abdominal pregnancies, where the placenta is implanted outside the uterus, for instance, in one case where the placenta was attached to the broad ligament of the uterus and the fetus was carried to 26 weeks, surgically delivered, and survived (Dahab et al. 2011). Another case of successful abdominal pregnancy is that of a 37-year-old woman who carried an abdominal pregnancy to 29 weeks, when the

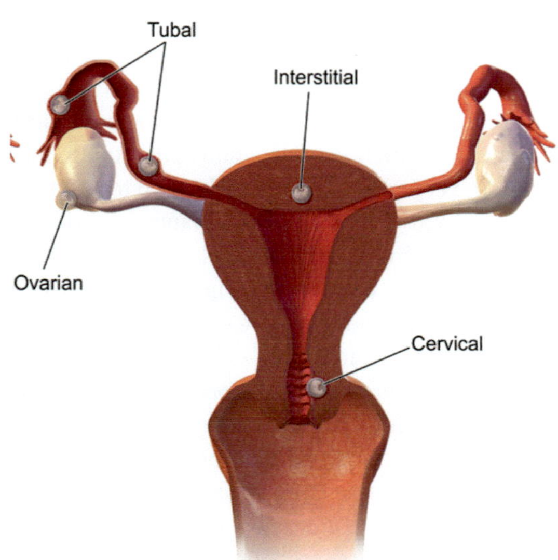

FIGURE 5.4 Typical locations of ectopic pregnancies in humans. (Image by Bruce Blaus - Own work, CC BY-SA 4.0, via Wikimedia.)

baby was surgically delivered and survived (Gorincour and Boukerrou 2023). How is this possible? Can these clinical facts be compatible with the decidua hypothesis?

Full-term abdominal pregnancies are rare and result in a dramatic emergency because removing the placenta is inevitably associated with massive hemorrhage that needs immediate attention. In this situation, it is understandable that no one considers preserving the placental attachment tissue for further examination. We could not find investigations describing the nature of the placental attachment site in full-term abdominal pregnancies. In contrast, the more frequent tubal pregnancies are, when diagnosed in time, removed and sometimes histologically examined. Before we proceed to what is known about the tubal implantation sites, we need to discuss the nature of the stromal tissue of the organs where ectopic implantation happens.

It has been known since the late 19th century that parts of the female reproductive tract can undergo changes that resemble decidual differentiation (Walker 1887). In one study, the fallopian tubes were examined in the context of post-partum sterilization, and it was found that 12% of patients showed histological signs of decidual transformation of the tubal stromal tissue (Tilden and Winstedt 1943). Also, the peritoneum of pregnant women can show signs of decidualization, a condition called deciduosis. One clinical study secondary to cesarian deliveries detected macroscopically visible and histologically confirmed decidual lesions of the abdominal serosa in 10% of the patients (Markou et al. 2016). What do we know about these cells that can undergo apparent decidual differentiation, and what do we know about the putative decidual cells during ectopic pregnancy?

The stromal cells of the tubal mucosa have a remarkable cell biology: they express smooth muscle actin (aSMA) and display primary cilia. Their ultra-structural features, together with the aSMA identify them as myofibroblasts (Oliver et al. 1999, Hagiwara et al. 2008), the kind of stromal cell typical for wound healing and also as a transient state in decidual differentiation (see Chapter 6). Interestingly, during ectopic pregnancy, the glandular epithelia express estrogen receptor in about 50% of cases examined, but progesterone receptor was detected neither in the epithelium nor in the stroma (Land and Arends 1992). This seems to contradict the decidual nature of these cells, but to our knowledge, this finding has not been replicated. Tubal implantation sites also show a normal complement of immune cells comparable to eutopic implantation sites, with the remarkable exception of natural killer cells (uNK cells), which are absent in the stroma of tubal implantation sites (Rango et al. 2001). Invasiveness of the trophoblast is more intense, or better, the invasibility of the tubal stroma is higher than than that of the uterine mucosa (Gao et al. 2018).

During human pregnancy, decidual-like reactions of stromal cells in the female reproductive tract are not rare, but also not a universal feature. This fact raises a number of questions. For one, why would cells undergo a decidual-like differentiation if no implantation should take place in these locations normally? Can the ectopic formation of decidual cells explain the remarkable ability of the human embryo to implant and, in very rare cases, even develop to full term?

The fact that extra-uterine stromal cells during pregnancy can occasionally differentiate into decidua-like cells can be understood by remembering that gene regulatory evolution of one cell type can have "spill-over" (pleiotropic) effects on gene expression of other, related cell types. Comparative studies of cell type evolution have shown evolutionary evidence for correlated gene expression evolution (Liang et al. 2018). That at least some of that correlated gene expression evolution can be due to pleiotropic effect has been shown experimentally (Dighe et al. 2024). Hence, the most likely explanation is that stromal cells in the female reproductive tract and even in the peritoneum are closely related cell types, and thus selection on uterine endometrial stromal cells likely leads to similar gene regulatory changes at least in stromal cells of other female reproductive tract tissues. After all, the fallopian tubes and the uterus are different parts of the same embryonic anlagen, the Müllerian ducts, that attract similar mesenchymal cells from the lateral plate mesoderm to form the mucosa. Tubal and uterine stromal cells are developmentally similar. This very similarity makes pleiotropic effects of changes to the uterine stroma likely to also cause similar effects in extra-uterine stromal cells. Deciduosis of the peritoneum may be related to the ability of embryos to implant in the abdominal cavity, which is not based on mesenchymal decidualization, but that of the peritoneum, which is a cell type with a hybrid epithelial/mesenchymal character, expressing, for instance, both vimentin, a mesenchymal intermediate fiber, and cytokeratin, typically found in epithelial cells. It is also noteworthy that uterine endometrial mesenchyme has the ability to implant into the peritoneum, leading to a condition called endometriosis, suggesting a biological affinity between uterine mucosa and the peritoneum.

Whether the ectopic decidual cells enable the extra-uterine survival and implantation of embryos is, to our knowledge, not known. The problem is that, at least in the case of tubal pregnancies, the decidual reaction is not particularly strongly developed, although the clinical literature is sometimes hard to assess. Reports of the tubal stroma associated with tubal implantation often do not report the gestational age of the conceptus. It is thus not clear whether the degree of tubal decidualization relates to the age until which embryos can survive. In any case, the biology of ectopic implantation sites should be recognized as an important system to test ideas about the cell biological requirements for the establishment of a stable fetal-maternal interface.

TAKE HOME AND CARRY OVER MESSAGES

Decidual cells are known only from eutherian mammals and likely evolved once in the stem lineage of eutherian mammals, coincidental with the evolution of invasive placentation. Of the eutherian species without reported decidual cells, the hoofed animals and the Galago represent cases of genuine loss of decidualization, while other species, where a lack of decidual cells is suggested, require additional investigation. The limited evidence available from comparative single-cell data suggests a two-step process of decidual cell evolution. The first step leads to immunomodulatory decidual cells (similar to "pre-decidual" cells from the human luteal phase endometrium). This stage is represented by the decidua of the afrotherian *Tenrec ecaudatus* (Stadtmauer et al. 2025). Within the Boreoeutheria, the decidual cells acquired an endocrine module, expressing genes like PRL or a paralog of PRL and/or OXT and similar. This scenario is also consistent with the observation that decidual cells in Afrotheria and Xenarthra (Atlantogenata) are present during early gestation, while in Euarchonotoglires, where present, they are necessary until the end of pregnancy, like in humans. These observations suggest that the physiological role of decidual cells in early branching lineages is more limited than the roles DSCs play in primates and rodents. A putative list of projectable criteria for decidual cell identity is proposed, consisting of edema and leukocyte recruitment during the process of decidual cell differentiation, as well as morphological and gene expression changes. The decidua, denoting the tissue rather than the cell type, includes, in addition to decidual cells, uterine natural killer cells, uterine macrophages, and extra-placental trophoblast cells.

NOTES

1. To be more precise: all species with spontaneous decidualization (as far as we know) menstruate, but not all menstruating species have spontaneous decidualization, as for instance some old-world monkeys.
2. Note also the presence of a quasi-inflammatory reaction during the attachment phase of pig pregnancy (see later in this chapter).
3. Technically, one does distinguish between different degrees of invasion of the placenta into the myometrium, with "*placenta increta*" representing a situation where the placenta invades the myometrium, and "*placenta percreta*" where the placenta perforates the uterine wall. All of these conditions, however, can be seen as belonging to the "placenta accreta spectrum."
4. Although the generality of that pattern among Atlantogenata species still needs to be assessed more rigorously.
5. Decidual prolactin is the same as pituitary prolactin at the level of the molecular structure of the peptide but its transcript has a different 5'UTR because it is regulated by an alternative promoter (Gerlo, S., J. R. Davis, D. L. Mager and R. Kooijman (2006). "Prolactin in man: a tale of two promoters." *Bioessays* **28**(10): 1051–1055).

6. A PubMed search in April 2024 with the parameters: (epithelial polarity[Title/Abstract]) AND (trophoblast[Title/Abstract]), only yielded three references, of which only one (Ozguldez et al., 2023) actually speaks of trophoblast cell polarity. From this, we infer that the question of trophoblast epithelial polarity has not attracted much attention until recently.
7. The clade of apes includes humans.
8. Note that eutherian epitheliochorial placentation is derived from invasive placentation (see Chapter 2).
9. This point was brought up by a student at the 2023 EMBO Venice Summer School, Eva Zaffarini, during a small group discussion with GPW. I appreciate the point she raised.

REFERENCES

Antczak, D. F. and W. R. T. Allen (2021). "Placentation in equids." *Adv Anat Embryol Cell Biol* **234**: 91–128.

Arendt, D., J. M. Musser, C. V. H. Baker, A. Bergman, C. Cepko, D. H. Erwin, M. Pavlicev, G. Schlosser, S. Widder, M. D. Laubichler and G. P. Wagner (2016). "The origin and evolution of cell types." *Nat Rev Genet* **17**(12): 744–757.

Arutyunyan, A., K. Roberts, K. Troule, F. C. K. Wong, M. A. Sheridan, I. Kats, L. Garcia-Alonso, B. Velten, R. Hoo, E. R. Ruiz-Morales, C. Sancho-Serra, J. Shilts, L. F. Handfield, L. Marconato, E. Tuck, L. Gardner, C. I. Mazzeo, Q. Li, I. Kelava, G. J. Wright, E. Prigmore, S. A. Teichmann, O. A. Bayraktar, A. Moffett, O. Stegle, M. Y. Turco and R. Vento-Tormo (2023). "Spatial multiomics map of trophoblast development in early pregnancy." *Nature* **616**(7955): 143–151.

Bazer, F. W. and G. A. Johnson (2014). "Pig blastocyst-uterine interactions." *Differentiation* **87**(1–2): 52–65.

Bellofiore, N., S. J. Ellery, J. Mamrot, D. W. Walker, P. Temple-Smith and H. Dickinson (2017). "First evidence of a menstruating rodent: the spiny mouse (*Acomys cahirinus*)." *Am J Obstet Gynecol* **216**(1): 40.e41–40.e11.

Bernischke, K. (2015). "Nine-banded armadillo, *Dasypus novemcinctus*." *Comparative Placentation*, 2025, from https://placentation.ucsd.edu/indxfs.html.

Brandley, M. C., R. L. Young, D. L. Warren, M. B. Thompson and G. P. Wagner (2012). "Uterine gene expression in the live-bearing lizard, *Chalcides ocellatus*, reveals convergence of squamate reptile and mammalian pregnancy mechanisms." *Genome Biol Evol* **4**(3): 394–411.

Brosens, J. J., M. S. Salker, G. Teklenburg, J. Nautiyal, S. Salter, E. S. Lucas, J. H. Steel, M. Christian, Y. W. Chan, C. M. Boomsma, J. D. Moore, G. M. Hartshorne, S. Sucurovic, B. Mulac-Jericevic, C. J. Heijnen, S. Quenby, M. J. Koerkamp, F. C. Holstege, A. Shmygol and N. S. Macklon (2014). "Uterine selection of human embryos at implantation." *Sci Rep* **4**: 3894.

Cain, J. W., H. Seo, K. Bumgardner, C. Lefevre, R. C. Burghardt, F. W. Bazer and G. A. Johnson (2024). "Pig conceptuses utilize extracellular vesicles for interferon-gamma-mediated paracrine communication with the endometriumdagger." *Biol Reprod* **111**(1): 174–185.

Carter, A. M., T. N. Blankenship, H. Kunzle and A. C. Enders (2004a). "Structure of the definitive placenta of the tenrec, *Echinops telfairi*." *Placenta* **25**(2–3): 218–232.

Carter, A. M., A. C. Enders, H. Kunzle, D. Oduor-Okelo and P. Vogel (2004b). "Placentation in species of phylogenetic importance: the Afrotheria." *Anim Reprod Sci* **82–83**: 35–48.

Carter, A. M., T. N. Blankenship, H. Kunzle and A. C. Enders (2005). "Development of the haemophagous region and labyrinth of the placenta of the tenrec, *Echinops telfairi*." *Placenta* **26**(2–3): 251–261.

Carter, A. M. (2005). "Placentation in an American mole, *Scalopus aquaticus*." *Placenta* **26**(8–9): 597–600.

Casey, M. L. and P. C. MacDonald (1988). "Biomolecular processes in the initiation of parturition: decidual activation." *Clin Obstet Gynecol* **31**(3): 533–552.

Cha, J., X. Sun and S. K. Dey (2012). "Mechanisms of implantation: strategies for successful pregnancy." *Nat Med* **18**(12): 1754–1767.

Chau, Y. M., S. Pando and T. H. S (2002). "HOXA11 silencing and endogenous HOXA11 antisense ribonucleic acid in the uterine endometrium." *J Clin Endocrin Metabol* **87**: 2674–2680.

Chavan, A. R., B.-A. S. Bhullar and G. P. Wagner (2016). "What was the ancestral function of decidual stromal cells? A model for the evolution of eutherian pregnancy." *Placenta* **40**: 40–51.

Chavan, A. R. and G. P. Wagner (2016). "The fetal-maternal interface of the nine-banded armadillo: endothelial cells of maternal sinus are partially replaced by trophoblast." *Zoological Lett* **2**: 11.

Chen, S. T., W. W. Shi, Y. Q. Lin, Z. S. Yang, Y. Wang, M. Y. Li, Y. Li, A. X. Liu, Y. Hu and Z. M. Yang (2023). "Embryo-derive TNF promotes decidualization via fibroblast activation." *Elife* **12**:e82970.

Dahab, A. A., R. Aburass, W. Shawkat, R. Babgi, O. Essa and R. H. Mujallid (2011). "Full-term extrauterine abdominal pregnancy: a case report." *J Med Case Rep* **5**: 531.

Davenport, H. (1971). "Why the stomach does not digest itself." *Scientific American* **226**(1): 86–93.

Denker, H. W. (1974). "Trophoblastic factors involved in lysis of the blastocyst coverings and in implantation in the rabbit: observations on inversely orientated blastocysts." *J Embryol Exp Morphol* **32**(3): 739–748.

Denker, H. W. (1977). "Implantation. The role of proteinases, and blockage of implantation by proteinase inhibitors." *Adv Anat Embryol Cell Biol* **53**(5): 3–123.

Denker, H. W. and C. H. Tyndale-Biscoe (1986). "Embryo implantation and proteinase activities in a marsupial (*Macropus eugenii*). Histochemical patterns of proteinases in various gestational stages." *Cell Tissue Res* **246**(2): 279–291.

Dighe, A., J. Maziarz, A. Ibrahim-Hashim, R. A. Gatenby, Kshitiz, A. Levchenko and G. P. Wagner (2024). "Experimental and phylogenetic evidence for correlated gene expression evolution in endometrial and skin fibroblasts." *iScience* **27**(1): 108593.

Dudley, J. S., M. B. Renfree, G. P. Wagner and O. W. Griffith (2024). "The extension of mammalian pregnancy required taming inflammation: independent evolution of extended placentation in the tammar wallaby." *Proc Natl Acad Sci U S A* **121**(42): e2310047121.

Elliot, M. G. and B. J. Crespi (2009). "Phylogenetic evidence for early hemochorial placentation in eutheria." *Placenta* **30**(11): 949–967.

Elmoheen, A., W. Salem, M. Eltawagny, R. Elmoheen and K. Bashir (2020). "The largest tubal pregnancy: 14th week." *Case Rep Obstet Gynecol* **2020**: 4728730.

Emera, D., C. Casola, V. J. Lynch, D. E. Wildman, D. Agnew and G. P. Wagner (2011). "Convergent evolution of endometrial prolactin expression in primates, mice, and elephants through the independent recruitment of transposable elements." *Mol Biol Evol* **29**(1): 239–247.

Emera, D. and G. P. Wagner (2012). "Transposable element recruitments in the mammalian placenta: impacts and mechanisms." *Brief Funct Genomics* **11**(4): 267–276.

Enders, A. C., G. D. Buchanan and R. V. Talmage (1958). "Histological and histochemical observations on the armadillo uterus during the delayed and post-implantation periods." *Anat Rec* **130**(4): 639–657.

Enders, A. C. and R. K. Enders (1969). "The placenta of the four-eye opossum (Philander opossum)." *Anat Rec* **165**(3): 431–449.

Erlebacher, A. (2013). "Immunology of the maternal-fetal interface." *Annu Rev Immunol* **31**: 387–411.

Gao, T., Y. Liang, H. Tang and L. Quan (2018). "The increased level of Tspan5 in villi suggests more proliferation and invasiveness of trophoblasts in tubal pregnancy." *Eur J Obstet Gynecol Reprod Biol* **228**: 38–42.

Garcia-Alonso, L., L. F. Handfield, K. Roberts, K. Nikolakopoulou, R. C. Fernando, L. Gardner, B. Woodhams, A. Arutyunyan, K. Polanski, R. Hoo, C. Sancho-Serra, T. Li, K. Kwakwa, E. Tuck, V. Lorenzi, H. Massalha, M. Prete, V. Kleshchevnikov, A. Tarkowska, T. Porter, C. I. Mazzeo, S. van Dongen, M. Dabrowska, V. Vaskivskyi, K. T. Mahbubani, J. E. Park, M. Jimenez-Linan, L. Campos, V. Y. Kiselev, C. Lindskog, P. Ayuk, E. Prigmore, M. R. Stratton, K. Saeb-Parsy, A. Moffett, L. Moore, O. A. Bayraktar, S. A. Teichmann, M. Y. Turco and R. Vento-Tormo (2021). "Mapping the temporal and spatial dynamics of the human endometrium in vivo and in vitro." *Nat Genet* **53**(12): 1698–1711.

Gellersen, B. and J. J. Brosens (2014). "Cyclic decidualization of the human endometrium in reproductive health and failure." *Endocr Rev* **35**(6): 851–905.

Gerlo, S., J. R. Davis, D. L. Mager and R. Kooijman (2006). "Prolactin in man: a tale of two promoters." *Bioessays* **28**(10): 1051–1055.

Goetz, R. H. (1938). "Studien zur Placentation der Centetiden I. Eine Neu-Untersuchung der Centetesplacenta." *Z f Anat u Entwicklungsgesch* **106**: 315–342.

Gorincour, G. and M. Boukerrou (2023). "Abdominal ectopic pregnancy." *N Engl J Med* **389**(24): e51.

Green, J. A., R. D. Geisert, G. A. Johnson and T. E. Spencer (2021). "Implantation and placentation in ruminants." *Adv Anat Embryol Cell Biol* **234**: 129–154.

Griffith, O. W., A. R. Chavan, M. Pavlicev, S. Protopapas, R. Callahan, J. Maziarz and G. P. Wagner (2019). "Endometrial recognition of pregnancy occurs in the grey short-tailed opossum (*Monodelphis domestica*)." *Proc Biol Sci* **286**(1905): 20190691.

Griffith, O. W., A. R. Chavan, S. Protopapas, J. Maziarz, R. Romero and G. P. Wagner (2017). "Embryo implantation evolved from an ancestral inflammatory attachment reaction." *Proc Natl Acad Sci U S A* **114**(32): E6566–E6575.

Hagiwara, H., N. Ohwada, T. Aoki, T. Suzuki and K. Takata (2008). "Immunohistochemical and electron microscopic observations of stromal cells in the human oviduct mucosa." *Med Mol Morphol* **41**(4): 221–226.

Huang, Y., Q. Zhu and Y. Sun (2025). "Glucose metabolism and endometrium decidualization." *Front Endocrinol (Lausanne)* **16**: 1546335.
Jia, Z., Y. Wei, Y. Zhang, K. Song and J. Yuan (2024). "Metabolic reprogramming and heterogeneity during the decidualization process of endometrial stromal cells." *Cell Commun Signal* **22**(1): 385.
Johns, D. N., C. G. Lucas, C. A. Pfeiffer, P. R. Chen, A. E. Meyer, S. D. Perry, L. D. Spate, R. F. Cecil, M. A. Fudge, M. S. Samuel, C. M. Spinka, H. Liu, M. C. Lucy, K. D. Wells, R. S. Prather, T. E. Spencer and R. D. Geisert (2021). "Conceptus interferon gamma is essential for establishment of pregnancy in the pig." *Biol Reprod* **105**(6): 1577–1590.
Johnson, G. A., F. W. Bazer and H. Seo (2021). "The early stages of implantation and placentation in the pig." *Adv Anat Embryol Cell Biol* **234**: 61–89.
Johnson, G. A., R. C. Burghardt, M. M. Joyce, T. E. Spencer, F. W. Bazer, C. Pfarrer and C. A. Gray (2003). "Osteopontin expression in uterine stroma indicates a decidualization-like differentiation during ovine pregnancy." *Biol Reprod* **68**(6): 1951–1958.
Kellas, L. M. (1966). "The placenta and foetal membranes of the antelope *Ourebia ourebi* (Zimmermann)." *Acta Anat* **64**: 390–445.
Kim, J. J., R. C. Jaffe and A. T. Fazleabas (1999). "Blastocyst invasion and the stromal response in primates." *Hum Reprod* **14 Suppl 2**: 45–55.
Kin, K., J. Maziarz and G. P. Wagner (2014). "Immunohistological study of the endometrial stromal fibroblasts in the opossum, *Monodelphis domestica*: evidence for homology with eutherian stromal fibroblasts." *Biol Reprod* **90**(5): 111.
Kurman, R. J., L. H. Ellenson and B. M. Ronnett (2019). *Blauenstein's Pathology of the Female Genital Tract.* New York, Springer.
Land, J. A. and J. W. Arends (1992). "Immunohistochemical analysis of estrogen and progesterone receptors in fallopian tubes during ectopic pregnancy." *Fertil Steril* **58**(2): 335–337.
Liang, C., J. M. Musser, A. Cloutier, R. O. Prum and G. P. Wagner (2018). "Pervasive correlated evolution in gene expression shapes cell and tissue type transcriptomes." *Genome Biol Evol* **10**(2): 538–552.
Lynch, V. J., K. Brayer, B. Gellersen and G. P. Wagner (2009). "HoxA-11 and FOXO1A cooperate to regulate decidual prolactin expression: towards inferring the core transcriptional regulators of decidual genes." *PLoS One* **4**(9): e6845.
Lynch, V. J., G. May and G. P. Wagner (2011). "Regulatory evolution through divergence of a phosphoswitch in the transcription factor CEBPB." *Nature* **480**(7377): 383–386.
Lynch, V. J., A. Tanzer, Y. Wang, F. C. Leung, B. Gellersen, D. Emera and G. P. Wagner (2008). "Adaptive changes in the transcription factor HoxA-11 are essential for the evolution of pregnancy in mammals." *Proc Natl Acad Sci USA* **105**(39): 14928–14933.
Markou, G. A., I. Goubin-Versini, O. M. Carbunaru, C. Karatzios, J. M. Muray and M. Fysekidis (2016). "Macroscopic deciduosis in pregnancy is finally a common entity." *Eur J Obstet Gynecol Reprod Biol* **197**: 54–58.
Martin, J. F. and G. P. Wagner (2019). "The origin of platelets enabled the evolution of eutherian placentation." *Biol Lett* **15**(7): 20190374.
Martin, R. D. (2008). "Evolution of placentation in primates: implications of mammalian phylogeny." *Evol Biol* **35**(2): 125–145.
McLendon, B. A., H. Seo, A. C. Kramer, R. C. Burghardt, F. W. Bazer and G. A. Johnson (2020). "Pig conceptuses secrete interferon gamma to recruit T cells to the endometrium during the peri-implantation perioddagger." *Biol Reprod* **103**(5): 1018–1029.
Meng, X., C. Chen, J. Qian, L. Cui and S. Wang (2023). "Energy metabolism and maternal-fetal tolerance working in decidualization." *Front Immunol* **14**: 1203719.
Mess, A. and A. M. Carter (2006). "Evolutionary transformation of fetal membrane characters in Eutheria with special reference to Afrotheria." *J Exp Zool Part B (Mol Dev Evol)* **306B**: 140–163.
Milroy, C. L., D. Richards, V. L. Wilding and K. H. Wong (2005). "Expression of oviduct specific genes in the uteri of Hoxa10 and Hoxa11 mutant mice." *Fertil Steril* **84, Suppl. 1**: S60.
Mossman, H. W. (1937). "Comparative morphogenesis of the foetal membranes and accessory uterine structures." *Contr Embyol* **26**: 129–246.
Mossman, H. W. (1987). *Vertebrate Fetal Membranes.* New Brunswick, NJ, Rutgers University Press.
Nancy, P., J. Siewiera, G. Rizzuto, E. Tagliani, I. Osokine, P. Manandhar, I. Dolgalev, C. Clementi, A. Tsirigos and A. Erlebacher (2018). "H3K27me3 dynamics dictate evolving uterine states in pregnancy and parturition." *J Clin Invest* **128**(1): 233–247.

Nnamani, M. C., S. Ganguly, E. M. Erkenbrack, V. J. Lynch, L. S. Mizoue, Y. Tong, H. L. Darling, M. Fuxreiter, J. Meiler and G. P. Wagner (2016). "A derived allosteric switch underlies the evolution of conditional cooperativity between HOXA11 and FOXO1." *Cell Rep* **15**(10): 2097–2108.

Okada, H., T. Tsuzuki and H. Murata (2018). "Decidualization of the human endometrium." *Reprod Med Biol* **17**(3): 220–227.

Oliver, C., M. J. Montes, J. A. Galindo, C. Ruiz and E. G. Olivares (1999). "Human decidual stromal cells express alpha-smooth muscle actin and show ultrastructural similarities with myofibroblasts." *Hum Reprod* **14**(6): 1599–1605.

Osokine, I., J. Siewiera, D. Rideaux, S. Ma, T. Tsukui and A. Erlebacher (2022). "Gene silencing by EZH2 suppresses TGF-beta activity within the decidua to avert pregnancy-adverse wound healing at the maternal-fetal interface." *Cell Rep* **38**(5): 110329.

Ozguldez, H. O., N. Govindasamy, R. Fan, H. Long, K. Mildner, D. Zeuschner, B. Trappmann, A. Ranga and I. Bedzhov (2023). "Polarity inversion reorganizes the stem cell compartment of the trophoblast lineage." *Cell Reports* **42**(4): 112313.

Pavličev, M. and G. P. Wagner (2024). "Reading the palimpsest of cell interactions: what questions may we ask of the data?" *iScience* **27**(5): 109670.

Prasad, M. R., H. W. Mossman and G. L. Scott (1979). "Morphogenesis of the fetal membranes of an American mole, *Scalopus aquaticus*." *Am J Anat* **155**(1): 31–68.

Rango, U. v., I. Classen-Linke, S. Kertschanska, B. Kemp and H. M. Beier (2001). "Effects of trophoblast invasion on the distribution of leukocytes in uterine and tubal implantation sites." *Fert Steril* **76**(1): 116–124.

Riedelsheimer, B., P. Unterberger, H. Hünzle and U. Welsch (2007). "Histological study of the cloacal region and associated structures in the hedgehog tenrec *Echinops telfairi*." *Mamm Biol* **72**(6): 330–341.

Roth, J. J., M. Breitenbach and G. P. Wagner (2005). "Represson domain and nuclear localization signal of the murine Hoxa-11 protein are located in the homeodomain: no evidence for role of poly-Alanine stretches in transcriptional repression." *J Exp Zool Part B (Mol Dev Evol)* **304B**: 468–475.

Schmid-Schonbein, G. W. (2008). "Biomechanical aspects of the auto-digestion theory." *Mol Cell Biomech* **5**(2): 83–95.

Seo, H., G. D. Melo, R. V. Oliveira, G. A. Franco-Johannsen, F. W. Bazer, K. G. Pohler and G. A. Johnson (2024). "Immunohistochemical examination of the uteroplacental interface of cows on days 21, 31, 40, and 67 of gestation." *Reproduction* **167**(2): e230444.

Siniza, S., D. G. Lupianez, R. Jimenez and U. Zeller (2012). "Morphology and ultrastructure of the chorioallantoic placenta of the Iberian mole (*Talpa occidentalis*) with special reference to heterophagous areolas and the nature of interhaemal barrier." *J Anat* **221**(2): 164–173.

Soares, M. J. (2004). "The prolactin and growth hormone families: pregnancy-specific hormones/cytokines at the maternal-fetal interface." *Reprod Biol Endocrinol* **2**: 51.

Stadtmauer, D. J., S. Basanta, J. D. Maziarz, A. G. Cole, G. Dagdas, G. R. Smith, F. van Breukelen, M. Pavlicev and G. P. Wagner (2025). "Cell type and cell signalling innovations underlying mammalian pregnancy." *Nat Ecol Evol* **9**: 1469–1486.

Stadtmauer, D. J. and G. P. Wagner (2021). "Single-cell analysis of prostaglandin E2-induced human decidual cell in vitro differentiation: a minimal ancestral deciduogenic signal." *Biol Reprod* 106: 155-172.

Stock, R. J. (1991). "Tubal pregnancy. Associated histopathology." *Obstet Gynecol Clin North Am* **18**(1): 73–94.

Suryawanshi, H., P. Morozov, A. Straus, N. Sahasrabudhe, K. E. A. Max, A. Garzia, M. Kustagi, T. Tuschl and Z. Williams (2018). "A single-cell survey of the human first-trimester placenta and decidua." *Sci Adv* **4**(10): eaau4788.

Taylor, H. S., P. Igarashi, D. L. Olive and A. Arici (1999). "Sex steriods mediate HOXA11 expression in human peri-implantation endometrium." *J Clinical Endocrin Metabol* **84**: 1129–1135.

Tian, Q., J. P. He, C. Zhu, Q. Y. Zhu, Y. G. Li and J. L. Liu (2022). "Revisiting the transcriptome landscape of pig embryo implantation site at single-cell resolution." *Front Cell Dev Biol* **10**: 796358.

Tilden, I. L. and R. Winstedt (1943). "Decidual reactions in fallopian tubes: histologic study of tubal segments from 144 post-partum sterilizations." *Am J Pathol* **19**(6): 1043–1055.

Vento-Tormo, R., M. Efremova, R. A. Botting, M. Y. Turco, M. Vento-Tormo, K. B. Meyer, J. E. Park, E. Stephenson, K. Polanski, A. Goncalves, L. Gardner, S. Holmqvist, J. Henriksson, A. Zou, A. M. Sharkey, B. Millar, B. Innes, L. Wood, A. Wilbrey-Clark, R. P. Payne, M. A. Ivarsson, S. Lisgo, A. Filby, D. H. Rowitch, J. N. Bulmer, G. J. Wright, M. J. T. Stubbington, M. Haniffa, A. Moffett and S. A. Teichmann (2018). "Single-cell reconstruction of the early maternal-fetal interface in humans." *Nature* **563**(7731): 347–353.

Wagner, G. P. (2014). *Homology, Genes and Evolutionary Innovation*. Princeton, NJ, Princeton University Press.

Walker, A. (1887). "Der Bau der Eihäute bei Graviditas abdominalis." *Virchows Arch f Path Anat* **107**: 72–99.

Wang, W., F. Vilella, P. Alama, I. Moreno, M. Mignardi, A. Isakova, W. Pan, C. Simon and S. R. Quake (2020). "Single-cell transcriptomic atlas of the human endometrium during the menstrual cycle." *Nat Med* **26**(10): 1644–1653.

Wildman, D. E., C. Chen, O. Erez, L. I. Grossman, M. Goodman and R. R (2006). "Evolution of the mammalian placenta revealed by phylogenetic analysis." *Proc Natl Acad Sci USA* **103**: 3203–3208.

Xie, M., Y. Li, Y.-Z. Meng, P. Xu, Y.-G. Yang, S. Dong, J. He and Z. Hu (2022). "Uterine natural killer cells: a rising star in human pregnancy regulation." *Front Immunol* **13**. https://doi.org/10.3389/fimmu.2022.918550

Yang, M., J. Ong, F. Meng, F. Zhang, H. Shen, K. Kitt, T. Liu, W. Tao and P. Du (2023). "Spatiotemporal insight into early pregnancy governed by immune-featured stromal cells." *Cell* **186**(20): 4271–4288. e4224.

Younesi, F. S., A. E. Miller, T. H. Barker, F. M. V. Rossi and B. Hinz (2024). "Fibroblast and myofibroblast activation in normal tissue repair and fibrosis." *Nat Rev Mol Cell Biol* **25**(8): 617–638.

Yu, J., S. L. Berga, E. B. Johnston-MacAnanny, N. Sidell, I. C. Bagchi, M. K. Bagchi and R. N. Taylor (2016). "Endometrial stromal decidualization responds reversibly to hormone stimulation and withdrawal." *Endocrinology* **157**: 2432–2446.

Zhang, X.-H., X. Liang, X.-H. Liang, T. S. Wang, Q.-R. Qi, W.-B. Deng, A.-G. Sha and Z.-M. Yang (2013). "The mesenchymal—epithelial transition during in vitro decidualization." *Reprod Sci* **20**: 354–360.

6 A Synthetic Scenario For the Origin of Decidual Cells

HOW TO INVESTIGATE THE MOLECULAR BIOLOGY OF A NOVEL CELL TYPE?

In this chapter, we want to approach the question of how we can understand the evolutionary origin of the decidual cell type, and the decidua as a novel tissue type in general, from a molecular, mechanistic point of view. This raises a wide array of questions, since the difficulty of identifying the critical molecular innovations underlying a cell type also applies to all the other cell types that originated in the evolution of animal life.[1] Novel cell types originate from previously existing cell types, either by sister-cell type differentiation (Arendt 2008) or by cell type "hybridization" (pages 65 to 66 in Schlosser 2021). As a consequence, all cell types in an organism are, to various degrees, related to each other, forming a hierarchy of cell type families (Arendt 2008, Wagner 2014, Liang et al. 2015, Musser and Wagner 2015, Arendt et al. 2016, Oakley 2017, DiFrisco et al. 2023). That fact further implies that all cell types within an animal share a considerable amount of their molecular biology. This extends not only to the most basic cellular functions, such as genes for "household" enzymes, generic stress reactions, and proliferation, but also includes mechanisms shared among more closely related cell types, i.e., members of a "cell type family." An example for the latter would be those shared among all different kinds of fibroblasts or macrophages. This fact poses constraints on how experimental evidence can inform the origin of a novel cell type or, really, any evolutionary innovation.

The fact that cell types in an animal share molecular mechanisms implies that classical experimental strategies, such as "slash and burn"[2] experiments of various sorts, do not help with identifying cell-type-specific mechanisms. The reason is that any functionally important molecular mechanism (and which ones would not be important?), if knocked down or knocked out, would affect the cell under investigation in one way or another.[3] If we interfere with protein biosynthesis, any function of the cell will be affected. The same is true for most metabolic enzymes. Would we not expect the same for neurons if we interfere with the function of a "pan-neuronal" gene or pathway, if they exist? This means that classical experimental approaches will not be able to distinguish between plesiomorphic mechanisms shared with other cell types and those that are specific to the cell type identity and the cell type-specific function, unless these experiments are systematically done on all related cell types in a species.[4] For that reason, the investigation of the mechanistic basis of any cell type's identity should combine experimental data with comparative phylogenetic evidence, or better: experiments need to be done in a comparative context. What that means will be discussed below, but a brief outline will be presented in the next paragraph.

Given that cell types in an organism share large parts of their biochemical and gene regulatory networks, the question of what is specific for a given cell type has to be answered by two kinds of comparisons. On the one hand, any cell type in the body is a member of a cell type family resident in the same organism. For instance, macrophages are tissue-resident cells that are specialized for the tasks in those specific tissues, such as microglia in the brain and alveolar macrophages in the lung. Hence, hypothesized cell-type-specific mechanisms need to be tested against their presence in other cell types in the same cell type family for their specificity. Only if the mechanism is only active in the specific cell type but not in others in the same cell type family have we found the cell type-specific identity mechanisms. On the other hand, cell types arise, most often, by differentiation into two sister cell types from an ancestral cell type. If we are lucky, we can find the ancestral cell

DOI: 10.1201/9781032717777-6

type in an extant outgroup species. Again, a cell type identity mechanism for a derived cell type is predicted to be absent in the ancestral cell type present in an outgroup species. These two criteria are common sense but need to be enforced when potential mechanisms for the origin of a cell type are presented in the scientific literature.

Another difficulty in reconstructing and explaining the way a novel cell type or any novelty (Type 1 novelty in the sense of Wagner 2014) arose in evolution is that we do not have, in most cases, the pure ancestral character available for experimentation. Hence, the animals and cells we can investigate are a palimpsest of their original structure plus a large number of later modifications that evolved in all lineages of descent, including the one from the ancestor to the specific derived species and that from the ancestor to the outgroup species (Hallgrimsson et al. 2009). An obvious example of this problem is that most of what we know about the biology of the decidual cells comes from the investigation of human decidual cells (summarized in Gellersen and Brosens 2014). Not only are humans, as all other eutherian mammals, at least 60+ Mio years removed from the eutherian ancestor, but humans and other catarrhine animals acquired menstruation, which is largely (but not strictly) associated with spontaneous decidualization, i.e., decidual cell differentiation without an embryo. Other differences among mammalian decidua have been discussed before, which also support the notion that the decidual cells of recent species are a collection of more or less modified forms of this cell type. Of course, there is the chance, and we have to make this assumption, that some aspects of the ancestral cell type and its mechanisms are preserved in one or the other way among the diversity of recent species. The question of how these features can be extracted is the question pursued in this chapter. The proposal is that information about the cell biology of embryo implantation helps focus attention on the causal constraints on that evolutionary process. These constraints then scaffold the interpretation of empirical data into a causal and historical narrative.

BRIEF OVERVIEW OF THE HUMAN DECIDUAL CELL DIFFERENTIATION

In spite of the arguments put forward in the previous section against human ESF/DSC as a model of decidual cells, knowledge from studies on human cells provides the basis for much of what we know about ESF/DSC biology. For that reason, we start here with a (very) brief overview of what is known about human decidualization, much of it from *in vitro* studies, as *in vivo* experimentation is out of the question in humans and even higher primates.

The standard protocol for *in vitro* human DSC differentiation is treatment with a progesterone analog and a chemically modified cAMP. The most often used progesterone analog is MPA, standing for Medroxy-Progesterone-Acetate, a chemically more stable derivative of progesterone than progesterone itself. The cAMP derivative is most often 8-bromo cAMP, which is a form of cAMP that is able to cross the cell membrane more easily than cAMP. Extracellular cAMP is not a physiological signal but is normally produced inside the cell as a result of the stimulation of a G-protein-coupled receptor activating the ATP cyclase, leading to cAMP production. cAMP, in turn, is responsible for activating the protein kinase A (PKA), which exerts its effect by phosphorylating some protein substrates (Figure 6.1). The question of which extracellular signal is responsible for activating the cAMP/PKA pathway is still unanswered, or at least there is no broad consensus about it. There are several candidates discussed below as we consider the ancestral decidualizing signals. For now, the standard model states that decidualization is the result of the convergence of at least two signaling pathways, the progesterone signal via the nuclear receptor isoform A and the cAMP/PKA pathway (Figure 6.1). Activation of these two is at least sufficient *in vitro*, although there is the possibility that some factors in the serum are released from carrier proteins, such as TGFb. Nevertheless, there is evidence for the participation of other signaling pathways, such as ROS/NOX4 signaling (Al-Sabbagh et al. 2011), BMP/Wnt (Li et al. 2013), as well as the MAPK pathway (Vallejo et al. 2011, Sheller-Miller et al. 2018). How these mechanisms are integrated into a unitary cellular identity is largely unknown.

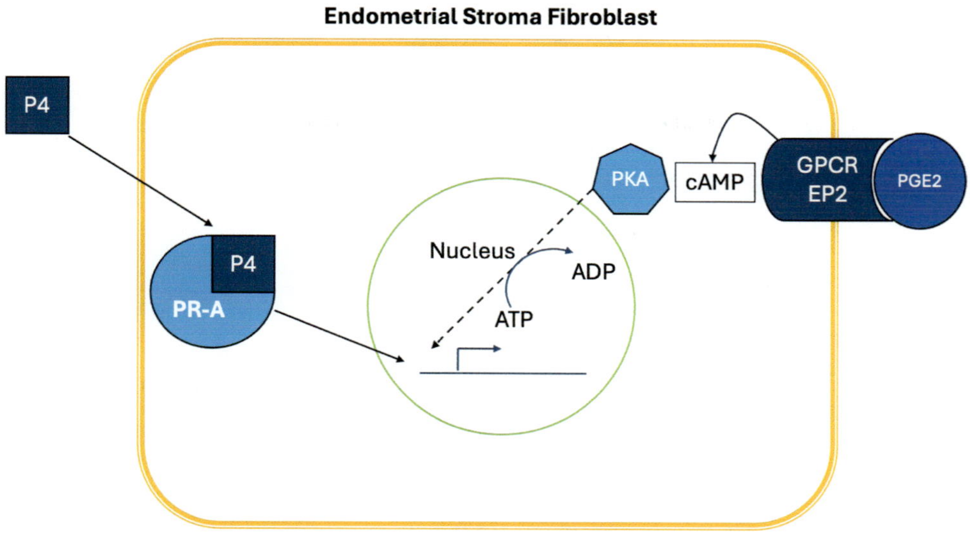

FIGURE 6.1 Schematic representation of the classical "converging two-signaling-pathways" model of the differentiation of decidual cells in humans. The two signaling pathways are progesterone via its nuclear receptors, PGR-A, and G-protein-coupled receptor cAMP PKA pathway. The ligand for activating the cAMP pathway is likely prostaglandin E2, PGE2. (Figure composed by GPW, CC BY NC.)

DECIDUALIZING SIGNALS AND THEIR "SEMANTICS"

Here, we use the term "semantics" to refer to the physiological information the signals are conveying to their target cells. The semantics of the progesterone and cAMP signals are to indicate the coincidence of two physiological events (Figure 6.2). Progesterone indicates that an ovulation has occurred, as its primary source is the corpus luteum, which forms after ovulation.[5] This requirement reflects the fact that decidual cells are only needed if ovulation has taken place, and thus a fertilized egg or an embryo can be expected to arrive in the uterus. The second signal, working through cAMP and PKA, is not that straightforward to understand, but we will argue below that it originally was a signal indicative of the arrival of an invasive blastocyst.

Progesterone owes its name to the fact that it is a necessary factor to maintain pregnancy in placental mammals (progesterone is short for pro-gestational steroidal ketone). It is important to remember, however, that progesterone is not necessary for the continuation of marsupial gestation, and thus this role is derived in placental mammals (on the evolution of the corpus luteum and progesterone function see Basanta and Pavlicev 2025). The role of progesterone for placental gestation is paralleled by its role in maintaining the differentiated state of decidual stromal cells, which is largely non-controversial. In fact, decidualization is reversible *in vitro* when cAMP and progesterone are withdrawn (Yu et al. 2016) (Pavličev, unpublished observation). It is also clear that progesterone, during decidualization, acts through its nuclear receptor A rather than through one of the membrane-bound progesterone receptors. As mentioned, its role in the initiation of decidualization is more controversial, from which Gellersen and Brosens (2014) concluded that there have to be additional factors to *initiate* DSC differentiation, while progesterone is responsible for *maintaining* the differentiated state.

While it is clear that full decidualization requires the activation of the cAMP/PKA signaling pathway, a consensus about which extracellular signal[s] are responsible for this event has still not been reached. We will argue below that the lack of clarity may result from the possibility that the regulation of decidualization is not a unitary mechanism, but has been modified in different placental lineages, in particular in the primate lineage, which includes species with spontaneous

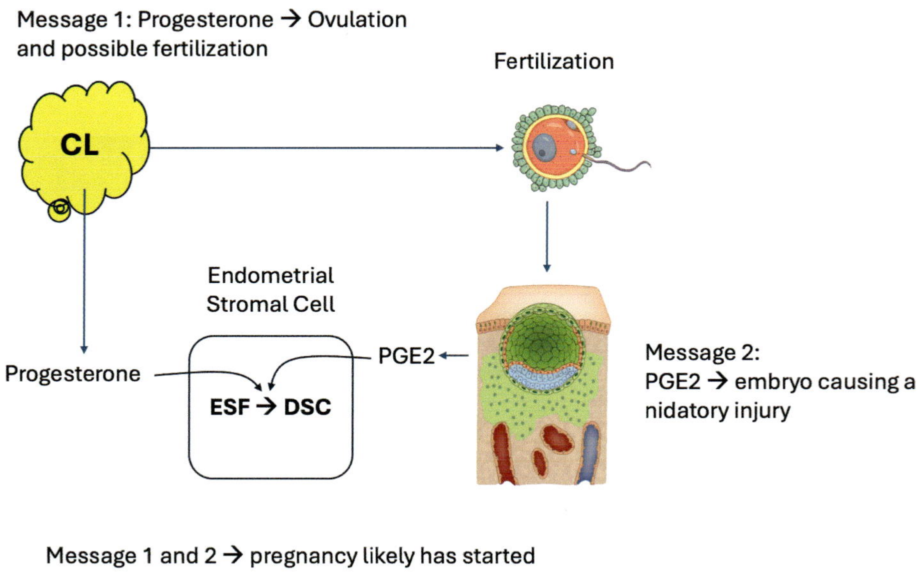

FIGURE 6.2 The "meaning" or "semantic" of the two signals causing the differentiation of the decidual cell. An increase in the systemic level of progesterone indicates that an ovulation has occurred, and thus it is possible that a fertilized ovum and ultimately an early embryo is on its way toward the uterus. Prostaglandin signaling is a generic signal activated during an inflammatory response, indicating an injury. In conjunction with progesterone, the injury is most likely caused by the arriving embryo rather than by other external causes. Together, these two signals tell the endometrial stromal fibroblasts that it is time to differentiate into a decidual cell to engage with the implanting embryo. (Figure composed by GPW, CC BY NC, fertilized ovum and blastocyst invasion icons from anatomytool.org/content/slagter-drawing-implantation-blastocyst-and-formation-embryonic-disc-no-labels.)

decidualization. Candidate ligands must be able to activate the GPCR–cAMP pathway, leading to PKA activation, and be available during implantation. The list of candidates considered in the literature includes relaxin (RLN), corticotropin-releasing hormone (CRH), prostaglandin E2 (PGE2, via its receptors EP2 and EP4), as well as the gonadotropic hormones follicle-stimulating hormone (FSH), luteinizing hormone (LH), and chorionic gonadotropin (CG).

We may first ask what the putative ancestral decidual signals may be. To identify a candidate, one can first eliminate all signals that have a more restricted taxonomic distribution than placental mammals. This argument assumes that the ancestral signal was not frequently replaced by others during the evolution of placental mammals. Signals with restricted taxonomic distribution are the placentally expressed CRH, which is only found in primates, as well as CG. The former is expressed under the influence of a cis-regulatory element derived from a transposable element (THE1B) only found in primates (prosimians) (Dunn-Fletcher et al. 2018). CG belongs to the glycoprotein hormones that consist of two peptide chains, a conserved alpha-chain, shared among all the glycoprotein hormones, and a beta chain that is specific for the particular hormone. The beta chain of CG arose from a gene duplication of the LH beta chain in the stem lineage of the Catarrhini, and thus also is not a candidate for the ancestral decidualizing signal. One also needs to keep in mind that *CG-B* genes have been further duplicated in the primate lineage, such that humans have 6 paralogs (Talmadge et al. 1984, Maston and Ruvolo 2002).

Relaxin is disqualified as an ancestral decidualizing signal because of its expression dynamics in humans. Its expression peaks 9 to 10 days after ovulation, i.e., after decidualization was initiated in the human menstrual cycle (Stewart et al. 1990, Johnson et al. 1993). Furthermore, although RLN is able to activate the adenosine cyclase (Palejwala et al. 2002), this signal is short-lived and not able to induce decidual marker gene expression in human ESF (Brighton et al. 2024).

LH-B and CG-B are closely related peptides, and the corresponding LH and CG hormones are often considered functionally equivalent or nearly so because they act through the same receptor, called LHCGR. The role of LHCGR in placental mammalian reproduction is complicated, which has led to controversies about the potential role of these hormones in decidualization. To start with, Pakarainen and colleagues have shown that an LHCGR-KO mouse can reproduce normally if its ovaries are replaced by wild-type ovaries (Pakarainen et al. 2005). This means that any extra-ovarian LHCGRs are not essential for reproduction and, by implication, also not for decidualization, as decidual cells are essential for implantation also in mice. In humans and baboons, however, there is more evidence for a role of LHCGR in reproduction and decidualization, which will be discussed below, in the context of the evolution of spontaneous decidualization.

This leaves us with prostaglandins. It is known that PGE2, PGD2, and PGI2 are produced at implantation sites. Many prostaglandin receptors signal through adenyl cyclase/cAMP and may thus be able to cause PKA activation that is generically assumed to be essential for DSC differentiation. In particular, this is the case for the PGD2 receptor DP, the PGI2 receptor IP, and the EP2 receptor of PGE2. The situation is a little more complicated with PGE2 signaling, since PGE2 has four different receptors, called EP1, EP2, EP3, and EP4. EP1 and EP3 do not signal through cAMP and PKA and are, in fact, inhibitory to cAMP signaling. EP4 is able to signal through cAMP, but, in contrast to EP2, has also the ability to signal through PI3K, ERK, and other signaling pathways. Hence, the expression of EP4 protein or *PTGER4* mRNA does not uniquely indicate the kind of signaling happening in a cell with that receptor.

The expression dynamics and species differences in the endometrium of prostaglandin receptors are complicated, and a review of these facts goes beyond the scope of this chapter. Nevertheless, what can be said is that adenylate cyclase activation is likely mediated through various prostaglandin receptors during the peri-implantation period and associated with decidualization. The complication is the expression and function of EP4, which is often expressed in endometrial stromal cells, but its function is impossible to determine without knowledge of the associated G-proteins and downstream signaling effects. In contrast, the remaining three are definitely signaling through cAMP/PKA: EP2 is induced in human stromal cells *in vitro* by progesterone (Brar et al. 1997, Stadtmauer and Wagner 2021), DP is expressed in stromal cells during the mouse peri-implantation period (Negishi et al. 1995) and is also involved in human decidualization (Sakamoto et al. 2024), and IP is involved in mouse decidualization (Lim et al. 1999). Hence, prostaglandin signaling, through one of the several cAMP/PKA activating receptors, is a highly likely ancestral decidualizing signal. This model is also attractive because of the known role of PGE2 during inflammation, and hence it is a molecule likely present at the site of the nidatory injury, i.e., implantation site. In fact, our lab has shown that the inflammatory state of the late pregnant opossum is associated with PGE2 expression (Griffith et al. 2017), and thus, PGE2 was present at the location of the embryo in the uterus, even before the evolution of implantation and decidua cells. This fits the general pattern that "specific signals" are ancestrally present before the response in the target cells evolved (Wagner 2014).

Assuming that the above inference of an ancestral role of prostaglandins at the site of embryo attachment and nidatory injury is correct, one is led to the suggestion that the semantics of prostaglandin signaling indicate the presence of a blastocyst in the uterus, secondary to the nidatory injury (Figure 6.2). This inference is based on the fact that PGE2 is part of a mucosal inflammatory response and can be triggered by the presence of a protease-secreting blastocyst. Hence, decidualizing signals indicate the coincidence of two events: the presence of an inflammatory stimulus in the uterus (PGE2 or similar) after ovulation (progesterone). This coincidence suggests that the inflammatory stimulus is due to a blastocyst rather than an infection.

AN ARGUMENTATIVE STRATEGY

In the previous section, we proposed a risky strategy to approach the question of how mammalian embryo implantation and decidual cells may have originated. It is based on a speculative framework, trying to constrain the likely possibilities to eventually arrive at testable hypotheses. To manage the risks, or at least make the risks transparent, we will employ an argumentative strategy that will be alien to many of our colleagues. It is inspired by the way mathematics was taught at the University of Vienna in the 1970ies and also inspired by the style of writing, typical for the early Ludwig Wittgenstein. The characteristic of this approach is to clearly identify assumptions and facts entering the argument by labeling them as "Axioms," and statements directly and easily derived from axioms, as "Corollaries," and numbering them to highlight their logical dependencies. Transparency is thus achieved at the cost of a pleasing narrative flow, as the latter easily hides logical and causal discontinuities. Preferring transparency over narrative pleasantry, we will proceed despite knowing that not everyone will like it.

An axiom is a statement that is taken as a starting point for further argumentation. It does not mean that we assume it is true *a priori*, as the axioms of Euclidean geometry were perceived to be until Hilbert and others constructed non-Euclidean geometries. We mean only a statement that we believe is (or should be) uncontroversial, but still is empirically fallible, and it is used as a starting point for an inference.

In mathematics, a corollary is usually a statement that directly or easily follows from a previous statement without much effort. In our case, we list the most likely inferences following from one of the "axioms" under normal physiological conditions. These are generic biological reactions and processes that occur under normal circumstances, as "injury leads to inflammation". No logical derivation is implied, only a bio-"logical" connection.

Many of the arguments discussed below build on the facts reviewed in Chapter 5. Thus, in this part of the chapter, we will minimize direct citations and point to Chapter 5 for details and focus on the structure of the argument.

THE "AXIOMS" OF EMBRYO IMPLANTATION

In what follows, we will condense much of what has been said in previous chapters on the evolutionary and molecular biology of embryo implantation and decidualization. Highlighting some of these facts here signals the assumption that they are critical for understanding the evolution of decidua and implantation.

Axiom 1: *In eutherian mammals with invasive placenta, the embryo hatching from its zona pellucida, or shell coat, causes a nidatory injury or at least an irritation to the uterine endometrium.*

In both "primitive" marsupials (e.g., opossums and dunnarts) and eutherians, the embryo or fetus hatches from its coverings (zona pellucida or eggshell or egg coat) by secretion of proteases. This has been shown in human blastocysts as well as opossum (Brosens et al. 2014, Griffith et al. 2017). The irritation to the uterine endometrium is thus a side effect of continued expression of these enzymes by the trophoblast after hatching. The "decision" to be made by further evolution is whether to accept a short fetal-maternal contact, expel the fetus, and expand the post-partum development and growth of an altricial neonate, as is the case in most marsupials. One alternative is to extend gestation, for which the expression of proteases has to be reduced, leading to a non-invasive and non-irritant embryo, as seems to be the case in macropodids, e.g., wallaby (Dudley et al., 2024). In the third alternative, invasiveness may have advantages, perhaps by creating a more intimate contact between fetus and mother. If these advantages outweigh the negative consequences of nidatory injury, then extended gestation becomes possible through the suppression of the nidatory inflammation after the establishment of the fetal-maternal interface. The latter is the direction the eutherian lineage has gone (Figure 6.3).

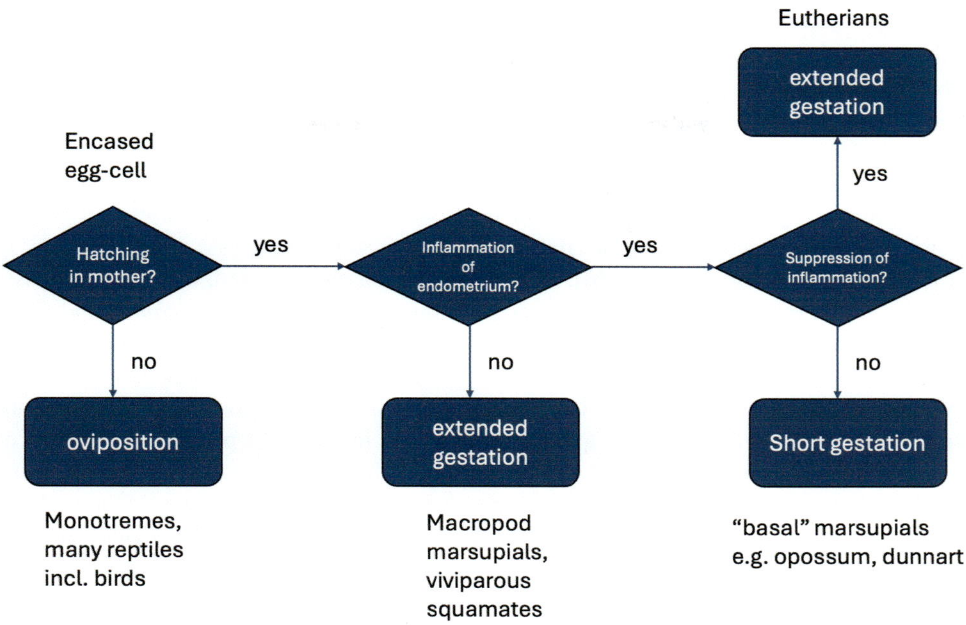

FIGURE 6.3 Decision tree of the evolution of the fetal-maternal relationship in the uterus: if the embryo retains its covers until it is delivered, we have oviposition, like in monotremes and many reptiles, including birds. If the egg coverings are lost while in the Müllerian tube, the further development depends on whether the loss of the egg covering causes endometrial inflammation. If it does not, gestation can continue as exemplified in macropods and viviparous reptiles. If inflammation is caused by the embryo, it either can lead to a short gestation, like in the opossum, or it is actively suppressed extended pregnancy can evolve, like in eutherian mammals. (Figure composed by GPW, CC BY-NC.)

Of course, we need to remember here again that the non-invasive (e.g., pigs) or minimally invasive placentation in eutherians (horses, cows, etc.) is secondarily evolved (Mess and Carter 2006, Wildman et al. 2006, Elliot and Crespi 2009) and thus represents a different chapter in the evolution of the fetal-maternal relationship. In all other eutherians, embryo implantation involves the local destruction of the luminal epithelium of the endometrium and thus matches the definition of an epithelial injury. This then leads to the "corollaries" of Axiom 1:

Corollary 1.1: *At least ancestrally, embryo implantation was associated with the activation of the endometrial fibroblasts.*

In mammals and perhaps in all vertebrates, disruption of epithelia initiates a wound-healing reaction in the associated stroma, specifically a process called *fibroblast activation* (Younesi et al. 2024). We argue that the same has to be expected for endometrial fibroblasts of animals in the stem lineage of eutherians. Fibroblast activation has been studied extensively in the medical sciences, not only because it is part of the healing process but also because it can, when misregulated, lead to permanent impairments of the affected organ by producing fibrosis, the overproduction of collagen. The most broadly recognized signal received by the stromal cells from the injured epithelium is TGFb1, which is then also expressed by the fibroblasts acting in an autocrine fashion, may be to lock in the activated state. On the phenotype level, the most obvious change in activated fibroblasts is the expression of alpha smooth muscle actin (aSMA, *ACTA2*) and an associated contractile phenotype, which is said to help in closing the wound. Gene expression in activated fibroblasts is mediated by SMAD transcription factors induced by the TGFb signaling pathway, cooperating with STAT3 (Chakraborty et al. 2017). Hence, it is to be expected that these same pathways would have been activated in the animals in which embryo implantation first occurred. Fibroblast activation thus is likely the foundation upon which the decidual cell identity has evolved.

Corollary 1.2: *At least ancestrally, irritation or injury by the embryo elicited an inflammatory reaction in the uterine endometrium, what we may want to call "nidatory inflammation."*

Any kind of compromised tissue integrity, be it due to infection, sterile injury, or physiological stress (e.g., Type II diabetes), elicits an inflammatory reaction (see chapter 5). This includes the innate immune system, the recruitment of neutrophils, edema, and the activation of macrophages with subsequent activation of the adaptive immune system (in the case of an infection). If we accept Axiom 1, it is natural to infer that, as embryo implantation evolved, it was initially associated with an inflammatory reaction in the endometrium. In opossum (*Monodelphis*) and Dunnart (*Sminthopsis*), the nidatory inflammation of the uterus (including neutrophil recruitment) is followed by parturition in short order (see Chapter 5). In the opossum at least, the fetus is contributing inflammatory mediators, such as IL1A, IL6, IL17, and PGE2, and thus cooperates with the mother (Stadtmauer and Wagner 2020), likely to ensure the timely initiation of parturition (Hansen et al. 2017). In humans, it has been known for a long time that embryo implantation activates at least part of an inflammatory cascade, which, however, is resolved as pregnancy continues (Mor et al. 2011). Hence, *inflammation, in addition to fibroblast activation, was likely the physiological status from which sustained embryo implantation evolved.*

Axiom 2: *Decidua and the decidual cell type originated during the evolution of extended placentation in eutherian mammals and were instrumental in the evolution of a sustained fetal-maternal unit.*

Marsupial and eutherian reproduction most clearly differ in the duration of pregnancy and, more importantly, in the duration of direct fetal-maternal contact. Marsupials have short gestation, except for macropods and some of their close relatives, the possums[6] (Phalangeridae), which evolved a non-invasive form of placentation (see Chapter 5). In contrast, the eutherians tend to have longer pregnancies, such as up to two years in elephants, 9 months in humans, and 16.5 weeks in pigs, for instance. At some point, or in parallel in many lineages, gestational length must have increased. A likely scenario is an adaptation driven by natural selection on gestational length, directly or indirectly due to selection for increased body size (Basanta and Pavlicev 2025). In either case, evolutionary changes to the fetal-maternal interface were necessary to sustain an extended placentation, in particular in lineages that remained hemochorial.

Some support for a causal role of the decidua and decidual cells in the extended eutherian pregnancy can be derived from the fact that decidual integrity and, in particular, the absence of inflammation are essential for the continuation of pregnancy in humans (Romero et al. 2014). This, however, needs to be contextualized with the fact that the continuous presence of decidua is not necessary in at least some Atlantogenata (see above, Chapter 5), but is only present at the beginning of pregnancy. The most parsimonious interpretation is thus that the ancestral decidual function was to enable the transition from the nidatory inflammation to inflammatory quiescence till the end of pregnancy.

Nevertheless, the core assumption of this "Axiom" should be subjected to additional scrutiny. What direct evidence can be mustered to support the notion that decidua and decidual cells evolved once in the stem lineage of eutherians, "in order" to allow the extension of pregnancy? One unsolved problem is that we do not know what the gestational length was of the common eutherian ancestor. Studies based on conventional ancestral state reconstruction methods come to estimates that are implausibly long, e.g., 125 days for an animal of the size of a small rat (Werneburg et al. 2016), a gestation time longer than that of the domestic pig. The difficulty seems to arise from an evolutionary innovation at the root of eutherians, consisting in the decoupling of the length of the luteal phase and that of pregnancy (Basanta and Pavlicev 2025). For a single evolutionary origin of decidual cells, it is at least required that the ancestral eutherian had a gestation time that required accommodations to attenuate the nidatory inflammation. Addressing this issue requires experimental evidence from basally branching lineages about the role of decidual cells in the establishment of pregnancy in these animals. For instance, one should test whether implantation is possible while decidualization is inhibited. At least in mice, the answer is "no," but we do not know what the case is in, say, tenrecs, hyrax, or armadillos (Atlantogenata). Answers to these questions are achievable but will require a research program of broad taxonomic scope.

Despite these uncertainties, a role of decidua in sustaining implantation typical for eutherians is suggested by the fact that all species with invasive placentation have at least a temporary presence of decidual cells (see Chapter 5). This correlation has been noted early in the history of reproductive biology and was used to argue that decidua are a "maternal defense" against placental invasion (see Chapter 10). Furthermore, the evolutionary loss of decidual cells is associated with a loss of invasive placentation (see Chapter 5).

Corollary 2.1: *Decidual cells and decidua evolved to attenuate and control the nidatory inflammation.*

This corollary is supported by the anti-inflammatory activities found for the human decidual cells discussed below. Among them is the suppression of Th17 cell differentiation by decidual cell secretions (Chavan et al. 2021), and others. Again, the uncertainty is that we know virtually nothing about the biology of the decidual cells of basally branching lineages such as hyrax, tenrec, or armadillo. We can, at this point, only speculate that the biological role of human decidual cells in implantation is not too different from that of the decidual cells of other eutherians.

Corollary 2.2: *The differentiation of decidual cells needs to be coordinated with the onset of pregnancy.*

Corollary 2.2.1: *The signals triggering decidualization should, at a minimum, reflect the recent occurrence of ovulation and the arrival of the embryo in the uterus.*

As discussed at the beginning of this chapter, the two signals known to be involved in decidualization, progesterone and PGE2, PGD2, or PGI2/cAMP/PKA, would fit that bill. Progesterone indicates a recent ovulation, and prostaglandin the arrival of the embryo via the effects of the nidatory injury. Again, the weakness of this inference is the lack of experimental data about animals other than humans and mice as the model species with invasive placentation.

INTERLUDE 1: FIBROBLAST ACTIVATION AND ITS RESOLUTION

Fibroblast activation was introduced and mentioned briefly in previous chapters and paragraphs. Here, we want to discuss this concept a little more to prepare for the section on the evolutionary scenario for the origin of decidual cells. Fibroblasts are one of the main cell types in the stroma of many tissues and organs (Adler et al. 2020). They provide the collagenous matrix that gives tissues their mechanical integrity, and also have many other, less obvious functions. Fibroblasts are, like macrophages, sentinels of tissue integrity, meaning that they sense violations of tissue integrity and transduce the information to the innate immune system, leading to the recruitment and activation of neutrophils, macrophages, and other immune cell types. They also participate in tissue repair (Krausgruber et al. 2020). In response to tissue injury, fibroblasts assume a different cell state, that of "activated fibroblast." The "hallmark" of fibroblast activation is the expression of smooth muscle actin (SMA, *ACTA2*), such that activated fibroblasts become contractile cells, quite similar to smooth muscle cells (with which they are closely related). In addition, activated fibroblasts produce collagen (Col1a1/2, Col3, Col6), although there is a question whether the ACTA2 expression and the Collagen production phenotype are present in the same cells simultaneously, or are mutually exclusive activities of the same cell population, but not the same cells (Umbarkar et al. 2021). In the medical field, fibroblast activation has attracted considerable interest, since uncontrolled activated fibroblasts are the cellular mediators of tissue fibrosis. Fibrosis is the overproduction of collagenous ECM, which can, in the worst case, substantially hinder or even replace the functional (parenchymatic) cells of an organ or tissue, leading to organ failure (e.g., cirrhosis). As a consequence, the medical literature on fibroblast activation is often formulated in terms of "mechanisms contributing to fibrosis," even though it is clear that what is described is also part of a normal wound healing response. Fibrosis is an extension of processes that are fundamental to wound healing, not a different biological phenomenon. Many diseases are (extreme) states of a physiological trait or process, rather than a distinct trait in itself, i.e., they are often not a meaningful independent biological entity (Pavlicev and Wagner 2022). Hence, when reading the literature on fibroblast activation, one has to remember that the mechanisms described can contribute to a pathological outcome but are not "disease mechanisms" as such. Only the loss of control over fibroblast activity leads to fibrosis. But what, in brief, do we know about fibroblast activation?

The best investigated signal leading to fibroblast activation is TGFb1. TGFb1 is secreted by injured epithelia and initiates the wound healing process. According to the accepted model, TGFb1 acts through a receptor tyrosine kinase, phosphorylating the transcription factors SMAD2 and SMAD3, which, through interaction with the "co-SMAD" SMAD4, are translocated into the nucleus, where they regulate the transcription of its target genes, such as *ACTA2* (for smooth muscle actin) and collagens. It has been established for a long time that other signaling pathways are also "contributing to fibrosis," meaning that they contribute to fibroblast activation. These are SMAD-independent pathways of TGFb1 signaling, such as focal adhesion kinase (FAK), hinting at a connection between cytoskeletal gene expression and function. Others are early growth response 1, mitogen-activated protein kinases (MAPK), and tyrosine kinase c-ABL. In a relatively recent paper, Chakraborty and colleagues have shown that the activities of various fibrotic signaling pathways are integrated through the phosphorylation of STAT3 by JAK, SRC, c-ABL, and JNK (Chakraborty et al. 2017). Activated fibroblasts also produce TGFb1 themselves, leading to an autocrine feedback loop which makes activated fibroblasts independent of the initial stimulus.

Another pro-fibrotic factor acting downstream of TGFb1 is IL11 (Schafer et al. 2017), reviewed in (Corden et al. 2020). In human fibroblasts, TGFb1 stimulation leads to strong upregulation of IL11, establishing an autocrine loop as fibroblasts express IL11 receptor, upon which the stromal cells activate ERK signaling and STAT3. Interestingly, the main effect of IL11 in fibroblasts is on the rate of translation of mRNA of fibrotic genes, such as collagen I, rather than on gene transcription. IL11 is also induced by other profibrotic stimuli, like PDGF, angiotensin II, bFGF, IL13, and others (Wynn 2008).

When it comes to other factors affecting fibroblast activation and potentially fibrosis, it is useful to identify the role of the factor relative to the TGFb1 pathway (MacLean and Pasumarthi 2014). For instance, Angiotensin II (AngII) has been identified as a contributing factor in heart muscle fibrosis by inducing TGFb1 expression. The role of AngII is downstream of its role in the regulation of systolic blood pressure and a factor in leading to stress-induced hardening of the heart muscle. Similarly, Wnt3a is also a fibroblast-activating factor, because it induces TGFb1 expression in embryonic fibroblasts. Mechanical stress and ECM stiffness also have the ability to induce TGFb1 expression and thus to activate fibroblasts.

On the other hand, there are factors that either enhance the TGFb1 signaling, similar to IL11, such as for instance NOX4 and ROS, which enhance P-SMAD effects (MacLean and Pasumarthi 2014, Schafer et al. 2017), or also further upregulate TGFb1 expression.[7] Furthermore, Endothelin 1 (ET1) is a known transcription factor induced by TGFb1, which itself targets ACTA2, forming a coherent feed-forward loop with TGFb1-SMAD.

As decidualization is likely derived from fibroblast activation but normally does not lead to wound healing (during pregnancy) or a permanent fibrotic state (after parturition or menstruation), the question is, how is fibroblast activation resolved before a fibrotic state is reached or how incipient fibrosis can be reverted. This problem thus affects the process of decidualization but also the post-partum repair and, where present, the post-menstrual repair (Ang et al. 2023). In fact, we will encounter here a number of genes that also play central roles in decidualization.

One molecule that is able to cause the reversion of activated fibroblasts to "quiescent" fibroblasts is PGE2 (Garrison et al. 2013). This effect is mediated through the PGE2 receptor 2 (*PTGER2*, EP2) via the cAMP/PKA pathway. Huang and collaborators have shown that the PGE2→EP2→cAMP pathway acts through at least two pathways further downstream to revert fibroblast activation

(Huang et al. 2008). On the one hand, there is the PKA pathway already mentioned, which inhibits collagen 1 expression, and on the other hand, there is the Epac1 pathway, which is responsible for the anti-proliferative role of PGE2. At the same time, PGE2/EP2 inhibits the activity of the PI3K/Akt pathway, which, in fibroblasts, inhibits the expression of EP2. This is achieved via the upregulation of PTEN, which is a direct inhibitor of the PI3K activity through the dephosphorylation of phosphatidylinositol triphosphate (PIP3), which is necessary for the activation of PI3K. In fact, in PTEN -/- cells, PGE2 becomes pro-fibrotic via signaling through EP1, which activates the PI3K pathway. The reader may remember the role of EP2 induction by progesterone during decidualization of human endometrial fibroblasts (Frank et al. 1994, Stadtmauer and Wagner 2021).

The summary above is more detailed than would be expected in a monograph on a more general topic, but this detail is necessary for the reader to appreciate the relationship to the molecular pathways of decidualization.

INTERLUDE 2: RESOLUTION OF INFLAMMATION

Another concept with a central role in understanding the evolution of mammalian implantation is inflammation, which arises as a natural consequence of nidatory injury. A logical consequence of this process is that the extension of pregnancy requires the resolution of nidatory inflammation. To contextualize the question of how this resolution has evolved, we want to have a look at how inflammation is resolved in wound healing and infection.

For a long time, it was thought that the resolution of inflammation was a passive consequence of the removal of the inflammatory stimulus, i.e., infection or other irritants. However, it turned out that the resolution of inflammation is an active process, directly triggered by, and mechanistically connected to, the initiation of inflammation (Serhan and Savill 2005). Under favorable conditions, inflammation is an actively self-limiting process. But what are the pathways through which inflammation is resolved? Below, we will mostly follow the review by Sugimoto and colleagues (Sugimoto et al. 2016).

A key event in the initiation of inflammation is the recruitment of neutrophils to the place of infection or injury. As a consequence, one of the main variables affected by the pro-resolution mechanisms is the recruitment and survival of leukocytes, in particular neutrophils. This can be achieved by decreasing the availability of signals for leukocyte recruitment and survival. An additional dimension is the clearance of apoptotic cells by macrophages. The latter process triggers the transformation of the macrophages from a pro-inflammatory phenotype, called M1, to an anti-inflammatory phenotype, called M2. M2 macrophages secrete IL10, TGFb1, and express arginase 1. The expression of arginase 1 is particularly interesting as it converts arginine into ornithine and is thus at the beginning of the polyamine synthesis pathway. One product of this pathway is spermine, which in turn can prevent the formation of the inflammasome and has other anti-inflammatory and antifibrotic effects (Chia et al. 2022, Gao et al. 2024).

A particularly interesting mechanism that illustrates the self-limiting nature of inflammation is the shifting role of NFkB. NFkB is a family of transcription factor complexes consisting of pairwise combinations of five proteins: p50, p52, p65, cRel, and RelB. The main driver of pro-inflammatory gene expression is p50::p65[8]. In contrast, other dimers have pro-resolution activities. For instance, p50 has no transactivation domain, and p50::p50 homodimers compete with p50::p65 for binding to cis-regulatory elements and thus act as antagonists of p50::p65-induced pro-inflammatory gene transcription. Heterodimers with cRel, such as p50::cRel and p65::cRel, are involved in inducing genes related to the resolution of inflammation. Interestingly, cRel expression is induced by p50::p65, providing a direct link between initiation of inflammation and its eventual resolution (Figure 6.4).

Surprisingly, the most inflammatory cell type, neutrophils, is also involved in the resolution of inflammation. Secretions produced by neutrophils not only attack infectious agents (bacteria, fungi, etc.) but also degrade cytokines involved in recruiting more neutrophils. Already mentioned

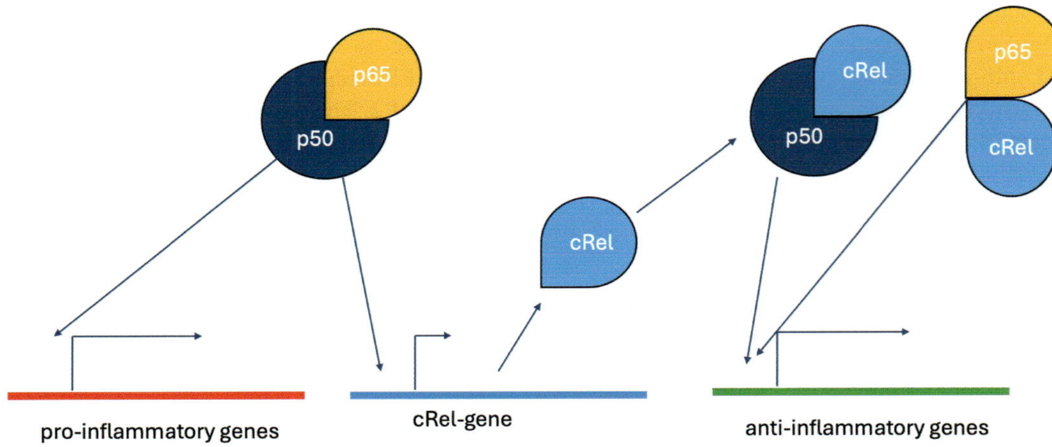

FIGURE 6.4 Example of how mechanisms of inflammation can be self-limiting: the transcription factors p50 and p65 are part of the NFkB pathway, where the p50::p656 heterodimer induces the expression of pro-inflammatory genes. In addition, the expression of cRel is induced, which can disrupt the p50::p656 heterodimers, leading to the formation of p50::cRel and p65::cRel heterodimer transcription factor complexes. These induce the expression of anti-inflammatory signals. (Figure composed by GPW, CC BY-NC.)

is the conversion of M1 pro-inflammatory macrophages to M2 anti-inflammatory macrophages. This conversion is in part driven by the efferocytosis of apoptotic immune cells, i.e., the ingestion of dead cells as they arise during the inflammatory and immune reaction. M2 macrophages repress the expression of IL6 and promote the expression of IL10 and TGFb1 and are thus anti-inflammatory. In addition, the reprogramming of macrophages is guided by PGE2, produced by both the macrophages themselves and fibroblasts. PGE2 induces the expression of M2 marker genes such as Arginase1, LIGHT, and SPHSK1, as well as being implicated in wound healing.

PHYLOGENETIC CONTEXT

Now we want to reflect upon an evolutionary scenario based on the background of facts and assumptions outlined above, as well as in previous chapters, and explore what implications these have for understanding the structure of the gene regulatory network, supporting decidualization.

As discussed in Chapter 5, decidual cells only exist in eutherian species. In these, decidual cells differentiate from endometrial stromal fibroblasts as well as from pericytes. However, the endometrium, or rather more precisely, the mucosa of the Müllerian duct, exists also in all other amniotes, if not all tetrapods, and hence there are endometrial fibroblasts even in animals that are primarily non-deciduate or even oviparous. The most informative non-deciduate outgroup of eutherians are the marsupials. In fact, there is no doubt that the marsupial ESF and those of eutherians are homologous (Kin et al. 2014, Erkenbrack et al. 2018). Nevertheless, marsupial ESF differ from eutherian ESF by their inability to differentiate into decidual cells. For that reason, it is helpful to call the ESF in marsupials, as well as those of other primarily[9] non-deciduate animals, as "paleo-ESF" and those of eutherians as "neo-ESF." Since there is agreement that DSC evolved in the stem lineage of eutherians, it follows that neo-ESF are also an apomorphy (shared derived character) of eutherians (Figure 6.5). However, it is not clear whether neo-ESF of all eutherians share the ability to differentiate into DSC. For instance, it is unclear whether the ESF of the pig endometrium has a cryptic capability to differentiate into DSC homologs. Phylogenetically, ESF of the pig and those of other non-deciduate eutherians are neo-ESF by descent but may fundamentally differ from other neo-ESF because they normally do not differentiate into decidual cells. An interesting experimental approach to test the deciduogenic potential of these cells is to investigate whether a deciduoma can be induced in these

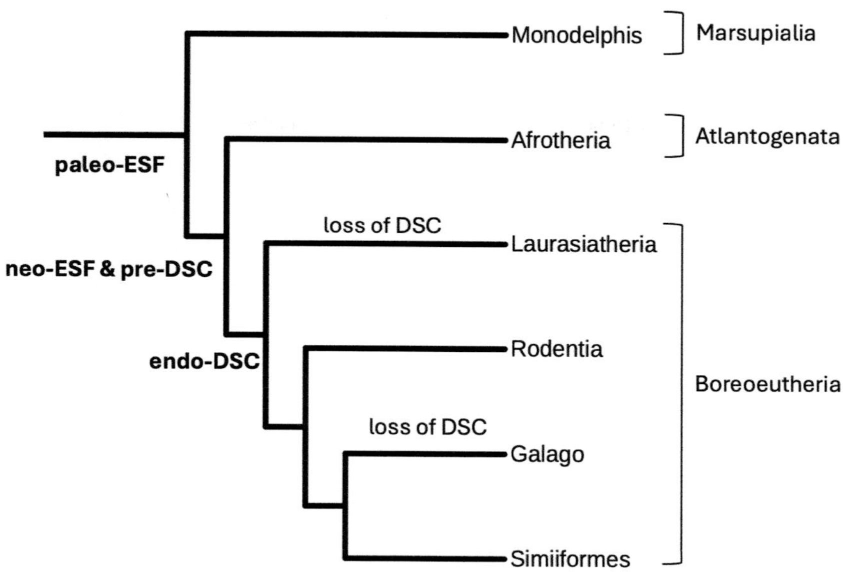

FIGURE 6.5 Scenario for the origin and secondary loss of decidual cells in therian mammals. Endometrial stromal fibroblasts (ESF) exist in all therian mammals. In marsupials, these cells can not differentiate into decidual stromal cells (DSC) and are thus called paleo-ESF. In the stem lineage of eutherian mammals, the ESF acquire the ability to differentiate into DSC and are then called neo-ESF. The first kind of DSC evolving is called predecidual cells, pre-DSC, because of the similarity with predecidual cells from the human menstrual cycle. These cells are the only ones expected in the Atlantogenata, such as afrotherians. In the stem lineage of Boreoeutheria, a second kind of DSC evolved with endocrine secretions, thus called endo-DSC. In the Laurentiatheria, some lineages lose DSC in the context of evolving a non-invasive placentation. (Figure composed by GPW, CC BY-NC.)

animals, i.e., decidual capability can be elicited experimentally through a minor injury or irritation of the luminal epithelium during the secretory phase of the ovarian cycle, even though they do not differentiate during normal pregnancy.

From the above considerations, a key source of information is the comparison of marsupial paleo-ESF and eutherian neo-ESF. Among marsupials, the species from basally branching lineages are likely most informative, since these have retained more ancestral features in their reproductive biology (Freyer et al. 2003). These are opossums, dunnarts, and others. Of course, there is no guarantee that the cells from these animals faithfully represent the biology of the ESF that was present at the ancestral therian node, i.e., are ancestral to the eutherian neo-ESF. The question is whether the biology of the endometrium has undergone relevant independent (marsupial-specific) changes that would render them misleading as an outgroup model. However, the important issue here is that paleo-ESFs do not have the gene regulatory network that allows neo-ESFs to differentiate. In other words, we want to know what neo-ESF has that is necessary for DSC differentiation, which, at the same time, is absent in paleo-ESF. Formulated that way, it is unlikely that any marsupial-specific evolutionary changes would mislead the investigation.

A bigger issue is the question of which eutherian species are most informative to understand the origin of the DSC. Not only are there species with non-invasive placenta, which clearly are not similar to the initial stages of the evolution of eutherian fetal-maternal interface, but there are other derived physiologies to consider even in species with invasive placenta. Most notable is the fact that Catarrhini menstruate, a condition only represented in a minority of about 4 to 5% of eutherian species, as far as we can tell (Critchley et al. 2020). That makes research on human ESF/DSC problematic. This is unfortunate in the light of a great number of resources existing for research on human ESF. The alternative is mouse, which is non-menstruating with an invasive placenta, or an even better alternative would be the cells from basally branching lineages that retained many primitive features but also have decidual cells. Among them, an interesting group is the tenrecs, which belong to the Afrotheria, and have a number of primitive features, like a cloaca (Riedelsheimer et al. 2007) and a blastula rather than a blastocyst (Nicoll and Racey 1985), and a seemingly primitive inventory of decidual cells (Stadtmauer et al. 2025).

There are several obvious methods to approach this goal, such as comparative studies of transcriptomes, but to our knowledge, there is no broadly accepted paradigm of how to do that, which also affects the aim of this chapter. For this reason, we want to systematically review what is known about the decidual cell and how this knowledge can be assembled toward a deeper understanding of the specific molecular features and mechanisms of the decidual cells. Doing so may suggest a research strategy that might be transferable to other cell types as well. In order to aid in disentangling the ancestral and derived features of decidual cells, we want to approach the problem by discussing molecular and cell biological constraints and opportunities for the evolution of these structures. As discussed above, the functional/cell biological context is the fact that embryo attachment involves a nidatory injury to the uterine endometrium and thus needs to be thought of as *occurring in the context of nidatory inflammation and fibroblast activation.*

DECIDUAL STROMAL CELLS PLAY AN IMMUNE-MODULATORY ROLE

The functional role of decidual cells, in particular in humans, is complex; not surprisingly, given their more than 65 million-year history since their origin. Hence, controversies about the functional role of decidual cells are frequent. However, here the question is rather specific. According to our starting assumptions ("Axiom 2"), the original and thus presumably most fundamental role of decidual cells is the regulation of the inflammatory and immune environment. But what is the evidence that decidual cells play such a role, and how are they doing it?

According to the reproductive immunology literature, the immune regulatory role of decidua is based on regulating effector cell types of the immune system, in particular macrophages and regulatory T cells (Treg). As mentioned above, the decidua is home to a specialized population of macrophages, so-called decidual macrophages, dMph. These cells are related to the anti-inflammatory kind of macrophages, generally called M2 macrophages. It has been shown that conditioned media of cultured decidual cells can induce the M2 phenotype (Lindau et al. 2021). This implies that decidual cells secrete some molecules that induce the M1 to M2 transition. A partial analysis of the DSC secretome identified CSF1 (colony-stimulating factor 1) as at least partially responsible for this effect. CSF1 is able to overcome the pro-inflammatory effect of CSF2 (Lindau et al. 2021). Another study has shown that conditioned media from DSC are able to block the differentiation of naïve T cells into Th17 cells (Chavan et al. 2021). The latter play a major role in the recruitment of neutrophils via the secretion of IL17 and thus are key players in the inflammatory reaction. Naïve T cells can be induced to become Th17 cells by IL6, IL23, and TGFb1, and this effect can be suppressed by DSC conditioned media. Which molecule mediates this effect is not known.

The other important role of DSC is related to their ability to induce the differentiation of regulatory T cells (Treg) (Lindau et al. 2021), which are known as negative regulators of an over-reacting adaptive immune system. This shows that DSC also has a role in regulating the adaptive immune system, not only during the initial nidatory inflammation. The evolutionary history of regulatory T cells in the placental bed is particularly interesting. In eutherian mammals, there are two types of Treg cells: those developing in the thymus (tTreg) and those induced in the periphery (i.e., not in the thymus, pTreg). The differentiation of pTreg is controlled by a cis-regulatory element called CNS1 (conserved non-coding sequence 1) and is responsive to TGFb1 signaling via SMAD3 and retinoic acid (RA) signaling via RXR nuclear receptor. CNS1 only exists in eutherian mammals, and not in marsupials or say zebra fish (Samstein et al. 2012)[10]. The CNS1 and supposedly pTreg cell type evolved coincidentally with the evolution of invasive placentation, and their role in modulating the immune response at the fetal-maternal interface was likely the driving force for their origin. Lindau and colleagues (2021) have shown that conditioned media from DSC induce pTreg differentiation and DSC express two of the key signals important for pTreg development: TGFb1 and RA (retinoic acid), although other cell types in the decidua are also contributing RA. In fact, decidual macrophages produce the largest amount of RA in the decidua (Rajakumar et al. 2020) and thus seem to cooperate with DSC and other cell types in inducing pTregs at the fetal-maternal interface.

Overall, it is clear that DSC participate in the local moderation of innate immunity (inducing M2 phenotype, suppressing Th17 differentiation) as well as the adaptive immune response (pTreg differentiation), at least in human and mouse. What is noteworthy, with respect to the activated fibroblast origin of DSC, is that, in the case of Treg differentiation, one part of the mediating signals is closely related to fibroblast activation, namely TGFb1, and retinoic acid-producing enzyme ALDH1A3 is highly expressed in late gestation opossum ESF (Stadtmauer unpublished). Hence, the evolution of pTreg differentiation likely occurred in an environment in which the relevant ligands were already expressed, and the new cell type arose by evolving a response to a pre-existing ligand environment. This seems to be a frequent pattern involved in the origin of evolutionary innovations, where inducing ligands are older than the induced novel character (and may have other causes of expression), the novel character evolving via the evolution of receptors for these ligands and downstream signal transduction (Wagner 2014), a fact that was also mentioned in the case of reproductive biology by Paul Medawar (Medawar 1953).

DECIDUAL CELLS ARE DERIVED FROM ACTIVATED ENDOMETRIAL FIBROBLASTS

The evolutionary inference starts with the assumption that decidua evolved at the root (=stem lineage) of eutherian mammals as a device to support extended gestation via suppression or modification of the nidatory inflammation ("Axiom 2"). It is thus plausible that the first evolutionary steps in the evolution of eutherian implantation were the cooption of genes that resolve nidatory inflammation, since inflammation is incompatible with sustained pregnancy, at least in humans and likely for eutherian mammals in general. Accordingly, these changes in the ESF should have happened in the context of fibroblast activation ("Corollary 1.1"), a natural consequence of breaching the epithelial barrier of the endometrium or any violation of tissue integrity. The core of the decidual gene regulatory network should be derived from (= homologous to) that which, in other fibroblasts, controls fibroblast activation. What is the evidence for this proposal?

To reach the perspective of fibroblast activation as the starting point for the evolution of decidual cells, a single-cell study of human decidual cell differentiation was very helpful (Stadtmauer and Wagner 2021). When a population of cells is exposed to decidualizing stimuli for a few days, cells will be found in different stages of differentiation. Not every cell is instantaneously transforming into a decidual cell. There is a large measure of stochasticity in the time course of cellular differentiation. Due to this stochasticity, and the large number of individual cells analyzed in an SC study, a "snapshot" of the population can provide information about different stages of decidualization, recapitulating an entire trajectory of cell differentiation (Figure 6.6).

Some cells will remain at an undifferentiated proliferative state, some will be in transit, and others will have fully differentiated. This fact can be used to infer the direction of gene expression change during decidual cell differentiation ("RNA velocity inference"; Figure 6.6A). Using this approach, it was discovered that proliferative cells undergo a transformation toward a cell state that has the hallmark of an activated fibroblast (aESF), namely the expression of smooth muscle actin (Figure 6.6B). From there, the differentiation bifurcates to a small population of senescent cells (snESF) and, along another trajectory, toward cells that express markers of mature decidual cells, such as prolactin (PRL). This bifurcation was also found in an independent SC study from the Jan Brosens laboratory at the University of Warwick Medical School (Lucas et al. 2020). The transition

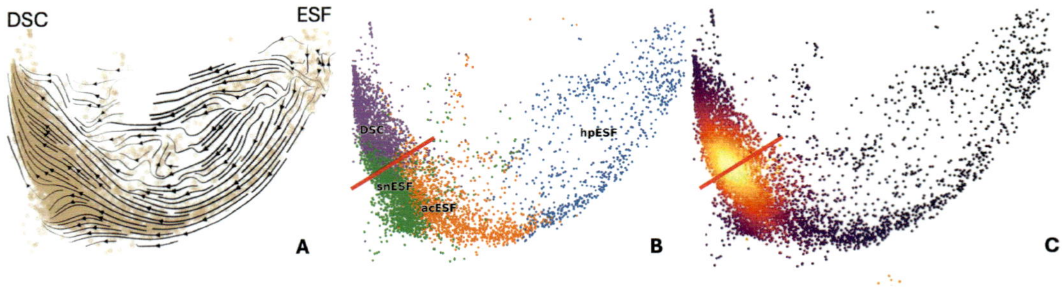

FIGURE 6.6 Single cell analysis of *in vitro* decidualization: (A) vector field that shows the direction of transformation of ESF into DSC under the influence of progesterone and prostaglandin E2. (B) Cell clusters were identified among the transcriptomes of single cells. To the right are proliferative endometrial stromal fibroblasts, hpESF, which are transformed into a population that resembles activated fibroblasts, acESF. The remaining two clusters consist of senescent cells, snESF, and mature decidual cells, DSC. (C) Heat map that indicates the transcriptome complexity of the cells. Note the peak of transcriptome complexity at the transition toward mature DSC, which is an indication of a differentiation event. (Images from Stadtmauer and Wagner (2021) reproduced with permission.)

from what looks like activated fibroblasts toward mature DSC is marked by a point of increased "intrinsic dimensionality" (Figure 6.6C), that is, a transient peak in the number of different genes expressed, which can be taken as a signature of cell type differentiation,[11] i.e., a transition between two stable regimes of gene expression. From this data, the scenario arises that, during decidualization, endometrial fibroblasts first enter a phase that resembles fibroblast activation, and only the activated fibroblast commits to the decidual cell identity or undergoes senescence:

ESF → aESF→ DSC + snESF

The natural question is this: is this pattern an artifact of *in vitro* decidualization, where the ESF are treated in the absence of other cells that could have an influence on their differentiation trajectory? *In vivo* data have been supplied by several single-cell studies of the human fetal-maternal interface. The most accessible data is from the first trimester of human pregnancy by Vento-Tormo and colleagues (Vento-Tormo et al. 2018). In this study, the authors identified three endometrial stromal cell populations in the pregnant decidua called by the authors, dS1, dS2, and dS3 (Figure 6.7A). dS1 and dS2 are poorly differentiated with respect to each other and likely represent "pre-decidualized" cell states. dS3 are by all likelihood mature decidual cells, as indicated by their expression of PRL (dS3 = DSC; Figure 6.7B). The transition from the dS1/2 cluster to dS3 is marked by an abrupt loss of *ACTA2* (SMA) expression (Figure 6.7C), consistent with the pattern seen in the *in vitro* single cell study outlined above. This pattern is consistent with a scenario where, also *in vivo*, mature decidual cells differentiate from cells that carry the hallmark of activated fibroblasts.

The idea that decidualization is a two-step process with an SMA expressing intermediary can also be found in the older literature. For instance, Kim, Jaffe, and Fazleabas, reviewing their work on baboon decidualization, proposed such a scenario (Kim et al. 1999). The ESF first undergo a transformation to a SMA expression cell that they call pre-decidualized[12] and only then differentiate into mature decidual cells under the influence of signals from the embryo. In their work, IGFBP1 was used as a marker for mature decidual cells. They emphasized that SMA and IGFBP1 expression are exclusive, i.e., do not, or only briefly, occur in the same cell. They also cite preliminary experimental evidence that these two states are mechanistically incompatible.

From the evolutionary perspective, the SMA-expressing state identified by Kim et al., Stadtmauer and Wagner, as well as Vento Tormo et al. is likely homologous to the activated endometrial fibroblasts induced by the nidatory injury, although the experimental literature does not spell this out explicitly. A recent paper on mouse implantation and decidualization goes a step further by investigating additional markers of fibroblast activation (Chen et al. 2023). From the pathology literature,

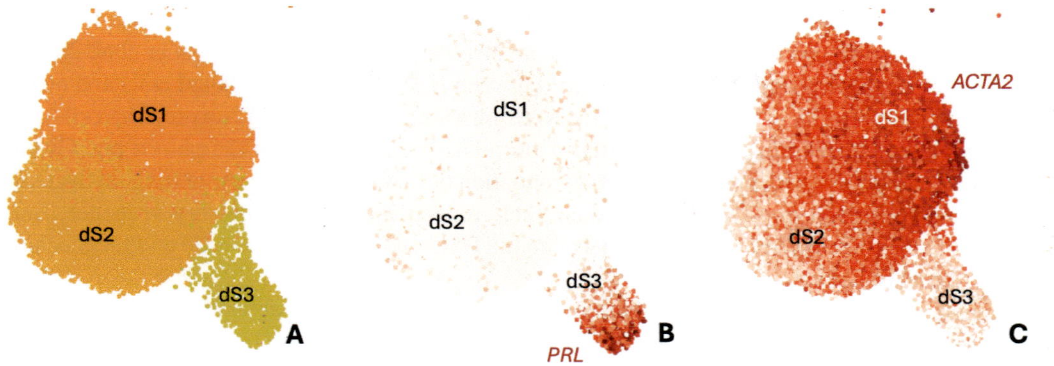

FIGURE 6.7 Single-cell transcriptomic analysis of human fetal-maternal interface by Vento-Tormo and collaborators (2018). The three clusters of endometrial fibroblasts identified in mid-gestational endometrium are dS1, dS2, and dS3. (B) Expression of prolactin (PRL) identifies dS3 as the mature DSC. (C) Expression of smooth muscle actin (ACTA2) identifies dS1 and dS2 as similar to the activated fibroblasts that were found during *in vitro* differentiation (see Figure 6.6B). This data shows that expression of ACTA2 and PRL is locally exclusive and thus reflects distinct cell states, namely activated ESF and mature DSC. (Images generated from the Reproductive Cell Atlas provided under CC BY-NC-ND 4.0 license; https://www.reproductivecellatlas.org/ and annotated by GPW.)

they identified eight markers of fibroblast activation: smooth muscle actin (SMA, *ACTA2*), fibroblast activation protein (FAP), S100A4 (=FSP1, ferroptosis suppressing protein 1), tenascin C (TNC), Vimentin[13] (Vim), Desmin (DES), Periostin (POSTN), and SPARC (Secreted Protein Acidic and Cysteine Rich) (Kuzet and Gaggioli 2016). The authors find, during the implantation phase of day 4 to day 6 after copulation, a transient stromal expression of SMAa, TNC, S100A4, and SPARC, and interpret this as evidence that endometrial fibroblasts undergo a process similar to fibroblast activation. They also document the expression of *ACTIVIN* A, which can induce expression of decidual genes *BMP2, WNT4,* and *Prl8A2*. They also provide evidence for the involvement of prostacyclin (PGI_2) and the nuclear receptor PPARD in these developments, proposing a mechanistic model that needs further testing.

The data summarized above about the differentiation of human, baboon, and mouse decidual cells is essentially a recapitulatory argument, i.e., claiming that the order of events in development (first fibroblast activation, then differentiation of decidual cells) indicates the order of events during evolution. There is a broad consensus that such a developmental-phylogenetic parallelism is not generally true (Nelson 1978, Olsson et al. 2017). However, it is also clear that there are certain circumstances in which developmental-phylogenetic parallelism can be expected and has evidential force. The paradigm for a justified developmental-phylogenetic parallelism is Richard Prum's model for the evolution of feathers in theropod dinosaurs (Prum 1999). If a developmental stage is causally necessary for a subsequent developmental stage, the inference is justified that, in evolution, the sequence of evolutionary innovations had to follow the same order as in development. For instance, the development of an epidermal tube is necessary before feather branches (rami) can develop by slicing the epidermal tube into individual feather structures (for details see Prum 1999 and Prum and Brush 2002).

In the case of decidual cell differentiation, the dependency of decidualization upon prior fibroblast activation is less obvious than in the case of feather development, and to our knowledge, this idea was never rigorously tested. We thus have to ask how well-founded is our assumption that an activated fibroblast state is a necessary precursor of decidual cell differentiation. Short of a detailed mechanistic understanding of decidual cell differentiation, we have to rely on comparative evidence of conservation. A useful data point in that respect is evidence from the most distantly related eutherian mammals (relative to human or any other boreoeutherian mammal) for which we have molecular single-cell data, the *Tenrec ecaudatus*, an afrotherian mammal (Stadtmauer et al. 2025). For *Tenrec,* it has been found that the difference between *IL15*-expressing decidual cells and other endometrial stromal cells is lower *ACTA2* (SMA) expression, and that *ACTA2*-expressing cells are precursors of *IL15*-expressing cells. A similar pattern has been observed in the guinea pig. Given the limited comparative data available, the differentiation of DSC from SMA-expressing (activated) ESC appears conserved in eutherians and thus likely reflects a causally necessary sequence. But how about a more mechanistic connection between the DSC differentiation cascade and the mechanisms of fibroblast activation?

As mentioned above, TGFb1 is considered a key signal for fibroblast activation, secreted from injured epithelia and inducing autocrine TGFb1 expression in fibroblasts. In the human endometrium, progesterone can induce the expression of TGFb1 in luminal epithelial cells (Kim et al. 2005) and induce endometrial stromal fibroblasts to express TGFb1 (Arici et al. 1996) as well as PRL, as a sign of decidualization. These studies were done with human cells, where some degree of predecidualization is induced by progesterone without the embryo. Hence, the progesterone-dependent release of TGFb1 by the luminal epithelial cells could be a mechanism to induce embryo-independent (spontaneous) decidualization, while any epithelial injury is the generic trigger, caused, for instance, by nidatory injury. This evidence, replicated by Longjun Wu in our laboratories, suggests an identical TGFb1 circuity exists in decidualization as implicated in fibroblast activation.

Another member of the TGF family of signaling molecules is Activin A. There is a moderate literature implicating Activin A in fibroblast activation (Aoki et al. 2005, Loomans and Andl 2014, Samain and Sanz-Moreno 2020, Tsai et al. 2024). A pro-decidual effect of Activin A on endometrial fibroblasts has been reported by Jones and collaborators (Jones et al. 2002a, Jones et al. 2002b), establishing an autocrine loop similar to what has been reported for TGFb1 (see previous paragraph). Similar effects were reported for mouse stromal cells (Chen et al. 2023).

As reviewed above, an important factor downstream of TGFb1 in fibroblast activation is IL11 (see above section on fibroblast activation), forming yet another autocrine feedback loop. IL11 has been found in mouse implantation to be expressed by stromal cells during the initiation of decidualization, and a KO of the IL11 receptor alpha chain, IL-11Ra, leads to infertility due to defective decidualization (Robb et al. 1998). In human endometrial stromal cells, IL11 is also transiently expressed during decidualization (Dimitriadis et al. 2000), and inhibition of IL11 signaling affects human ESF decidualization (Dimitriadis et al. 2005, Karpovich et al. 2005). Finally, we mentioned the role of NADPH oxidase 4, NOX4, in enhancing the TGFb1 signal in the activation of fibroblasts. A similar role has been documented for NOX4 in human decidual cell differentiation (Al-Sabbagh et al. 2011), although it is not clear whether the effect in decidual cells plays the same role as in activated fibroblasts.

So far, so good. The difficulty with affinities between decidualization and fibroblast activation is to assess how strong the evidence is that these similarities provide. Is this apparent affinity solely due to cherry picking, or does it reflect a deeper biological connection? One temptation is to consider this question from a straightforward statistical point of view, similar to the enrichment statistics used in functional genomics, where the frequency of genes belonging to a gene ontology category is compared with the total number of genes of the same gene ontology category in the genome. Hence, enrichment is treated as an "urn experiment," where we ask how likely it is to randomly draw a "black" ball out of an urn of "black" and "red" balls. However, the collection of genes expressed in a cell is not a collection of independent random events. Genes are interconnected in various ways through the gene regulatory network active in the cell, which makes the choice of an appropriate statistical null model difficult. We think, however, that the question of whether the facts discussed above are telling a biologically meaningful story is not a statistical issue at all, but one of phylogenetic inference.[14] The question rather is this: can we test the hypothesis that early stages of decidualization are homologous to the generic forms of fibroblast activation as seen in fibroblasts in other tissues? To address this question, we need information about the cell biology of endometrial stromal cells from a sample of mammalian species, and also the cell biology of fibroblast activation in different other tissues, and ask whether a model assuming historical continuity is better supported than one where the patterns of gene expression arose independently. Needless to say, our current knowledge base in comparative reproductive biology is inadequate to answer this question, but given current technologies, not impossible to attain. Despite these limitations, the evidence that in early stages of decidual stromal cell differentiation resemble and probably are homologous to fibroblast activation is as strong as it can be, given the limited number of species investigated.

INTERLUDE 3: THE CONTRIBUTIONS OF FIBROBLASTS TO THE RESOLUTION OF INFLAMMATION

In generic wound healing processes, fibroblasts have been found to contribute to the resolution of inflammation through several pathways (Le Blanc and Mougiakakos 2012). The two main ones are promoting the M1 to M2 transition and reducing the cytotoxicity of natural killer cells (NK). During the acute inflammatory phase, fibroblasts are exposed to a large number of pro-inflammatory signals. For their role in the resolution of inflammation, the most consequential pro-inflammatory signals are TNF and IFNG. TNF is expressed by activated M1 macrophages, and both TNF and IFNG are secreted by NK cells as well as inflammatory T cells (Th1). It is said that these two signals "license" the fibroblasts to start expressing anti-inflammatory mediators. According to Le Blanc and Mougiakakos (2012), the main ones are two small molecules, PGE2 (as well as other prostaglandins like PGD and PGI2) and kynurenine, KYN. PGE2, which we have encountered multiple times above and here, acts through its EP2 and EP4 receptors on the macrophages to support transition to the M2 phenotype. Kynurenine is a breakdown product of the amino acid tryptophan produced by the enzyme IDO (Indolamine-pyrrole 2,3-dioxygenase) and acts through the AHR (Aryl-Hydrocarbon Receptor) in macrophages to enhance the expression of TGFb1 and IL10 and other anti-inflammatory mediators (Figure 6.8). IL10 then inhibits the further recruitment of neutrophils. TGFb1 inhibits the recruitment of lymphocytes. PGE2, KYN, and TGFB1 are also responsible for decreasing the cytotoxicity of NK cells.

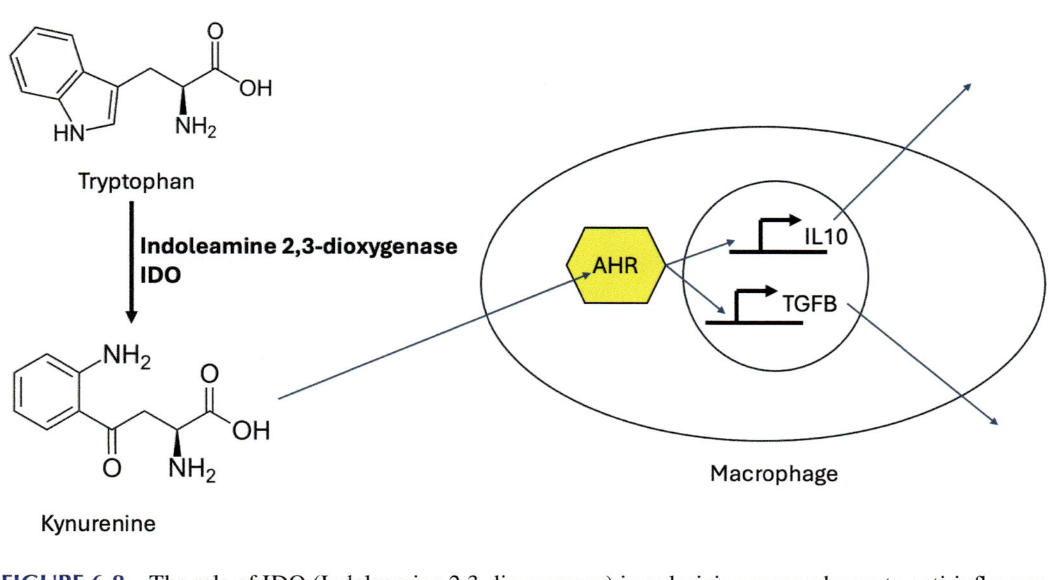

FIGURE 6.8 The role of IDO (Indoleamine 2,3-dioxygenase) in polarizing macrophages to anti-inflammatory role. IDO converts the amino acid tryptophan into kynurenine, and kynurenine attaches to the arylhydrocarbon receptor, AHR, which is a nuclear receptor that activates the expression of anti-inflammatory genes such as IL10 and TGFB1. (Image created by GPW, CC BY-NC.)

There are at least two other anti-inflammatory signals that "license" fibroblasts. One is TSG6 (TNF stimulated gene 6), which inhibits the TLR2-NFkB pathway in macrophages and thus their pro-inflammatory activation. The other is IL1Ra (IL1 receptor antagonist), which antagonizes the release of TNF from macrophages caused by IL1 stimulation. Given that fibroblasts contribute to the resolution of inflammation in normal wound healing, it seems plausible that the anti-inflammatory role of the decidual cells is derived from that generic activity. Now we want to put the pieces together to the extent we can, given what is known.

THE UNFINISHED STORY: FROM FIBROBLAST ACTIVATION TO DECIDUALIZATION

In the previous sections, we made the case that decidualization is developmentally secondary to activation of endometrial fibroblasts, because decidual cells evolved from fibroblasts that are activated due to the nidatory injury. Of course, decidual cells are more than just activated endometrial fibroblasts. The components of the fibroblast activation network have been identified in endometrial stromal cells, such as TGFb1, IL11, and Activin A, because of their effect on the expression of decidual effector genes such as IGFBP1 and PRL. This indicates that at least these effector genes are downstream of the putative fibroblast activation regulators. This is good, but it does not yet give us all the answers we need to understand the evolution of decidualization.

In contrast to the generic wound healing response, implantation does not lead to wound healing, as discussed in Chapter 4 under the "tissue biological paradox." Instead, implantation leads to a permanent wound, the placental bed, which nevertheless avoids the development of a fibrotic scar and suppresses inflammation. During generic fibroblast activation, a suite of genes related to anti-fibrotic deactivation of fibroblasts are epigenetically silenced (see review Younesi et al. 2024). Among those genes are *PPARG* along with its co-activator *Pgc1a*, as well as *PTGR2* (the gene for the EP2 prostaglandin receptor) and *PTGS2* (aka COX2, the rate-limiting enzyme of prostaglandin synthesis). During decidualization, a switchover occurs, where genes related to myofibroblast activation become silenced (Nancy et al. 2018) and anti-fibrotic genes are expressed, such as *PPARG* and *PTGER2* (Wu and Wagner, unpublished). Noteworthy is the fact that in the endometrial fibroblasts of opossum *PPARG* and *PTGER2* are downregulated under the influence of decidualizing signals but upregulated in human decidual cells (Erkenbrack et al. 2018). Note also that in neo-ESF progesterone induces the expression of PTGER2 (Stadtmauer and Wagner 2021). In mice, preventing the epigenetic silencing of myofibroblast genes reverts decidual cells into cells with the hallmarks of myofibroblasts (Osokine et al. 2022).

These experimental facts suggest that, in endometrial fibroblasts, the fibroblast activation module is under the control of pregnancy signals, i.e., most likely progesterone and PKA signaling (Figure 6.9). That appears to be one of the gene regulatory key innovations in the evolution of the decidual cell: the inversion of the regulation of fibroblast activation genes by signals from the ensuing pregnancy. The switch occurs even though the primary reason for fibroblast activation persists, i.e., the nidatory injury. But instead of returning to a quiescent state, as in normal wound healing, the cells assume an alternative identity compatible with the maintenance of an open wound and their primary function, the resolution of the nidatory inflammation.

Above, we have argued that for the evolution of DSC it was necessary for pregnancy signals to gain control over the transition from a myofibroblast phenotype to a non-fibrotic phenotype, essentially by upregulating anti-fibrotic genes such as *PPARG*. However, activated fibroblasts also play an important role in the resolution of inflammation by signaling to macrophages to assume an M2 phenotype (see above). In the endometrium, the anti-inflammatory support has to continue until the end of pregnancy and cannot end with the suppression of the myofibroblast state. In fact, key anti-inflammatory signals from fibroblasts in generic wound healing are expressed in mature decidual

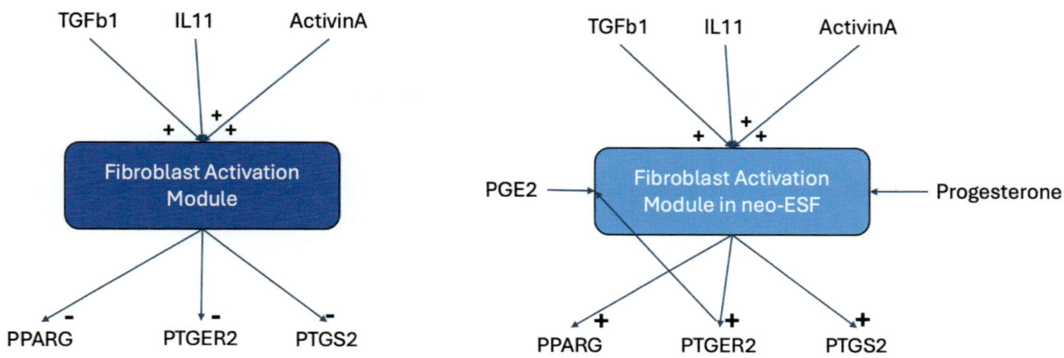

FIGURE 6.9 Comparison of two gene regulatory network modules in fibroblasts and endometrial fibroblasts. In normal tissue fibroblasts, TGFb1, IL11, and ActivinA cause a downregulation of PPARG, PTGER2, and PTGS2, while in neo-ESF, the same signals, under the additional influence of progesterone, upregulate the same genes, which in addition let PGE2 signal via the PTGER2 receptor of EP2. (Image created by GPW, CC BY-NC.)

cells from at least some species, such as IDO, a key enzyme for the production of Kynurenine, which has important anti-inflammatory effects, as well as prostaglandin E2[15].

But how, in evolution, could pregnancy signals gain control over the expression of anti-fibrotic as well as anti-inflammatory genes? A hint could come from the discovery that some transcription factors essential for the differentiation of human decidual cells have evolved their activity, such as Hoxa11 and CEBPB, in the stem lineage of eutherian mammals (Lynch et al. 2008, Lynch et al. 2011, Nnamani et al. 2016). In both cases, the transcription factor acts as a complex with FOXO1. The physical interaction between these transcription factors and FOXO1 evolved before the origin of decidual cells and thus is older and not the critical factor for the decidual cell-specific function (Brayer et al. 2011). It is also interesting that these transcription factor - FOXO1 complexes were ancestrally inhibitory. Amino acid substitutions in the stem lineage of eutherian mammals then made them activate transcription factor complexes. Could it be that the switch from inhibitory to activating transcription factor complex is responsible for the pregnancy-dependent expression of, say, PPARG and similar genes? In that case, the transcription factor complex with Hoxa11, CEBPB, and FOXO1 would be expected to be ancestrally responsible for the silencing of *PPARG* and other antifibrotic genes. Then the amino acid substitutions would directly be responsible for the derived expression of these genes in ESF and thus be critical for their expression in the context of decidual cell differentiation.

The above narrative links the re-wiring of the activated fibroblast regulation to pregnancy signals and could explain how pregnancy signals can switch the activated ESF into an alternative gene regulatory state that would eventually become the decidual cell type. What is missing here is an evolutionary and maybe adaptive reason for this evolutionary step. Above, we argued that the likely initial function of the decidual cell was to contribute to resolving the nidatory inflammation, since such an effect would have immediate benefits for the extension and maintenance of pregnancy, eventually leading to more mature neonates, should that be adaptively advantageous.

In "interlude 3" above, we summarized some of the knowledge about the anti-inflammatory role fibroblasts play in other tissues. While anti-fibrotic and anti-inflammatory pathways of fibroblasts have been investigated as independent phenomena, the question arises whether these are not two different effector arms of the same gene regulatory state of fibroblasts, i.e., the transcription factors controlling anti-fibrotic activities may also control the anti-inflammatory activities of fibroblasts. This seems plausible, since both activities play their roles in the same phase of wound healing. If this is true, the arguments made above for the control of anti-fibrotic genes by pregnancy signals may also extend to the genes responsible for the anti-inflammatory activity of endometrial fibroblasts. In other words, these genetic changes in the transcription factor activity discussed above would have directly precipitated the induction of an anti-inflammatory environment in the pregnant uterus and may thus be directly selectable if and when extension of pregnancy would convey a selective advantage. Furthermore, since the selectable effect may have been caused directly by a polarity switch of transcription factor proteins themselves (from inhibitory to activating) these changes would have also created a new transcription factor complex activity and thus fulfill the requirements for the origin of a new cell type, the evolution of a new cell type specific core regulatory complex regulating the cell type-specific effector gene expression (Arendt et al. 2016).

We are well aware that the speculative scenario outlined above can at best be a rather crude picture of the mechanistic underpinnings of the origin of DSC, if it has any resemblance to reality at all. In particular, the role of cell-cell interactions, likely critical for the decidual function and integrity, is largely ignored and will require a deeper dive into the cell communication networks of the endometrium of eutherian and non-eutherian animals. Despite these obvious shortcomings, which such a first attempt inevitably suffers from, we think that the model outlines the overall context within which any evolutionary, mechanistic narrative about the origin of decidual cells will have to show its explanatory power. We can be fairly confident that the starting point for an evolutionary explanation of DSC origins has to be the activated endometrial stromal cell. The physiological objective of the evolutionary process will have to be the control of anti-inflammatory and anti-fibrotic activities by physiological signals indicating an ensuing pregnancy (progesterone, PGE2/PGI2/PGD2 and others). How exactly this is achieved by modifying the gene regulatory network of activated endometrial fibroblasts is the open question. The above scenario, based on changes in transcription factor proteins, attempts to integrate, in this general framework, what is known about the evolution of transcription factors essential for human decidualization. But given how little we know about these evolutionary changes at the cellular level, this is at best an encouragement to find a more complete answer than being the definite answer itself.

CIRCLING BACK TO THE PARADOXA OF EUTHERIAN PREGNANCY

How, then, is the scenario outlined in this chapter related to the evolutionary paradoxa of the evolution of eutherian embryo implantation, as outlined in Chapter 4? All the paradoxa, from the cell-biological to the immunological paradoxon are related to the reactions of a mucosal tissue to irritation and injury. Loss or modification of epithelial polarity necessary for embryo attachment is most likely due to the inflammatory reaction of the uterine epithelium to irritants secreted by the embryo. The inflammation paradoxon is a consequence of the epithelial injury caused by embryo implantation. The tissue biological paradoxon is related to the initiation of the wound healing process, ultimately caused by the nidatory injury by the embryo, and the immunological paradoxon is due to the juxtaposition of genetically heterogeneous tissues as a consequence of implantation. Hence, the central biological issues in the evolution of eutherian embryo implantation are all related to the consequences of the nidatory injury caused by the allogeneic embryo, and the way the maternal organism is able to accommodate these consequences. It is thus plausible that this maternal accommodation of implantation is realized by the evolutionary changes in the maternal cells engaged at the site of the nidatory injury, that is, the cells of the mucosal stroma (endometrial fibroblasts) and the tissue resident cells of the innate immune system. In the scenario outlined here, the focus was on the evolutionary transformation of the mucosal fibroblasts, leading to the origin of the decidual cell type (or cell type family, as suggested by recent comparative single-cell data showing potentially multiple decidual cell types). The main objective for such a scenario is to explain how the processes of inflammation and wound healing were modified by changing the behavior of the maternal cells engaged in the wounding response. In that way, the biological paradoxa identified in chapter 5 define the agenda for a research program explaining the mechanistic underpinnings of the evolution of eutherian pregnancy. Hence, it is clear that even a complete model for the origin of the decidual cells is only partial, as we also need to understand the evolution of the immune cells in decidua, such as uterine macrophages, natural killer cells, and regulatory T cells, to provide a deeper understanding of eutherian embryo implantation.

NOTES

1. In principle, these questions also apply to cell type evolution in other multicellular clades such as plants, fungi, and various algae, but we are not certain that the cell biological considerations we will discuss here are transferable to other multicellular organisms. The skepticism is justified by the fact that multicellularity evolved several times independently and may be based on different kinds of cell biology. At least for plant cells, there is a strong case for expecting other features than in animals because of the immobility of plant cells, encased in a cell wall, and outfitted with extensive cytoplasmatic bridges between neighboring cells, a feature unusual in animals.
2. More charitably, these experimental strategies are called knock-down or knock-out experiments when done with genetic methods, or extirpation and transplantation experiments if done with surgical methods.
3. We are not aware of a formal test of this idea, but it is certainly the impression one gets when scanning the experimental literature on any cell type.
4. That applies not only to cell types but also to multicellular organs. For instance, a compilation of "feather" genes (Lowe, C. B., J. A. Clarke, A. J. Baker, D. Haussler and S. V. Edwards (2015). "Feather development genes and associated regulatory innovation predate the origin of Dinosauria." *Mol Biol Evol* **32**(1): 23–28.) turned out to include mostly genes involved in placodes and epidermal scales as well.
5. This is true for most mammals, with the possible exception of the standard rodents (e.g., not the spiny mouse), which have an abbreviated (non-pregnant) ovarian cycle with essentially no luteal phase.
6. Opossums and possums are different kinds of animals, even though the US vernacular sometimes calls opossums "possums." A deputy provost at Yale once joked that opossums are Irish possums: i.e., an O'Possum.
7. This role of NOX4 seems like a wrinkle not worth mentioning in a high-level summary of fibroblast activation, would it not also play a role in decidual cell differentiation.
8. This notation follows one that is used in parts of molecular biology, where X::Y means that X is physically but not covalently attached to Y.
9. "Primarily non-deciduate" means species that are non-deciduate and all their ancestors were non-deciduate. That term excludes non-deciduate eutherians, since decidual cells where present in the most recent common ancestor of eutherians.
10. CNS1 is derived from a transposable element, belonging to the MIR family, showing the importance of transposable elements in enabling evolutionary innovations.
11. The transition between two cell types is likely to represent a mixture of the transcriptomes of the two cell types, and thus, at the transition point, the number of different transcripts will be higher than before or after the transition.
12. There are several sources of the term pre-decidualized, but not all of them coincide. To sort through the various meanings of this term would be an interesting exercise.
13. The choice of Vimentin as a marker for activated fibroblasts is questionable as all mesenchymal cells express vimentin, including non-activated fibroblasts, all leukocytes, and endothelial cells.
14. Of course, phylogenetic inference can also be conceptualized as a form of statistical inference as shown by the work of Joe Felsenstein (Felsenstein, J. (1985). "Phylogenies and the Comparative Method." *American Naturalist* **125**(1): 1–15.). Here we make the difference between conventional statistical methods that most biologists are familiar with, which are based on statistically independent and identically distributed events, while phylogenetic methods that aim at identifying the most likely historical sequence of events are based on a given phylogenetic framework.
15. Whether IDO expression by DSC is due to cell-autonomous regulation or induced by paracrine signals from other cells is unclear. *In vitro* decidualized human ESF do not express IDO. A possible mechanism inducing IDO expression in the decidual tissue could be IFNG signaling from decidual NK cells, since IDO is a target gene of IFNG and IFNG is expressed in the mouse decidua by NK cells. Hence, some of the genes expressed by DSC could be due to stimulation from other cells in the decidual tissue rather than due to cell-autonomous gene regulation by the DSC itself.

REFERENCES

Adler, M., A. Mayo, X. Zhou, R. A. Franklin, M. L. Meizlish, R. Medzhitov, S. M. Kallenberger and U. Alon (2020). "Principles of cell circuits for tissue repair and fibrosis." *iScience* **23**(2): 100841.

Al-Sabbagh, M., L. Fusi, J. Higham, Y. Lee, K. Lei, A. C. Hanyaloglu, E. W. Lam, M. Christian and J. J. Brosens (2011). "NADPH oxidase-derived reactive oxygen species mediate decidualization of human endometrial stromal cells in response to cyclic AMP signaling." *Endocrinology* **152**(2): 730–740.

Ang, C. J., T. D. Skokan and K. L. McKinley (2023). "Mechanisms of regeneration and fibrosis in the endometrium." *Annu Rev Cell Dev Biol* **39**: 197–221.

Aoki, F., M. Kurabayashi, Y. Hasegawa and I. Kojima (2005). "Attenuation of bleomycin-induced pulmonary fibrosis by follistatin." *Am J Respir Crit Care Med* **172**(6): 713–720.

Arendt, D. (2008). "The evolution of cell types in animals: emerging principles from molecualr studies." *Nat Rev Genet* **9**: 868–882.

Arendt, D., J. M. Musser, C. V. H. Baker, A. Bergman, C. Cepko, D. H. Erwin, M. Pavlicev, G. Schlosser, S. Widder, M. D. Laubichler and G. P. Wagner (2016). "The origin and evolution of cell types." *Nat Rev Genet* **17**(12): 744–757.

Arici, A., P. C. MacDonald and M. L. Casey (1996). "Modulation of the levels of transforming growth factor beta messenger ribonucleic acids in human endometrial stromal cells." *Biol Reprod* **54**(2): 463–469.

Basanta, S. and M. Pavlicev (2025). "The shifting role and regulation of the corpus luteum in vertebrate reproduction: a synthetic review." *Q Rev Biol* **100**(3): 189–231.

Brar, A. K., G. R. Frank, C. A. Kessler, M. I. Cedars and S. Handwerger (1997). "Progesterone-dependent decidualization of the human endometrium is mediated by cAMP." *Endocrine* **6**(3): 301–307.

Brayer, K. J., V. J. Lynch and G. P. Wagner (2011). "Evolution of a derived protein-protein interaction between HoxA11 and Foxo1a in mammals caused by changes in intramolecular regulation." *Proc Natl Acad Sci U S A* **108**(32): E414–420.

Brighton, P. J., A. R. Walker, O. Mann, C. S. Kong, E. S. Lucas, P. Vrljicak, J. J. Brosens and A. C. Hanyaloglu (2024). "Spatial-temporal regulation of the prostanoid receptor EP2 co-ordinates PGE2-mediated cAMP signaling in decidualizing human endometrium." *iScience* **27**(11): 111170.

Brosens, J. J., M. S. Salker, G. Teklenburg, J. Nautiyal, S. Salter, E. S. Lucas, J. H. Steel, M. Christian, Y. W. Chan, C. M. Boomsma, J. D. Moore, G. M. Hartshorne, S. Sucurovic, B. Mulac-Jericevic, C. J. Heijnen, S. Quenby, M. J. Koerkamp, F. C. Holstege, A. Shmygol and N. S. Macklon (2014). "Uterine selection of human embryos at implantation." *Sci Rep* **4**: 3894.

Chakraborty, D., B. Sumova, T. Mallano, C. W. Chen, A. Distler, C. Bergmann, I. Ludolph, R. E. Horch, K. Gelse, A. Ramming, O. Distler, G. Schett, L. Senolt and J. H. W. Distler (2017). "Activation of STAT3 integrates common profibrotic pathways to promote fibroblast activation and tissue fibrosis." *Nat Commun* **8**(1): 1130.

Chavan, A. R., O. W. Griffith, D. J. Stadtmauer, J. Maziarz, M. Pavlicev, R. Fishman, L. Koren, R. Romero and G. P. Wagner (2021). "Evolution of embryo implantation was enabled by the origin of decidual stromal cells in eutherian mammals." *Mol Biol Evol* **38**(3): 1060–1074.

Chen, S. T., W. W. Shi, Y. Q. Lin, Z. S. Yang, Y. Wang, M. Y. Li, Y. Li, A. X. Liu, Y. Hu and Z. M. Yang (2023). "Embryo-derive TNF promotes decidualization via fibroblast activation." *Elife* **12**:e82970.

Chia, T. Y., A. Zolp and J. Miska (2022). "Polyamine immunometabolism: central regulators of inflammation, cancer and autoimmunity." *Cells* **11**(5): 896.

Corden, B., E. Adami, M. Sweeney, S. Schafer and S. A. Cook (2020). "IL-11 in cardiac and renal fibrosis: late to the party but a central player." *Br J Pharmacol* **177**(8): 1695–1708.

Critchley, H. O. D., E. Babayev, S. E. Bulun, S. Clark, I. Garcia-Grau, P. K. Gregersen, A. Kilcoyne, J. J. Kim, M. Lavender, E. E. Marsh, K. A. Matteson, J. A. Maybin, C. N. Metz, I. Moreno, K. Silk, M. Sommer, C. Simon, R. Tariyal, H. S. Taylor, G. P. Wagner and L. G. Griffith (2020). "Menstruation: science and society." *Am J Obstet Gynecol* **223**(5): 624–664.

DiFrisco, J., A. C. Love and G. P. Wagner (2023). "The hierarchical basis of serial homology and evolutionary novelty." *J Morphol* **284**(1): e21531.

Dimitriadis, E., L. A. Salamonsen and L. Robb (2000). "Expression of interleukin-11 during the human menstrual cycle: coincidence with stromal cell decidualization and relationship to leukaemia inhibitory factor and prolactin." *Mol Hum Reprod* **6**(10): 907–914.

Dimitriadis, E., C. Stoikos, M. Baca, W. D. Fairlie, J. E. McCoubrie and L. A. Salamonsen (2005). "Relaxin and prostaglandin E(2) regulate interleukin 11 during human endometrial stromal cell decidualization." *J Clin Endocrinol Metab* **90**(6): 3458–3465.

Dudley, J. S., M. B. Renfree, G. P. Wagner and O. W. Griffith (2024). "The extension of mammalian pregnancy required taming inflammation: independent evolution of extended placentation in the tammar wallaby." *Proc Natl Acad Sci U S A* **121**(42): e2310047121.

Dunn-Fletcher, C. E., L. M. Muglia, M. Pavlicev, G. Wolf, M. A. Sun, Y. C. Hu, E. Huffman, S. Tumukuntala, K. Thiele, A. Mukherjee, S. Zoubovsky, X. Zhang, K. A. Swaggart, K. Y. B. Lamm, H. Jones, T. S. Macfarlan and L. J. Muglia (2018). "Anthropoid primate-specific retroviral element THE1B controls expression of CRH in placenta and alters gestation length." *PLoS Biol* **16**(9): e2006337.

Elliot, M. G. and B. J. Crespi (2009). "Phylogenetic evidence for early hemochorial placentation in eutheria." *Placenta* **30**(11): 949–967.

Erkenbrack, E. M., J. D. Maziarz, O. W. Griffith, C. Liang, A. R. Chavan, M. C. Nnamani and G. P. Wagner (2018). "The mammalian decidual cell evolved from a cellular stress response." *PLoS Biol* **16**(8): e2005594.

Felsenstein, J. (1985). "Phylogenies and the comparative method." *Am Nat* **125**(1): 1–15.

Frank, G. R., A. K. Brar, M. I. Cedars and S. Handwerger (1994). "Prostaglandin E2 enhances human endometrial stromal cell differentiation." *Endocrinology* **134**(1): 258–263.

Freyer, C., U. Zeller and M. B. Renfree (2003). "The marsupial placenta: a phylogenetic analysis." *J Exp Zool A Comp Exp Biol* **299A**(1): 59–77.

Gao, Y., K. Y. Liu, W. Xiao, X. Xie, Q. Liang, Z. Tu, L. Yang, H. Yu, H. Guo, S. Huang, X. Han, J. Fu and Y. Zhou (2024). "Aryl hydrocarbon receptor confers protection against macrophage pyroptosis and intestinal inflammation through regulating polyamine biosynthesis." *Theranostics* **14**(11): 4218–4239.

Garrison, G., S. K. Huang, K. Okunishi, J. P. Scott, L. R. Kumar Penke, A. M. Scruggs and M. Peters-Golden (2013). "Reversal of myofibroblast differentiation by prostaglandin E(2)." *Am J Respir Cell Mol Biol* **48**(5): 550–558.

Gellersen, B. and J. J. Brosens (2014). "Cyclic decidualization of the human endometrium in reproductive health and failure." *Endocr Rev* **35**(6): 851–905.

Griffith, O. W., A. R. Chavan, S. Protopapas, J. Maziarz, R. Romero and G. P. Wagner (2017). "Embryo implantation evolved from an ancestral inflammatory attachment reaction." *Proc Natl Acad Sci U S A* **114**(32): E6566–E6575.

Hallgrimsson, B., H. Jamniczky, N. M. Young, C. Rolian, T. E. Parsons, J. C. Boughner and R. S. Marcucio (2009). "Deciphering the palimpsest: stydying the relationship between morphological integration and phenotypic covariation." *Evol Biol* **36**: 355–376.

Hansen, V. L., L. S. Faber, A. A. Salehpoor and R. D. Miller (2017). "A pronounced uterine pro-inflammatory response at parturition is an ancient feature in mammals." *Proc Biol Sci* **284**(1865):20171694.

Huang, S. K., S. H. Wettlaufer, J. Chung and M. Peters-Golden (2008). "Prostaglandin E2 inhibits specific lung fibroblast functions via selective actions of PKA and Epac-1." *Am J Respir Cell Mol Biol* **39**(4): 482–489.

Johnson, M. R., G. Carter, C. Grint and S. L. Lightman (1993). "Relationship between ovarian steroids, gonadotrophins and relaxin during the menstrual cycle." *Acta Endocrinol (Copenh)* **129**(2): 121–125.

Jones, R. L., L. A. Salamonsen and J. K. Findlay (2002a). "Activin A promotes human endometrial stromal cell decidualization in vitro." *J Clin Endocrinol Metab* **87**(8): 4001–4004.

Jones, R. L., L. A. Salamonsen, Y. C. Zhao, J. F. Ethier, A. E. Drummond and J. K. Findlay (2002b). "Expression of activin receptors, follistatin and betaglycan by human endometrial stromal cells; consistent with a role for activins during decidualization." *Mol Hum Reprod* **8**(4): 363–374.

Karpovich, N., P. Klemmt, J. H. Hwang, J. E. McVeigh, J. K. Heath, D. H. Barlow and H. J. Mardon (2005). "The production of interleukin-11 and decidualization are compromised in endometrial stromal cells derived from patients with infertility." *J Clin Endocrinol Metab* **90**(3): 1607–1612.

Kim, J. J., R. C. Jaffe and A. T. Fazleabas (1999). "Blastocyst invasion and the stromal response in primates." *Hum Reprod* **14 Suppl 2**: 45–55.

Kim, M. R., D. W. Park, J. H. Lee, D. S. Choi, K. J. Hwang, H. S. Ryu and C. K. Min (2005). "Progesterone-dependent release of transforming growth factor-beta1 from epithelial cells enhances the endometrial decidualization by turning on the Smad signalling in stromal cells." *Mol Hum Reprod* **11**(11): 801–808.

Kin, K., J. Maziarz and G. P. Wagner (2014). "Immunohistological study of the endometrial stromal fibroblasts in the opossum, Monodelphis domestica: evidence for homology with eutherian stromal fibroblasts." *Biol Reprod* **90**(5): 111.

Krausgruber, T., N. Fortelny, V. Fife-Gernedl, M. Senekowitsch, L. C. Schuster, A. Lercher, A. Nemc, C. Schmidl, A. F. Rendeiro, A. Bergthaler and C. Bock (2020). "Structural cells are key regulators of organ-specific immune responses." *Nature* **583**(7815): 296–302.

Kuzet, S. E. and C. Gaggioli (2016). "Fibroblast activation in cancer: when seed fertilizes soil." *Cell Tissue Res* **365**(3): 607–619.

Le Blanc, K. and D. Mougiakakos (2012). "Multipotent mesenchymal stromal cells and the innate immune system." *Nat Rev Immunol* **12**(5): 383–396.

Li, Q., A. Kannan, A. Das, F. J. Demayo, P. J. Hornsby, S. L. Young, R. N. Taylor, M. K. Bagchi and I. C. Bagchi (2013). "WNT4 acts downstream of BMP2 and functions via beta-catenin signaling pathway to regulate human endometrial stromal cell differentiation." *Endocrinology* **154**(1): 446–457.

Liang, C., A. R. Forrest and G. P. Wagner (2015). "The statistical geometry of transcriptome divergence in cell-type evolution and cancer." *Nat Commun* **6**: 60–66.

Lim, H., R. A. Gupta, W. G. Ma, B. C. Paria, D. E. Moller, J. D. Morrow, R. N. DuBois, J. M. Trzaskos and S. K. Dey (1999). "Cyclo-oxygenase-2-derived prostacyclin mediates embryo implantation in the mouse via PPARdelta." *Genes Dev* **13**(12): 1561–1574.

Lindau, R., S. Vondra, J. Spreckels, M. Solders, J. Svensson-Arvelund, G. Berg, J. Pollheimer, H. Kaipe, M. C. Jenmalm and J. Ernerudh (2021). "Decidual stromal cells support tolerance at the human foetal-maternal interface by inducing regulatory M2 macrophages and regulatory T-cells." *J Reprod Immunol* **146**: 103330.

Loomans, H. A. and C. D. Andl (2014). "Intertwining of Activin A and TGFbeta signaling: dual roles in cancer progression and cancer cell invasion." *Cancers (Basel)* **7**(1): 70–91.

Lowe, C. B., J. A. Clarke, A. J. Baker, D. Haussler and S. V. Edwards (2015). "Feather development genes and associated regulatory innovation predate the origin of Dinosauria." *Mol Biol Evol* **32**(1): 23–28.

Lucas, E. S., P. Vrljicak, J. Muter, M. M. Diniz-da-Costa, P. J. Brighton, C. S. Kong, J. Lipecki, K. J. Fishwick, J. Odendaal, L. J. Ewington, S. Quenby, S. Ott and J. J. Brosens (2020). "Recurrent pregnancy loss is associated with a pro-senescent decidual response during the peri-implantation window." *Commun Biol* **3**(1): 37.

Lynch, V. J., G. May and G. P. Wagner (2011). "Regulatory evolution through divergence of a phosphoswitch in the transcription factor CEBPB." *Nature* **480**(7377): 383–386.

Lynch, V. J., A. Tanzer, Y. Wang, F. C. Leung, B. Gellersen, D. Emera and G. P. Wagner (2008). "Adaptive changes in the transcription factor HoxA-11 are essential for the evolution of pregnancy in mammals." *Proc Natl Acad Sci USA* **105**(39): 14928–14933.

MacLean, J. and K. B. Pasumarthi (2014). "Signaling mechanisms regulating fibroblast activation, phenoconversion and fibrosis in the heart." *Indian J Biochem Biophys* **51**(6): 476–482.

Maston, G. A. and M. Ruvolo (2002). "Chorionic gonadotropin has a recent origin within primates and an evolutionary history of selection." *Mol Biol Evol* **19**(3): 320–335.

Medawar, P. B. (1953). Some immunological and endocrinological problems raised by the evolution of viviparity in vertebratges. *Evolution*. R. Brown and J. F. Danielli. New York, NY, Academic Press**:** 320–338.

Mess, A. and A. M. Carter (2006). "Evolutionary transformation of fetal membrane characters in Eutheria with special reference to Afrotheria." *J Exp Zool Part B (Mol Dev Evol)* **306B**: 140–163.

Mor, G., I. Cardenas, V. Abrahams and S. Guller (2011). "Inflammation and pregnancy: the role of the immune system at the implantation site." *Ann N Y Acad Sci* **1221**: 80–87.

Musser, J. M. and G. P. Wagner (2015). "Character trees from transcriptome data: origin and individuation of morphological characters and the so-called 'species signal'." *J Exp Zool B Mol Dev Evol* **324**(7): 588–604.

Nancy, P., J. Siewiera, G. Rizzuto, E. Tagliani, I. Osokine, P. Manandhar, I. Dolgalev, C. Clementi, A. Tsirigos and A. Erlebacher (2018). "H3K27me3 dynamics dictate evolving uterine states in pregnancy and parturition." *J Clin Invest* **128**(1): 233–247.

Negishi, M., Y. Sugimoto and A. Ichikawa (1995). "Molecular mechanisms of diverse actions of prostanoid receptors." *Biochim Biophys Acta* **1259**(1): 109–119.

Nelson, G. J. (1978). "Ontogeny, phylogeny, paleontology and the biogenetic law." *Syst Zool* **27**: 324–345.

Nicoll, M. E. and P. A. Racey (1985). "Follicular development, ovulation, fertilization and fetal development in tenrecs (Tenrec ecaudatus)." *J Reprod Fertil* **74**(1): 47–55.

Nnamani, M. C., S. Ganguly, E. M. Erkenbrack, V. J. Lynch, L. S. Mizoue, Y. Tong, H. L. Darling, M. Fuxreiter, J. Meiler and G. P. Wagner (2016). "A derived allosteric switch underlies the evolution of conditional cooperativity between HOXA11 and FOXO1." *Cell Rep* **15**(10): 2097–2108.

Oakley, T. H. (2017). "Furcation and fusion: the phylogenetics of evolutionary novelty." *Dev Biol* **431**(1): 69–76.

Olsson, L., G. S. Levit and U. Hossfeld (2017). "The 'Biogenetic Law' in zoology: from Ernst Haeckel's formulation to current approaches." *Theory Biosci* **136**(1–2): 19–29.

Osokine, I., J. Siewiera, D. Rideaux, S. Ma, T. Tsukui and A. Erlebacher (2022). "Gene silencing by EZH2 suppresses TGF-beta activity within the decidua to avert pregnancy-adverse wound healing at the maternal-fetal interface." *Cell Rep* **38**(5): 110329.

Pakarainen, T., F. P. Zhang, M. Poutanen and I. Huhtaniemi (2005). "Fertility in luteinizing hormone receptor-knockout mice after wild-type ovary transplantation demonstrates redundancy of extragonadal luteinizing hormone action." *J Clin Invest* **115**(7): 1862–1868.

Palejwala, S., L. Tseng, A. Wojtczuk, G. Weiss and L. T. Goldsmith (2002). "Relaxin gene and protein expression and its regulation of procollagenase and vascular endothelial growth factor in human endometrial cells." *Biol Reprod* **66**(6): 1743–1748.

Pavlicev, M. and G. P. Wagner (2022). "The value of broad taxonomic comparisons in evolutionary medicine: disease is not a trait but a state of a trait!" *MedComm (2020)* **3**(4): e174.

Prum, R. O. (1999). "Development and evolutionary origin of feathers." *J Exp Zool (Mol Dev Evol)* **285**: 291–306.

Prum, R. O. and A. H. Brush (2002). "The evolutionary origin and diversification of feathers." *Quart Rev Biol* **77**: 261–295.

Rajakumar, A., M. A. Kane, J. Yu, J. W. Jones, H. Qu, M. Badell, R. N. Taylor and N. Sidell (2020). "Alternatively activated macrophages are the primary retinoic acid-producing cells in human decidua." *Reprod Sci* **27**(1): 334–341.

Riedelsheimer, B., P. Unterberger, H. Künzle and U. Welsch (2007). "Histological study of the cloacal region and associated structures in the hedgehog tenrec Echinops telfairi." *Mamm Biol* **72**(6): 330–341.

Robb, L., R. Li, L. Hartley, H. H. Nandurkar, F. Koentgen and C. G. Begley (1998). "Infertility in female mice lacking the receptor for interleukin 11 is due to a defective uterine response to implantation." *Nat Med* **4**(3): 303–308.

Romero, R., S. K. Dey and S. J. Fisher (2014). "Preterm labor: one syndrome, many causes." *Science* **345**(6198): 760–765.

Sakamoto, R., T. Fujiwara, Y. Kawano, S. Aikawa, T. Inazumi, O. Nakayama, Y. Kawasaki-Shirata, M. Hashimoto-Iwasaki, T. Sugimoto, S. Tsuchiya, S. Nakao, T. Takeo, Y. Hirota and Y. Sugimoto (2024). "Uterine prostaglandin DP receptor-induced upon implantation contributes to decidualization together with EP4 receptor." *J Lipid Res* **65**(10): 100636.

Samain, R. and V. Sanz-Moreno (2020). "Cancer-associated fibroblasts: activin A adds another string to their bow." *EMBO Mol Med* **12**(4): e12102.

Samstein, R. M., A. Arvey, S. Z. Josefowicz, X. Peng, A. Reynolds, R. Sandstrom, S. Neph, P. Sabo, J. M. Kim, W. Liao, M. O. Li, C. Leslie, J. A. Stamatoyannopoulos and A. Y. Rudensky (2012). "Foxp3 exploits a pre-existent enhancer landscape for regulatory T cell lineage specification." *Cell* **151**(1): 153–166.

Schafer, S., S. Viswanathan, A. A. Widjaja, W. W. Lim, A. Moreno-Moral, D. M. DeLaughter, B. Ng, G. Patone, K. Chow, E. Khin, J. Tan, S. P. Chothani, L. Ye, O. J. L. Rackham, N. S. J. Ko, N. E. Sahib, C. J. Pua, N. T. G. Zhen, C. Xie, M. Wang, H. Maatz, S. Lim, K. Saar, S. Blachut, E. Petretto, S. Schmidt, T. Putoczki, N. Guimaraes-Camboa, H. Wakimoto, S. van Heesch, K. Sigmundsson, S. L. Lim, J. L. Soon, V. T. T. Chao, Y. L. Chua, T. E. Tan, S. M. Evans, Y. J. Loh, M. H. Jamal, K. K. Ong, K. C. Chua, B. H. Ong, M. J. Chakaramakkil, J. G. Seidman, C. E. Seidman, N. Hubner, K. Y. K. Sin and S. A. Cook (2017). "IL-11 is a crucial determinant of cardiovascular fibrosis." *Nature* **552**(7683): 110–115.

Schlosser, G. (2021). *Evolutionary Origin of Sensory and Neurosecretory Cell Types*. Boca Raton, London, New York, CRC Press.

Serhan, C. N. and J. Savill (2005). "Resolution of inflammation: the beginning programs the end." *Nat Immunol* **6**(12): 1191–1197.

Sheller-Miller, S., L. Richardson, L. Martin, J. Jin and R. Menon (2018). "Systematic review of p38 mitogen-activated kinase and its functional role in reproductive tissues." *Am J Reprod Immunol* **80**(6): e13047.

Stadtmauer, D. J., S. Basanta, J. D. Maziarz, A. G. Cole, G. Dagdas, G. R. Smith, F. van Breukelen, M. Pavlicev and G. P. Wagner (2025). "Cell type and cell signalling innovations underlying mammalian pregnancy." *Nat Ecol Evol* **9**: 1469–1486.

Stadtmauer, D. J. and G. P. Wagner (2020). "Cooperative inflammation: the recruitment of inflammatory signaling in marsupial and eutherian pregnancy." *J Reprod Immunol* **137**: 102626.

Stadtmauer, D. J. and G. P. Wagner (2021). "Single-cell analysis of prostaglandin E2-induced human decidual cell in vitro differentiation: a minimal ancestral deciduogenic signal." *Biol Reprod* **106**: 155–172.

Stewart, D. R., A. C. Celniker, C. A. Taylor, Jr., J. R. Cragun, J. W. Overstreet and B. L. Lasley (1990). "Relaxin in the peri-implantation period." *J Clin Endocrinol Metab* **70**(6): 1771–1773.

Sugimoto, M. A., L. P. Sousa, V. Pinho, M. Perretti and M. M. Teixeira (2016). "Resolution of inflammation: what controls its onset?" *Front Immunol* **7**: 160.

Talmadge, K., N. C. Vamvakopoulos and J. C. Fiddes (1984). "Evolution of the genes for the beta subunits of human chorionic gonadotropin and luteinizing hormone." *Nature* **307**(5946): 37–40.

Tsai, M. T., S. M. Ou, K. H. Lee, C. C. Lin and S. Y. Li (2024). "Circulating Activin A, kidney fibrosis, and adverse events." *Clin J Am Soc Nephrol* **19**(2): 169–177.

Umbarkar, P., S. Ejantkar, S. Tousif and H. Lal (2021). "Mechanisms of fibroblast activation and myocardial fibrosis: lessons learned from FB-specific conditional mouse models." *Cells* **10**(9):2412.

Vallejo, G., A. C. Mestre-Citrinovitz, V. Monckedieck, R. Grummer, E. Winterhager and P. Saragueta (2011). "Ovarian steroid receptors and activated MAPK in the regional decidualization in rats." *Biol Reprod* **84**(5): 1063–1071.

Vento-Tormo, R., M. Efremova, R. A. Botting, M. Y. Turco, M. Vento-Tormo, K. B. Meyer, J. E. Park, E. Stephenson, K. Polanski, A. Goncalves, L. Gardner, S. Holmqvist, J. Henriksson, A. Zou, A. M. Sharkey, B. Millar, B. Innes, L. Wood, A. Wilbrey-Clark, R. P. Payne, M. A. Ivarsson, S. Lisgo, A. Filby, D. H. Rowitch, J. N. Bulmer, G. J. Wright, M. J. T. Stubbington, M. Haniffa, A. Moffett and S. A. Teichmann (2018). "Single-cell reconstruction of the early maternal-fetal interface in humans." *Nature* **563**(7731): 347–353.

Wagner, G. P. (2014). *Homology, Genes and Evolutionary Innovation*. Princeton, NJ, Princeton University Press.

Werneburg, I., M. Laurin, D. Koyabu and M. R. Sanchez-Villagra (2016). "Evolution of organogenesis and the origin of altriciality in mammals." *Evol Dev* **18**(4): 229–244.

Wildman, D. E., C. Chen, O. Erez, L. I. Grossman, M. Goodman and R. Romero (2006). "Evolution of the mammalian placenta revealed by phylogenetic analysis." *Proc Natl Acad Sci USA* **103**: 3203–3208.

Wynn, T. A. (2008). "Cellular and molecular mechanisms of fibrosis." *J Pathol* **214**(2): 199–210.

Younesi, F. S., A. E. Miller, T. H. Barker, F. M. V. Rossi and B. Hinz (2024). "Fibroblast and myofibroblast activation in normal tissue repair and fibrosis." *Nat Rev Mol Cell Biol* **25**(8): 617–638.

Yu, J., S. L. Berga, E. B. Johnston-MacAnanny, N. Sidell, I. C. Bagchi, M. K. Bagchi and R. N. Taylor (2016). "Endometrial stromal decidualization responds reversibly to hormone stimulation and withdrawal." *Endocrinology* **157**: 2432–2446.

7 Recognition of Pregnancy
Coordinating Ovarian and Utero-Placental Function

So far, we viewed the evolution of the fetal-maternal relationship through a narrow focus on the cell biological events at the fetal-maternal interface. In fact, however, that utero-placental interaction is embedded and influenced, if not regulated, by a wider organismal context. The uterine events during pregnancy are integrated with the rest of the maternal organism, most directly with the ovarian cycle, but also with the broader physiology of the mother. The integration with the ovarian cycle also includes the central role of progesterone in regulating uterine responses to pregnancy, at least in eutherians.

THE OVARIAN CYCLE IN RELATION TO POST-FERTILIZATION EVENTS

All events of fetal development, and thus also all the events involved in viviparity, are downstream of ovulation. Consequently, all these events are related to, constrained by, and eventually integrated into the ovarian cycle (Basanta and Pavlicev 2025).

The least integration between ovarian and genital tract biology, naturally, is evident in species with external fertilization. Whatever the trigger is for ovulation and oviposition, often a large number of ova are released from the ovary and leave the maternal body before fertilization. In these species, the ovulation may be integrated with muscular contraction to achieve expulsion, but no further coordination is necessary. The further development happens outside the body, and only brood care, if it exists, may affect the physiology of the mother, or the father in some cases, such as pipefish (Stolting and Wilson 2007). In the case of birds, the situation is already more complicated. Birds have internal fertilization, and while the egg is traveling through the Müllerian ducts, it is vested with multiple layers of egg coverings, and the next ovulation is prevented until the egg is laid (Johnson 2011). So, not only is the production of egg covering materials coordinated by ovulation, but post-fertilization processing of the egg also feeds back to the ovary to delay subsequent ovulations and thus coordinates the ovarian cycle with the function of the Müllerian tract.

The ovarian cycle of vertebrates is roughly divided into two phases: the follicular phase where primary follicles grow and mature, eventually reaching the stage of the so-called Graafian follicle, just before ovulation (Figure 7.1). Ovulation is triggered by pituitary hormone signals, leading to the expulsion of the ova from the ovary with a few associated granulosa cells, called cumulus cells. The rest of the follicle stays behind and is transformed into an ephemeral endocrine organ, the *corpus luteum* (CL). The development of the CL initiates the post-ovulatory or luteal phase of the ovarian cycle. The principal hormonal signal of the CL is mostly progesterone, signaling to the organs derived from the Müllerian duct, i.e., oviduct, uterus, and cervix, if present. The CL has a finite lifetime, and its demise starts the follicular phase of the next cycle, if ovulation is cyclical rather than controlled by external clues, such as temperature, light period length, the presence of a male, or directly by copulation. The key question is how the length of the luteal phase is related to the length of postovulatory processes occurring in the reproductive tract (the egg or embryo internal development), and how this relationship is evolving to affect successful reproduction. This relation is less problematic in species where progesterone from the CL only plays a role in the initial portion of the internal development. This is mostly the case in oviparity and in nonmammalian viviparity. If so, the luteal phase can be much shorter than the internal development, as progesterone can be

DOI: 10.1201/9781032717777-7

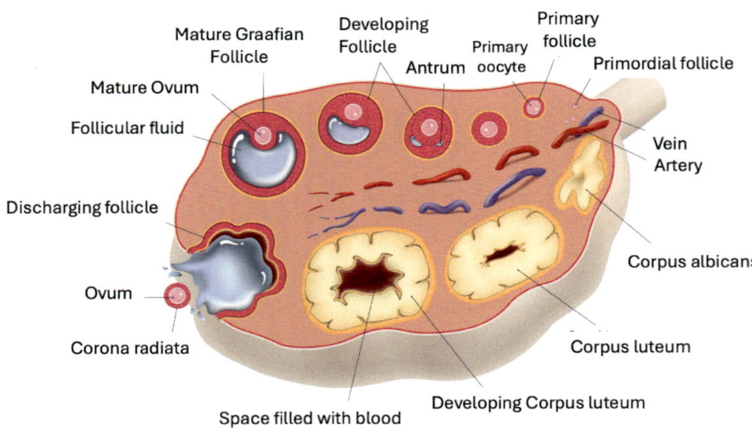

FIGURE 7.1 Human ovarian cycle and the development of the corpus luteum. (Image purchased by GPW from https://www.istockphoto.com under their standard license.)

withdrawn and the new follicular phase can start, before the egg or embryo is expelled. Eutherian viviparity is different, however, as it requires progesterone from the start to the end, and premature withdrawal would end it.

Gestation in eutherian species is initiated during the luteal phase, i.e., naturally after ovulation and internal fertilization. As it requires progesterone, the trademark of the luteal phase, there is a critical need for coordination between the length of the luteal phase and the length of internal development. Hence, the luteal phase and gestation are serially homologous processes. In order to allow the evolution of extended internal development of the fetus, these serial homologs needed to become independent in evolution, so as not to decrease the rate of reproduction by also prolonging the non-pregnant cycle (Basanta and Pavlicev 2025). The degree to which these two processes are coupled or independent from each other is the key to understanding the evolution of gestational regulation. Recognition of pregnancy is the physiological device that can switch from the luteal phase of the cycle to the gestational phase. More specifically, the term recognition of pregnancy (RoP) is used for the processes caused by the conceptus that change the survival period of the corpus luteum (Bazer et al. 1998). As we will see, there are also eutherian species with extended gestation but no RoP.

One situation where the length of the luteal phase and viviparous development are ancestrally in harmony is when the period of intra-uterine development is shorter than the luteal phase of the non-pregnant cycle. The classic example of this form of viviparity is the reproduction of the opossum, e.g., *Monodelphis domestica*. Ovulation in opossum is caused by male pheromones, which are produced by a skin gland on the chin of the male (Hinds et al. 1992). After ovulation, the corpus luteum survives for up to 27 days, although this is somewhat variable between cycles and individuals (Fadem and Rayve 1985). When fertilization occurs, gestation lasts for about 14 days and is thus substantially shorter than the luteal phase of non-pregnancy. In this situation, when intra-uterine development is shorter than the luteal phase, the ovarian cycle does not need to be modified to accommodate gestation. In fact, opossum has been recognized as a species without systemic recognition of pregnancy for a long time (Harder and Fleming 1981).

Gestation that is shorter than the luteal phase has been called "intra-cyclic gestation" (Chavan et al. 2016) because the gestational period fits within the unmodified luteal phase (Figure 7.2). On the other hand, a situation where the gestational length is longer than the luteal phase has been called "trans-cyclic gestation" by the same authors. It is plausible that intra-cyclic gestation was the ancestral form of viviparity in therian mammals, since it did not require additional modifications of the

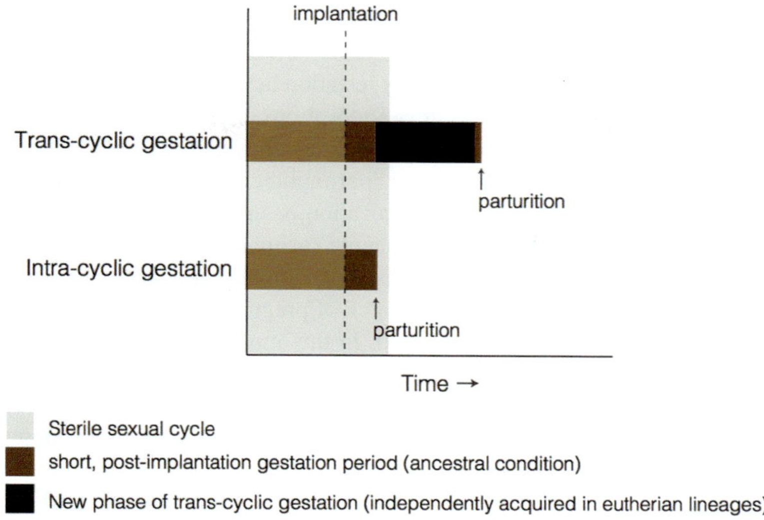

FIGURE 7.2 Illustration of the notion of trans- and intracyclic gestation. Transcyclic gestation is longer than the luteal phase of the non-pregnant ovarian cycle. Most eutherian mammals fall into this category. Intracyclic gestation is shorter than the luteal phase of the ovarian cycle. An example is the pregnancy of the opossum. (Figure 4 in Chavan et al. 2016.)

ovarian cycle, and may also be for other vertebrates, although to our knowledge this issue has not been systematically investigated. The other argument is that intra-cyclic gestation is found in those marsupials belonging to basally branching lineages in the marsupial clade, which have retained several primitive features of female reproduction [e.g., poly ovulation (Freyer et al. 2003)]. Also, stem eutherian fossils, as well as stem group members of the major lineages within eutherians, are all small compared to the average size of extant members of the clades (O'Leary et al. 2013). This is significant because data show that most of the time of trans-cyclic gestation is spent on fetal growth, and consequently, body size is positively correlated with gestational length (Martin and MacLaron 1985). This does not directly show that the gestation of the eutherian ancestor was intra-cyclic, but it is at least consistent with it. With a trend to body size increase within most eutherian lineages (dos Reis et al. 2012), however, the gestational length expanded up to the length of the luteal phase. Then, at least two types of constraints arose that likely were an obstacle to further increase in gestational length. These are the possibility of an ovulation happening while the uterus is still occupied with the previous litter, and the other is declining progesterone levels during gestation. The way these constraints have been overcome is key to understanding the evolution of viviparity at the systems level (Basanta and Pavlicev 2025).

Whether ovulation during pregnancy is problematic depends on several factors. Ovulation might, but does not need to be a problem for the extension of gestational length. For instance, if ovulation is triggered by external clues, such as male pheromones or copulation itself, like in the rabbit, gestation length that is longer than the luteal phase is not a problem, because ovulation is not directly triggered by the end of the luteal phase. In some cases, it might be even advantageous, namely if the fetus uses extra ova for nutrition, as in some sharks (see Chapter 3). But once spontaneous ovulation evolved, where ovulation directly follows the demise of the corpus luteum, and if the fetus relies on placental provisioning, rather than directly eating the contents and secretions of the female reproductive tract, pre-parturition ovulation is at least a waste of effort if not upsetting the delicate balance of fetal-maternal communication.

If the lifetime of the corpus luteum is shorter than the gestation length, one has to expect that the CL regresses during gestation, leading to declining progesterone levels. Declining progesterone levels also may or may not be a problem, depending on the role progesterone plays in female reproduction. In all eutherians tested, progesterone is essential for the maintenance of pregnancy (Spencer and Bazer 2002). If that is the case, then extending gestation beyond the length of the luteal phase is either impossible or requires some compensatory innovations. One such compensatory innovation is to expand the life span of the corpus luteum only in pregnancy. An example is human pregnancy. The corpus luteum of nonpregnancy survives for approximately 2 weeks, but its lifetime is about 7 weeks in pregnancy. Another compensatory innovation is an alternative source of progesterone. Examples are progesterone production by the placenta (primates and guinea pigs) or the adrenal gland (armadillo). In fact, in human gestation, it is well known that a luteo-placental shift in progesterone production occurs around the seventh week of pregnancy (Csapo 1969). In other viviparous vertebrates, the situation is more complicated. In the opossum, ovariectomy does not lead to abortion later in the gestation, and thus ovarian progesterone and other products of the CL are not necessary for the maintenance of pregnancy. Similarly, in viviparous reptiles, the requirement for progesterone is limited to initial stages of pregnancy, but overall, the situation is quite complicated (see chapters in Norris and Lopez 2024).

The above, somewhat associative reflections, suggest that the evolution of trans-cyclic gestation might not be problematic in some animals, where, for instance, progesterone is not required for the maintenance of pregnancy, such as squamates. In contrast, in eutherians, trans-cyclic gestation requires special innovations to (a) coordinate the next ovulation with parturition, if the ovarian cycle is spontaneous, and/or (b) secure the production of the necessary progesterone to maintain a functional fetal-maternal interface. The maternal processes that ensure the deployment of these mechanisms are called "recognition of pregnancy, if they are triggered by the presence of the conceptus.

RECOGNITION OF PREGNANCY IN A FEW EUTHERIAN SPECIES

Recognition of pregnancy are those physiological processes that support the continuation of pregnancy and are caused by the action of the conceptus, rather than other physiological pathways. In this section, we provide a few examples where the mechanisms triggered by the conceptus are known.

In humans, ovulation is spontaneous, and the menstrual cycle is 28 days. Counting from the first day of the menstrual bleeding, ovulation occurs around day 14, and implantation is possible between days 19 and 21. This means that in the menstrual cycle, the corpus luteum dies two weeks after ovulation. If implantation occurs, the corpus luteum has to support pregnancy until the 7th week, after which the placenta takes over the production of progesterone. The establishment and continuation of pregnancy is thus dependent on keeping the corpus luteum alive beyond the time at which it would normally degenerate. The prolongation of the lifetime of the CL is achieved through secretions from the embryo's trophoblast, in particular human chorionic gonadotropin (hCG), a paralog of luteinizing hormone (LH), the hormone secreted from the pituitary. Like maternal LH during the nonpregnant cycle, hCG produced by the trophoblast supports the persistence of the corpus luteum by binding to the same receptors and preventing the production of prostaglandin PGF2a in the ovary that otherwise would kill the corpus luteum.

The situation in humans and other great apes is one where, during the ovarian cycle, the signal causing the demise of the corpus luteum, prostaglandin PGF2a, is produced in the ovarian stroma. The hCG from the conceptus travels in the utero-ovarian portal vein, binds to the ovarian receptors, and maintains the functional corpus luteum. In other species, such as the pig and cattle, the luteolytic signal is also PGF2a, but it emanates from the uterine endometrium (McCracken et al. 1999). Consequently, in these species, the recognition of the pregnancy signal has to act on the endometrium to prevent sending the luteolytic signal to the ovary.

The short summary of pig RoP is based on the 2013 review by Fuller Bazer (Bazer 2013). During the ovarian cycle in the pig, the endometrium produces PGF2a, which reaches the ovary via the utero-ovarian portal vein, causing luteal decline. After fertilization, the conceptus signals to the endometrium by secreting estrogen, which changes the handling of PGF2a such that it does not enter the bloodstream. As a consequence, the uterine secretion of PGF2a switches from endocrine to exocrine. In the latter, the uterine glands secrete PGF2a into the uterine lumen, from where it does not reach the corpus luteum, thus preventing luteolysis. Besides estrogen, the blastocyst also secretes two interferons, IFNG and IFND, as well as prostaglandin E2 (Sullivan et al. 2004). IFNG and IFND are necessary for the establishment and maintenance of pregnancy, but whether they also have a role in the recognition of pregnancy is unclear. The porcine mode of pregnancy recognition is shared with other basally branching artiodactyl lineages, in particular the Tylopoda (camels and lama) (Bianchi et al. 2023), and is likely ancestral in artiodactyls.

In cattle and other ruminants, such as sheep and goats, the maternal luteolytic signal PGF2a also comes from the endometrium. The embryonic signal for pregnancy recognition, however, is not estrogen, but a special interferon, interferon tau (INFT) (Bazer 2013). INFT is only known from pecoran ruminants (deer, cattle, sheep) and inhibits the synthesis of PGF2a. The genome of an outgroup, the genus *Tragulina* (mouse-deer, not to be confused with deer mouse, *Peromyscus*), has been reported sequenced, but an annotated genome does not seem to be available. We thus do not know whether *Tragulus* has an *INFT* gene and whether INFT is a ruminant or a pecoran innovation (Roberts et al. 1998, Ealy and Wooldridge 2017). INFT is a paralog of interferon omega, and not closely related to those interferons reported to be expressed in the pig conceptus, IFNG and INFD, which makes the construction of an evolutionary scenario for the origin of the ruminant RoP mechanism more difficult.

Horses share with ruminants the endometrial production of PGF2a and the presence of a signal, emanating from the blastocyst, that prevents the production of PGF2a. However, what this blastocyst signals do to the uterus is, is not known. Finally, the rabbit seems to be similar to the pig in that the pregnancy recognition signal from the blastocyst is estrogen. The taxon sample of taxa where the RoP mechanisms are known is rather sparse (Braz et al. 2024), but the similarity between rabbit, pig, and camels suggests that fetal estrogen signaling could be relatively old.

EUTHERIAN SPECIES WITHOUT RECOGNITION OF PREGNANCY

As mentioned at the beginning of the last section, recognition of pregnancy is usually understood as those events that maintain the corpus luteum, are caused by the conceptus, and are thus directly dependent on the pregnancy having ensued. There are, however, other eutherian species where maintenance of the corpus luteum is possible without signals from the conceptus, and thus these species, technically, do not have a recognition of pregnancy.

One example is the house mouse, *Mus musculus*, and some of its relatives. The mouse has an extremely short ovarian cycle of four days, where the diestrus, or luteal phase, has been substantially shrunk. This might be an adaptation to increase the rate of reproduction in case of failing to become pregnant in one cycle. Hence, pregnancy requires some kind of mechanism to avoid the immediate demise of the CL. Note that because of the short diestrus, the signal to *maintain* CL cannot depend on the embryo arriving and doing its thing, because the functioning CL does not develop in the first place. The time between copulation and implantation is four days, way too long for "rescuing" the CL. Instead, in the mouse, the signal for developing the functional CL of pregnancy is stimulation of the uterine cervix during copulation. If one mates a receptive female with a vasectomized male, she will extend the luteal phase to almost the length of a normal pregnancy, a phenomenon called "pseudo-pregnancy." The mediator of the CL rescue is PRL (Soares et al. 2007), a pituitary hormone that is also released in humans upon orgasm (Komisaruk et al. 2006). The mouse cervico-pituitary reflex might be a homologue of the human female orgasm (Pavlicev and Wagner 2016).

One might speculate that the copulation-dependent rescue of the CL is necessary because implantation only happens on day 4 post copulation and thus later than the end of the sterile ovarian cycle. If this is true, this form of CL rescue has probably evolved secondarily in conjunction with the shortening of the ovarian cycle. How this may have worked is hard to reconstruct, as long as we do not know how the ovarian cycle was regulated before the ultra-short ovarian cycle evolved. If the ancestral condition required a RoP, then the evolutionary shortening of the luteal phase should have stopped at the time implantation would happen. Otherwise, the initiation of pregnancy would have been impossible, since RoP signals from the embryo would come too late, i.e., at a time when the corpus luteum would already be dead. This is an interesting problem to pursue.

To contextualize the above thoughts, one should add that the laboratory mouse (*Mus musculus*) is not entirely representative of rodents. Even within the superfamily Muroidea, which also contains rats, mice, and hamsters with shortened luteal phases, many species are reported to have longer luteal phases that are still shorter than their pregnancies. Examples are the Spinnifex hopping mouse (*Notomys alexis*), a member of the Muridae, that has an 8-day cycle (Breed 1975, Breed and Leigh 2011) or the African spiny mouse (*Acomys caharinus*), which has about 10-day estrus cycle (Peitz 1981). The clade that is most basally branching from the mouse lineage contains the guinea pig with a cycle of 15 days, as well as the Amazon spiny rat (*Proechimys guyannensis*) with a 10-day cycle (Sanabria et al. 2019). Hence, the ancestor of rodents likely had a normal cycle with likely some form of RoP. When and how often the ultra-short ovarian cycle evolved or was lost will require a focused research effort.

The other species known to lack conceptus-dependent recognition of pregnancy is the dog (Andersen and Simpson 1974). In the dog, the ovarian cycle has an extended luteal phase regardless of whether the female is pregnant or not. It might be noted that the dog is a mono-ovular seasonal breeder and thus extending the length of the non-pregnant cycle does not affect reproductive rate.

Marsupials are generally recognized as lacking recognition of pregnancy, as conceptualized in eutherians, i.e., a conceptus-dependent mechanism maintaining the CL (Harder and Fleming 1981). Nevertheless, there is still a local impact of the blastocysts on the endometrium, which changes in the morphology, secretory activity, and gene expression in the endometrium (Renfree 1972, Griffith et al. 2019). It is thus said that marsupials have "endometrial recognition of pregnancy," which, however, is unconnected to the maintenance of the CL. In fact, as mentioned above, the opossum pregnancy is shorter than the sterile ovarian cycle and thus does not really need a systemic recognition of pregnancy. Furthermore, progesterone is only necessary for the very early stages of pregnancy but is dispensable for most of the gestational period (Tyndale-Biscoe and Renfree 1987, Bradshaw and Bradshaw 2011). Only the macropodids have evolved an extended pregnancy (Tyndale-Biscoe and Renfree 1987). For instance, Wallaby is a seasonal mono-ovulatory species, where only one uterus is pregnant with associated changes in the ipsilateral ovary.

THE EVOLUTION OF RECOGNITION OF PREGNANCY MECHANISMS

Unfortunately, the number of species for which the mechanisms of recognition of pregnancy are known is small and very unequally distributed across the eutherian tree (Braz et al. 2024). Much is known about primates and a few rodents, as well as hoofed farm animals, but almost nothing outside these groups. This is not surprising, given the amount of experimental work necessary to establish the recognition of the pregnancy mechanism in any species. A consequence of that, however, is that very little can be inferred from a formal comparative analysis (see Braz et al. 2024). Nevertheless, let us see what can be said from the limited data we have.

On the broadest level, there is the fact that in all known cases, the luteolytic signal is PGF2a (McCracken et al. 1999). Next, we note the distinction between the source of the luteolytic signal. On the one hand, we have the primates that produce PGF2a in the ovary. On the other hand, we have the artiodactyls, where the PGF2a is produced by the uterine endometrium. This taxonomic and mechanistic pattern may be the sign of at least two independent origins of recognition of pregnancy. It is plausible for two reasons that the most basal eutherian mammals might not have had the need for a recognition of pregnancy mechanism. First, they seem to have been small, and therefore with a probably short gestation (Chavan et al. 2016, Basanta and Pavlicev 2025). Here, the argument is that gestation length scales with body size and thus a small body size of early eutherians could indicate short gestation length. Second, the earliest eutherians still shared with the marsupials an epipubic bone, which is incompatible with an expanding belly during pregnancy. So, arguably, the pregnancy of the eutherian ancestor was probably intra-cyclical, i.e., shorter than the non-pregnant ovarian cycle.

As argued at the introduction to this chapter, the need for recognition of pregnancy is particularly expected when the ovarian cycle is spontaneous or poly-estrous, i.e., not triggered by external signals, like male pheromones or the light cycle. We have argued in a different context that spontaneous ovulation is evolutionarily derived and has been independently evolved multiple times (Pavlicev and Wagner 2016). This argument, if correct (for a different perspective see Dixson 2021), suggests that RoP may have evolved several times in association with spontaneous ovulation, i.e., in conjunction with the evolution of a regular ovarian cycle.

The best taxon sample available for RoP mechanisms is in the artiodactyl animals. There, two modes of RoP have been described. One is based on estrogen signals from the blastocyst, found in tylopods and suids, and another is RoP signals to the uterus via IFNT in the ruminants. Given the structure of the phylogenetic tree (Figure 7.3), the most parsimonious interpretation of such a distribution is that the ruminant type of RoP has evolved from a porcine/tylopod type of mechanism, given that suids and tylopods are two consecutive outgroup lineages to ruminants. It is hard to imagine what could have driven this transition, but it is worth noting that the move from porcine to ruminant type of RoP is coincidental with a change in the character of the placenta. Suids and tylopods have a diffuse placenta with a smooth epitheliochorial fetal-maternal interface, while ruminants display a cotyledonary placenta together with the origin of the maternal caruncles (see Chapter 8). A cotyledonary placentation requires the coordinated development of the fetal cotyledon and the crypts of the caruncles, which may include the evolution of derived kinds of placental-uterine communication.

In the Archontoglires, the primates use chorionic gonadotropin with direct action on the ovary. This peptide evolved through a duplication of the LH-B gene in primates, consistent with an independent evolution of recognition of pregnancy in primates. The rest of the clade, lagomorphs and rodents, also support an independent origin of the primate and artiodactyl RoP. The clade contains the rabbit, which is a copulation-induced ovulator. Copulation with a sterile male does induce pseudo-pregnancy, although not as long as the full pregnancy. This also fits with the fact that mouse copulation also rescues the CL, via a pituitary PRL signal. This would be compatible with a scenario where the common ancestor of the Boreoeutherians, consisting of the Laurasiatheria (carnivores and hoofed animals) and the Archontoglires (primates, rodents, and lagomorphs), would have been an animal without RoP, as supported by extant lineages without RoP (carnivores in Laurasiatheria and some rodents in Archontoglires). Then we have to infer two independent origins of RoP in

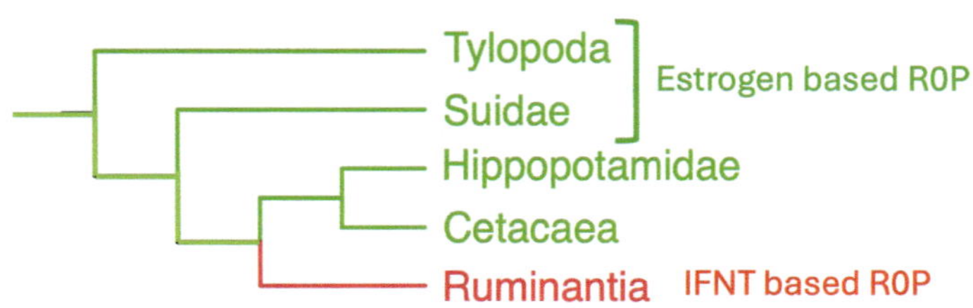

FIGURE 7.3 Taxonomic distribution of modes of recognition of pregnancy and phylogenetic relationships of taxa closely related to ruminants. The camels and the pigs share an estrogen-based recognition of pregnancy (RoP), while ruminants have an IFNT-based RoP. The recognition of pregnancy in hippopotamoids and whales is not known. This tree suggests that IFNT-based RoP evolved from estrogen-based RoP. (Image created by GPW, CC BY-NC.)

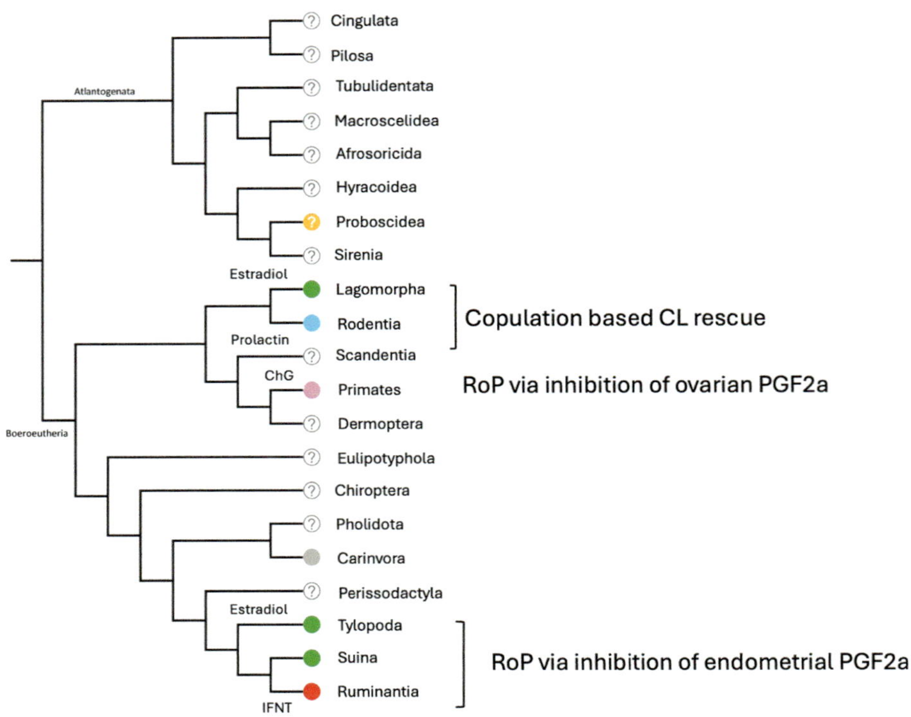

FIGURE 7.4 Taxonomic distribution of various mechanisms of recognition of pregnancy and the phylogenetic relationships among eutherian species. (Image modified from Braz et al. 2024, published under CC BY license.)

primates and artiodactyls (the situation in horses is still unclear) and a transformation of the tylopod/suid mechanism to the derived ruminant form based on IFNT (Figure 7.4).

Unfortunately, this speculative scenario excludes the most basally branching eutherian lineages, the Afrotheria and the Xenarthra, for the lack of detailed enough information about these animals. Overall, the messages of this chapter are (1) RoP is not a universal feature of eutherian pregnancy as there are animals without RoP, (2) it has evolved at least twice and likely more often, and (3) the ruminant RoP has evolved from the suid/tylopod form of RoP.

REFERENCES

Andersen, A. C. and M. E. Simpson (1974). *The Ovary and Reproductive Cycle of the Dog*. Los Altos, CA, Geron-X, Inc.

Basanta, S. and M. Pavlicev (2025). "The shifting role and regulation of the Corpus Luteum in vertebrate reproduction: a synthetic review." *Q Rev Biol* **100**(3): 189–231.

Bazer, F. W. (2013). "Pregnancy recognition signaling mechanisms in ruminants and pigs." *J Anim Sci Biotechnol* **4**(1): 23.

Bazer, F. W., T. L. Ott and T. E. Spencer (1998). "Maternal recognition of pregnancy: comparative aspects: a review." *Placenta* **19**: 375–386.

Bianchi, C. P., M. F. Gallelli, J. M. Herrera, M. A. Benavente, L. Rossetto and M. A. Aba (2023). "Current knowledge about the processes of luteolysis and maternal recognition of pregnancy in camelids." *Reprod Domest Anim* **58**(1): 3–9.

Bradshaw, F. J. and D. Bradshaw (2011). "Progesterone and reproduction in marsupials: a review." *Gen Comp Endocrinol* **170**(1): 18–40.

Braz, H. B., R. Barreto, L. N. D. Silva-Junior, B. O. Horvath-Pereira, T. S. D. Silva, M. D. D. Silva, F. Acuna and M. A. Miglino (2024). "Evolutionary patterns of maternal recognition of pregnancy and implantation in eutherian mammals." *Animals (Basel)* **14**(14): 2077.

Breed, W. G. (1975). "Environmental factors and reproduction in the female hopping mouse, Notomys alexis." *J Reprod Fertil* **45**(2): 273–281.

Breed, W. G. and C. M. Leigh (2011). "Reproductive biology of an old endemic murid rodent of Australia, the Spinifex hopping mouse, Notomys alexis: adaptations for life in the arid zone." *Integr Zool* **6**(4): 321–333.

Chavan, A. R., B.-A. S. Bhullar and G. P. Wagner (2016). "What was the ancestral function of decidual stromal cells? A model for the evolution of eutherian pregnancy." *Placenta* **40**: 40–51.

Csapo, A. (1969). "The luteo-placental shift, the guardian of pre-natal life." *Postgrad Med J* **45**: 57–64.

Dixson, A. F. (2021). *Mammalian Sexuality. The Act of Mating and the Evolution of Reproduction*. Cambridge, UK, Cambridge University Press.

dos Reis, M., J. Inoue, M. Hasegawa, R. J. Asher, P. C. Donoghue and Z. Yang (2012). "Phylogenomic datasets provide both precision and accuracy in estimating the timescale of placental mammal phylogeny." *Proc Biol Sci* **279**(1742): 3491–3500.

Ealy, A. D. and L. K. Wooldridge (2017). "The evolution of interferon-tau." *Reproduction* **154**(5): F1–F10.

Fadem, B. H. and R. S. Rayve (1985). "Characteristics of the oestrous cycle and influence of social factors in grey short-tailed opossums (Monodelphis domestica)." *J Reprod Fertil* **73**(2): 337–342.

Freyer, C., U. Zeller and M. B. Renfree (2003). "The marsupial placenta: a phylogenetic analysis." *J Exp Zool A Comp Exp Biol* **299A**(1): 59–77.

Griffith, O. W., A. R. Chavan, M. Pavlicev, S. Protopapas, R. Callahan, J. Maziarz and G. P. Wagner (2019). "Endometrial recognition of pregnancy occurs in the grey short-tailed opossum (Monodelphis domestica)." *Proc Biol Sci* **286**(1905): 20190691.

Harder, J. D. and M. W. Fleming (1981). "Estradiol and progesterone profiles indicate a lack of endocrine recognition of pregnancy in the opossum." *Science* **212**(4501): 1400–1402.

Hinds, L. A., M. Reader, S. Weinberg-Moller and N. R. Saunders (1992). "Hormonal evidence for induced ovulation in Monodelphis domestica." *J Reprod Fert* **95**: 303–312.

Johnson, A. I. (2011). Organization and functional dynamics of the arian ovary. *Hormones and Reproduction of Vertebrates*. D. O. Norris and K. H. Lopez. Amsterdam etc., Academic Press. **4: Birds:** 71–90.

Komisaruk, B. R., C. Beyer-Flores and B. Whipple (2006). *The Science of Orgasm*. Baltimore, The John Hopkins University Press.

Martin, R. D. and A. M. MacLaron (1985). "Gestation period, neonatal size and maternal investment in placental mammals." *Nature* **313**: 220–223.

McCracken, J. A., E. E. Custer and J. C. Lamsa (1999). "Luteolysis: a neuroendocrine mediated event." *Phys Rev* **79**: 263–323.

Norris, D. O. and K. H. Lopez, Eds. (2024). *Hormones and Reproduction of Vertebrates: Reptiles*. Hormones and Reproduction of Vertebrates. London, Academic Press.

O'Leary, M. A., J. I. Bloch, J. J. Flynn, T. J. Gaudin, A. Giallombardo, N. P. Giannini, S. L. Goldberg, B. P. Kraatz, Z. X. Luo, J. Meng, X. Ni, M. J. Novacek, F. A. Perini, Z. S. Randall, G. W. Rougier, E. J. Sargis, M. T. Silcox, N. B. Simmons, M. Spaulding, P. M. Velazco, M. Weksler, J. R. Wible and A. L. Cirranello (2013). "The placental mammal ancestor and the post-K-Pg radiation of placentals." *Science* **339**(6120): 662–667.

Pavlicev, M. and G. Wagner (2016). "The evolutionary origin of female orgasm." *J Exp Zool B Mol Dev Evol* **326**(6): 326–337.

Peitz, B. (1981). "The oestrous cycle of the spiny mouse (Acomys cahirinus)." *J Reprod Fertil* **61**(2): 453–459.

Renfree, M. B. (1972). "Influence of the embryo on the marsupial uterus." *Nature* **240**(5382): 475–477.

Roberts, R. M., L. Liu, Q. Guo, D. Leaman and J. Bixby (1998). "The evolution of the type I interferons1." *J Interferon Cytokine Res* **18**(10): 805–816.

Sanabria, V., S. Bittencourt, T. de la Rosa, J. Livramento, C. Tengan, C. A. Scorza, E. Cavalheiro and D. Amado (2019). "Characterization of the estrous cycle in the Amazon spiny rat (Proechimys guyannensis)." *Heliyon* **5**(12): e03007.

Soares, M. J., T. Konno and S. M. Alam (2007). "The prolactin family: effectors of pregnancy-dependent adaptations." *Trends Endocrinol Metab* **18**(3): 114–121.

Spencer, T. E. and F. W. Bazer (2002). "Biology of progesterone action during pregnancy recognition and maintenance of pregnancy." *Front Biosci* **7**: d1879–1898.

Stolting, K. N. and A. B. Wilson (2007). "Male pregnancy in seahorses and pipefish: beyond the mammalian model." *Bioessays* **29**(9): 884–896.

Sullivan, R. M., C. G. Lucas, M. Sponchiado, E. K. Eitel, L. D. Spate, M. C. Lucy, M. F. Smith, K. D. Wells, R. S. Prather and R. D. Geisert (2004). "Conceptus estrogen and prostaglandins provide the maternal recognition of pregnancy signal to prevent luteolysis during early pregnancyi n the pig." *Biol Reprod* **111**(4): 890–905.

Tyndale-Biscoe, C. H. and M. B. Renfree (1987). *Reproductive Physiology of Marsupials*. Cambridge, UK, Cambridge University Press.

8 "The Placenta" is Not a Unitary Character

The story of mammalian viviparity is often told as a story of the origin and evolution of the placenta. In these accounts, it is assumed that the placenta is the key innovation leading the way to the complex forms of eutherian viviparity. The preceding chapters should have made clear that the critical innovations are for the most part maternal, accommodating an invasive embryo, rather than fetal or placental. Only after the obstacles for the maintenance of an invasive fetus have been overcome (see Chapters 4, 5, and 6), the placenta, in particular the morphologically and physiologically complex placentae, could have evolved. Hence, the evolutionary elaboration of the placental structures was evolutionarily secondary to the evolution of a receptive endometrium that is able to form a "decidua" (Stadtmauer and Wagner 2020). Here, we will make the argument that the placenta, as a structured organ in many but not all eutherians, is not homologous across major eutherian lineages.

THE FORMAL DEFINITION OF A PLACENTA AND ITS LIMITATIONS

As briefly discussed in Chapter 3, the formal definition of a placenta essentially identifies as a placenta any contact between fetal and maternal structures dedicated to the exchange of nutrients, oxygen, signals, and waste products. For instance, Mossman writes in 1937: the placenta is "an intimate apposition or fusion of fetal organs to the maternal (or paternal, in the case of seahorses) tissues for physiological exchange" (Mossman 1937). Similarly, Grosser defines a placenta as "the intimate connection between the mucosa of the maternal genital tract with fetal appendage organs, primarily the chorion, [...] for enabling the transition of nutritional substances from the mother to the fetus"[1] (Grosser 1909). These definitions capture the essential functions of placentation and are broad enough to cover all different anatomical realizations of placentae. This covers, for instance, the placenta of marsupials that has few anatomical specializations beyond the plesiomorphic presence of the fetal membrane. But it also covers the case of the human placenta, which is a large, highly differentiated organ. Of course, the human placenta is homologous to parts of the fetal membrane from which it is formed but has a highly differentiated internal structure resembling a proper internal organ (see DiFrisco et al. 2020 and Parker 2024 for a discussion of organ identity, as well as Griffith and Wagner 2017 regarding the placenta as a model of organ origination). Explaining the origin of "the placenta" can be easy, if it is understood only as an apposition of fetal membranes to the uterine mucosa, or difficult, if we aim at explaining the origin and evolution of a discoidal placenta like that of humans, and even worse that of rodents, which is anatomically even more complicated than the human placenta. A model explaining the origin of the marsupial placenta does not explain the origin of the eutherian discoidal placenta. In that sense, the term "placenta" does not refer to a unitary biological entity even though, in mammals, all placentae are homologous via their common derivation from fetal membranes.

DIVERSITY AND EVOLUTION OF PLACENTAL MORPHOLOGIES

There are many excellent reviews, some book-length, of mammalian placental diversity. Such an overview goes beyond the scope of this chapter, and the interested reader is encouraged to consult the books by Ramsey (Ramsey 1982) and Wooding and Burton (Wooding and Burton 2008). Here, we limit ourselves to the description of some exemplary cases of placental morphologies that will serve in the discussion of the evolution of the mammalian placenta.

DOI: 10.1201/9781032717777-8

There are a number of classification schemes of placentae for eutherian mammals. They refer to the structure of the fetal-maternal interface, to the number and kinds of tissue layers separating maternal and fetal blood, or to the macroscopic shape of the fetal exchange organ. The structure of the fetal exchange surface can be villous, consisting of finger-like projections, or trabecular, consisting of folds or ridges, or a labyrinth. A labyrinth is a complex spongy system of blood spaces that develops when maternal blood capillaries are surrounded by trophoblast that removes the maternal endothelium. Within the fetal part of the labyrinth, fetal capillaries are developing, forming an interlaced system of fetal and maternal blood spaces (see Figure 3.1).

The classification of placentae by their micro-anatomy of the interhemal tissue layers goes back to Grosser (1909) and has been discussed in Chapter 3. Finally, the classification by macroscopic shape seems to be the least functionally and evolutionarily informative (Ramsey 1982). It includes four basic types: the discoidal placenta, where the placenta is a compact disc-shaped organ (Figure 8.1). It can come as a single disc, as in humans or mice, or two discs, as in some monkeys. A zonary placenta has the shape of a belt around an elongated embryo, which can be completely surrounding the embryo, as in the dog, or incomplete, as in the raccoon. There are cotyledonary placentae, where discrete tufts of villi are distributed all over the surface of the chorion. Finally, the morphologically least differentiated form is the diffuse placenta, as found in pigs, where more or less (see below) the whole surface of the chorion is covered with folds or villi that tightly interdigitate with the luminal epithelium. Below, we will have a closer look at the shape of the definitive placenta of humans, mice, pigs, and cattle as exemplars to discuss the evolution of the fetal-maternal interchange organs at the macroscopic level. We will ignore here the complicated story of how various placentae develop and refer the reader to the extensive literature on that subject.

At term, the human placenta is a disc with a diameter of about 22 cm with a shape vaguely resembling a classical apple pie,[2] and weighing about ½ kg, with the umbilical cord attached to the center of the "placental pie." The maternal-facing side is villous, with tree-like outgrowths, villi, most of which end freely floating in the space between maternal and fetal tissue, sealed off at the

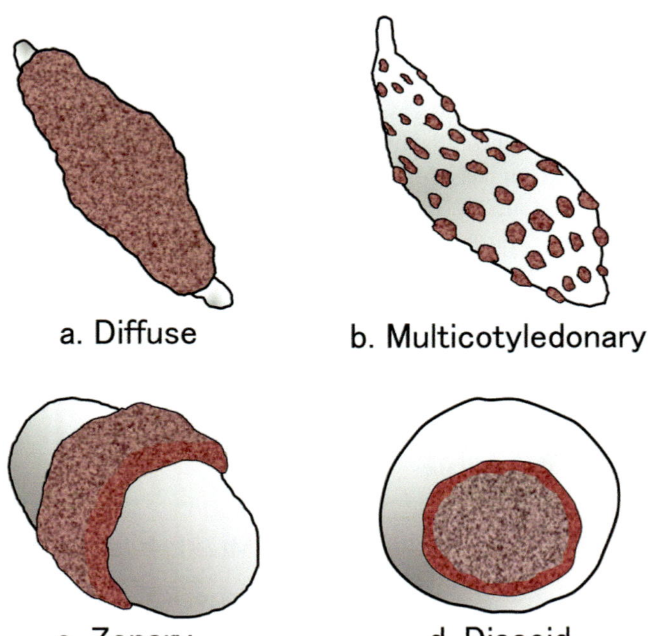

FIGURE 8.1 The most common morphological shapes of eutherian placentas. (Image from Furukawa et al. 2014, published under CC BY-NC-ND 3.0.)

edges, and filled with maternal blood. Some of the most distal villi anastomose, and some attach to the endometrium and are called anchoring villi. The villi are covered by one layer of syncytial trophoblast underlain by a layer of cellular cytotrophoblasts. At the anchoring villi, so-called villous cytotrophoblasts (VCT) detach and invade the endometrium, and some become extra-villous trophoblasts (EVT). EVTs either remain in the endometrium as interstitial EVTs or even migrate all the way to the muscular layer of the uterus, the myometrium. An important subpopulation of EVTs, with the help of uterine NK cells, erodes part of the maternal spiral arteries and inserts themselves in place of the endothelial cells, preventing vessel constriction and therefore increasing blood supply to the placenta. The placental disc is filled with highly vascularized extraembryonic mesenchyme. Overall, the human placenta is a compact organ with its own blood supply, and a dedicated "business end": the villous exchange surface.

The mouse placenta, similar to the human, is a compact disc attached to the umbilical cord and has a highly differentiated mother-facing surface (see Figure 3.1). The exchange surface of the placenta is a labyrinth of tunnels, through which flows the maternal blood, and is thus much more complicated than the human villous placenta. In addition, the placenta has yet another layer that has no counterpart in the human placenta, the spongiotrophoblast. It consists of a loose network of large cells with often large nuclei, which play a role in endocrine communication with the mother. The loose structure of the spongious layer allows maternal blood to reach and leave the labyrinth, which is the main exchange surface of the mouse placenta. As in humans, the placental interchange surface, in this case the lining of the tunnels in the labyrinth, is covered with trophoblast syncytium. In this case, however, it is two layers, rather than one.

Human and mouse placentae are presented as exemplars of the discoidal placenta type, but do not represent the limits of the diversity existing within this category. The guinea pig, for instance, being closely related to rodents (or belonging to the most basally branching lineage of rodents, depending on the definition of "Rodentia"), has a discoidal/labyrinthine placenta like the mouse, and, in addition, a so-called subplacenta. The subplacenta is a transient part of the guinea pig placenta located centrally in the maternal-facing surface and is villous rather than labyrinthine. Some other discoidal placentae have specialized hemophagous areas (as in *Tenrec ecaudatus*), as well as additional "para-placental" structures.

The other extreme of the placental shape, the diffuse placenta, seems to be primitive compared to the discoidal placenta. It is mostly known from pigs but is also found in hippopotamus, camels, and whales, i.e., all the artiodactyl relatives of pigs with the exception of ruminants. It lacks a compact organ-like organization, i.e., called "diffuse," but rather consists of folds and short villi that interdigitate with the luminal epithelium (Figure 8.2). The trophoblast remains cellular, and on the maternal side, no epithelial erosion has been observed. The two epithelia, the maternal luminal epithelium and the placental trophoblast, are tightly connected via intercellular molecular bridges. Nevertheless, the maternal and fetal blood vessels come as close to each other as biologically possible by indenting the fetal and maternal epithelia, at places reducing the diffusion distance down to 2 micro-meter. These apparent "penetrations" of the epithelia always respect epithelial integrity as the epithelial and endothelial cells remain separated by the basal membrane. In addition to the trophoblast-luminal interdigitation for hemotrophic nutrition, oxygen supply, and waste removal, there are also areas specialized for the uptake of histotrophic nutrition. These are the so-called areolae, which differentiate on the trophoblast side at locations opposite to the openings of uterine glands. The epithelium of the areolae is not attached to the luminal epithelium but leaves some open space between the fetal and maternal surfaces.

Cattle, and other ruminants have a cotyledon placenta, which consists of a large number of spatially limited smaller groups of villi, cotyledons (Figure 8.3A), interdigitating with permanent uterine structures, the caruncles (Figure 8.3B). A caruncle with the attached cotyledon is called a placentome. There are various contradictory uses of the term "placentome" which are clearly based on misunderstandings and loose talk, as discussed by Ramsey (1982, page 27).[3] The interhemal structure in cattle has been described as "synepitheliochorial" owing to the formation of bi-nuclear cells from

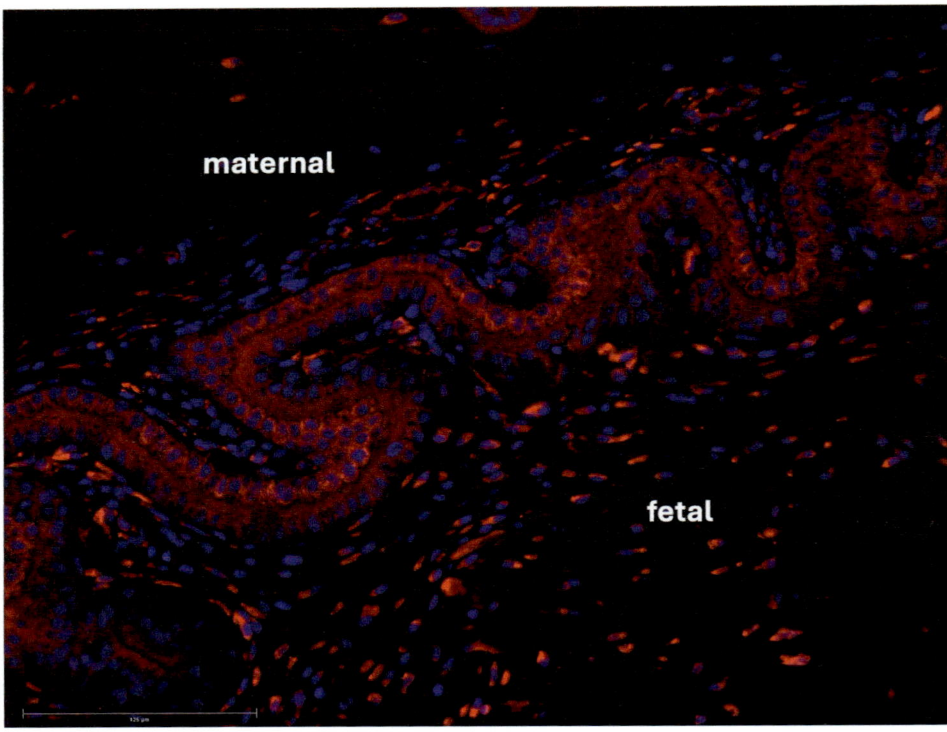

FIGURE 8.2 Fetal-maternal interface of a pig. The luminal (maternal) epithelium and the placental (fetal) epithelium are tightly attached and folded. The image shows a section stained for Foxa2, red, and DAPI, blue, for nuclei. (Image generated by GPW CC BY-NC.)

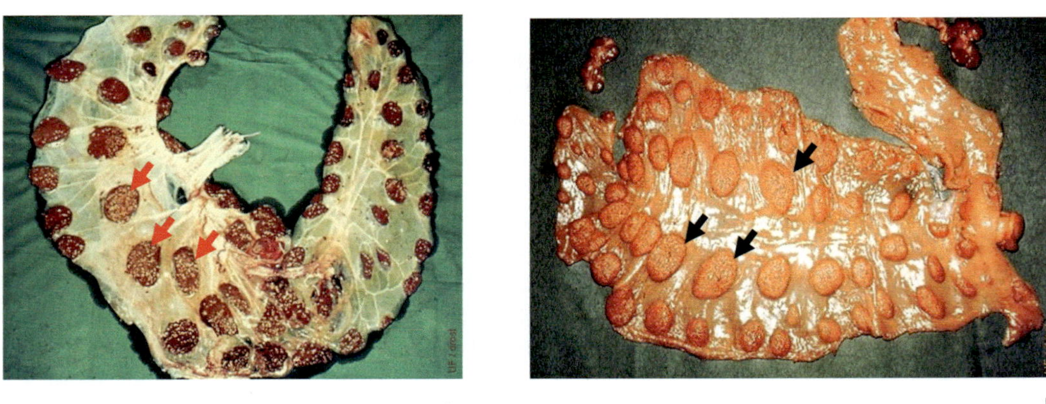

FIGURE 8.3 Macroscopic images of the fetal-maternal interface of a cow. (A) Maternal facing side of the placenta at or near term showing brown clusters of villi called cotyledons (red arrows). (B) Luminal surface of the uterus with caruncular bodies (black arrows). The cotyledons of the placenta match up and interdigitate with the caruncles, forming the placental-maternal exchange surface. (Images from The Visual Guides of Animal Reproduction, visgar.vetmed.ufl.edu, reproduced with permission.)

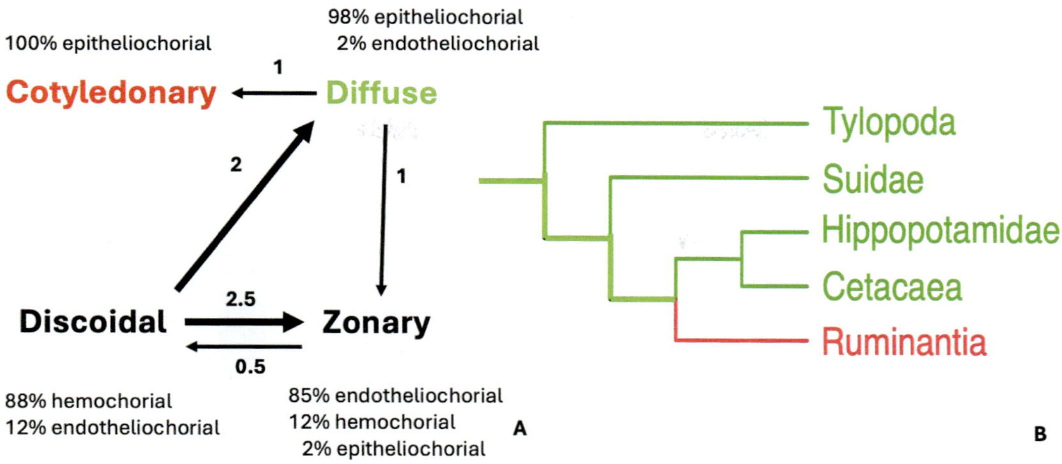

FIGURE 8.4 Evolutionary transitions in placental shape. (A) Estimated number of transitions between placental shapes according to Elliot and Crespi (2009), with the frequency of interhemal interface types for each placental shape. (B) Phylogenetic context of the single transition from diffuse and epitheliochorial placenta toward the cotyledonary placenta, only found in ruminants. Note that there are at least three independent outgroup clades with diffuse placenta, showing that the cotyledonary placenta is derived from diffuse placenta. (Images by GPW CC BY-NC.)

the fusion of trophoblast and luminal epithelial cells (Wooding and Burton 2008). More recent investigations, however, showed that the interhemal structure is much more polymorphic and dynamic, including periods of gestation and locations in the placentomes where the luminal epithelium is lacking and where even signs of trophoblast invasion into the endometrial stroma can be observed (Seo et al. 2024). The details of the cattle maternal-fetal interface thus remain a site of active research.

Phylogenetic reconstructions unambiguously suggest that the ancestral eutherian placenta was discoidal and labyrinthic, which is surprising given that the discoidal placenta is morphologically so much more complex than the diffuse placenta (Elliot and Crespi 2009) (Figure 8.4A). To the contrary, diffuse placenta originated twice, once in the artiodactyls and once in strepsirhine primates from the discoidal placenta, in both cases coincidental with the evolution of epitheliochorial placentation. The cotyledonary placenta originated once, derived from a diffuse placenta, in the stem lineage of ruminants. This conclusion is plausible, given that the ruminants are deeply nested within the artiodactyls (Figure 8.4B) and all non-ruminant artiodactyls have a diffuse placenta.

There is a strong correlation between the nature of the interhemal barrier and the shape of the placenta, where most of the discoidal placentas are hemochorial (or sometimes endotheliochorial) and diffuse placentas are in almost all cases epitheliochorial. Both diffuse and cotyledonary placentae are never hemochorial, as far as we could find. Zonary placentae are mostly associated with endotheliochorial placentation (Figure 8.5).

WHY IS THE DISCOIDAL PLACENTAL ANCESTRAL?

To recapitulate the results of the phylogenetic analysis, one can note that there is strong evidence that the ancestral eutherian placenta was a discoidal, labyrinthine, and hemochorial (Elliot and Crespi 2009) (Figure 8.4A). Hence, it was already a much more complex organ than the fetal membranes that constitute the marsupial placenta. In contrast, morphologically simpler eutherian placentae, such as the diffuse placenta of pigs and camels, are reconstructed to be derived from discoidal or zonary placentae. How is it that a more morphologically complex organ was the ancestral state for crown group eutherian mammals, and simpler placental morphology evolved later?

When we reviewed the comparative evidence for the ancestral nature of the discoidal placenta, we noted that there is a strong correlation between this form of the placenta and the nature of the

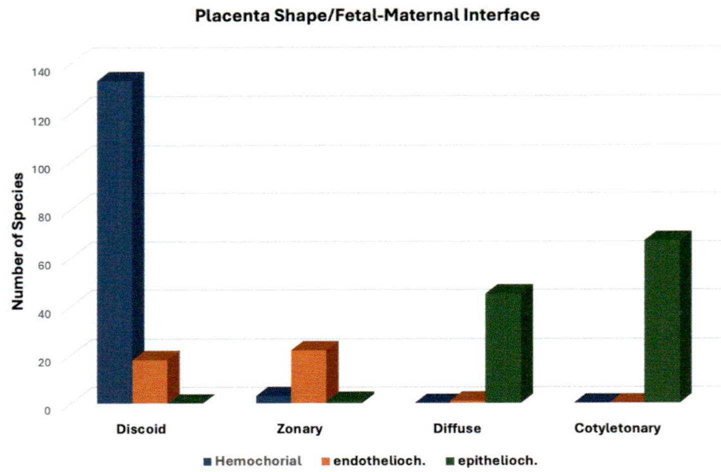

FIGURE 8.5 Correlation between placental shape and interhemal barrier based on the data assembled by Elliot and Crespi (2009). Discoidal placentas are overwhelmingly hemochorial, while diffuse and cotyledonary placentas are overwhelmingly or exclusively epitheliochorial, respectively. (Image generated by GPW CC BY-NC.)

interhemal barrier, with the overwhelming majority of animals with discoidal placenta also being hemochorial, while the diffuse and the cotyledonary placentae are overwhelmingly associated with epitheliochorial placentation (Figure 8.5). What could be the reason for that association?

Let us consider the facts of hemochorial placentation as it exists in eutherians. By definition, it includes the destruction of a part of the maternal blood vessels, that is, the opening of some of the endometrial arteries. This naturally leads to a local hemorrhage, quite literally (see implantation stage mouse uterus in Figure 8.6), and the placenta is in direct contact with the maternal blood. To make this into a sustainable configuration, the maternal blood needs to be contained within the placental bed. It is thus tempting to speculate that the local differentiation of the fetal membranes, which eventually will be the discoidal placenta, had the role of containing the nidatory hemorrhage,

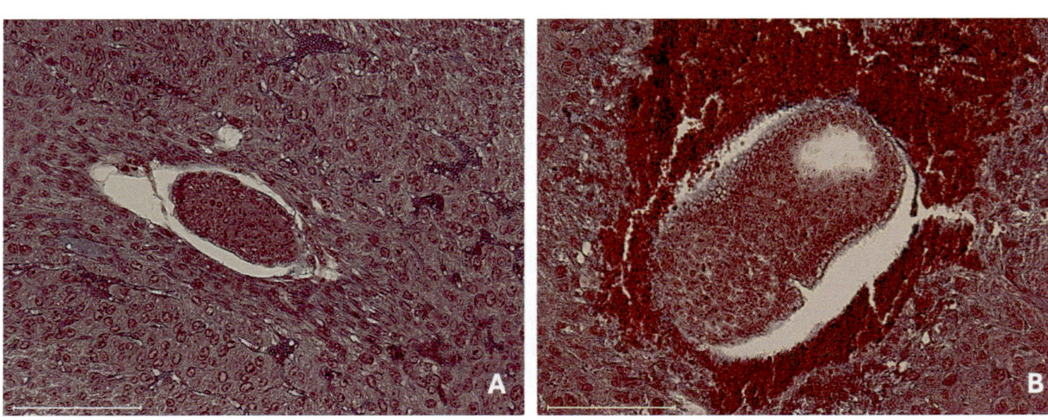

FIGURE 8.6 Early stages of implantation of a mouse embryo. (A) Day 5.5 pc embryo, where the luminal epithelium is already eroded. (B) Day 6.5 embryo where the maternal blood vessels are already compromised, leading to a massive but physiological hemorrhage at the site of implantation. (Images generated by GPW CC BY-NC based on histological preparations produced by Dr. Manfred Walzl, University of Vienna, and donated to MP.)

with specializations for chemical exchange (such as a labyrinth or villi) added later. Even with more sophisticated chemical exchange specializations, like the labyrinth, containing the endometrial hemorrhage, still plays a major role in the placenta for extant hemochorial species. Hence if hemochorial placentation is ancestral, as all indications suggest (Mess and Carter 2006, Wildman et al. 2006, Elliot and Crespi 2009), and if the above argument about containing the endometrial hemorrhage is correct, hemochorial placentation had to arise coincidentally with discoidal placentation, where the discoidal placenta is the "lid on top of the pot of the placental bed, filled with maternal blood" a metaphor used by Grosser monograph on fetal membranes (Grosser 1909).

To build on the above speculation, one may say that with the evolution of an endometrial hemorrhage, specializations to contain the maternal blood had to evolve first. At the same time, this very reason led to the individuation of a part of the fetal membranes first as a containment organ and later acquiring further specializations for chemical exchange. This is mostly the chorioallantois, which had privileged access to oxygen and blood-borne nutrients and thus was the preferred place to enhance the chemical exchange between the mother and the fetus. These then result into the various specializations like labyrinths, villi, and trabeculae. It is also the preferred place to produce and secrete hormones to communicate with the mother. This model, thus, posits that the initial step toward the evolution of a distinct organ-like differentiation, the discoidal placenta, was the need to contain endometrial hemorrhage, caused by the embryo.

Again, as mentioned previously, the discoidal placenta of the armadillo is an interesting exception in that there is no placental bed with an open blood space that needs to be contained. According to the phylogenetic reconstruction, the ancestral Xenarthra had a discoidal placenta, and yes, the placental villi are in direct contact with the maternal blood, but that is achieved by a rather minimally invasive form of placentation (Enders et al. 1958, Enders 1960). The villi grow into preformed maternal blood sinuses and partially replace the maternal endothelium (Chavan and Wagner 2016). At this point, the best accommodation of these facts is to assume that this situation evolved secondarily as a way to further contain maternal blood. The discoidal morphology of the placenta may be a phylogenetic carryover from a time when their ancestors had a more conventional hemochorial placenta.

Phylogenetic evidence further suggests that the evolution of non-invasive placentation was associated with the loss of the distinct discoidal morphology, such as in pigs and all other artiodactyls. How this can be achieved in a gradual transformation is an interesting and yet unanswered question. But it is also evident that the functional need for a discoidal placental morphology would disappear with the prevention of endometrial hemorrhage, due to the evolution of the epitheliochorial interhemal barrier. A more detailed analysis of the phylogenetic distribution of intermediary morphologies, such as endothelial placenta and zonary placental shape, would be an interesting pursuit.

CRITIQUE OF PLACENTAL TYPOLOGY

In the above discussion, we followed the tradition of discussing placental variation and evolution more or less in isolation from the mother, as if the placenta is a "stand-alone" organ, like the heart or the lung, even though connected to the rest of the fetal body, but nevertheless self-contained in its functional performance. Such an approach is, of course, completely wrong-headed, given the fundamental functional role of the placenta as an organ of communication between the mother and the fetus. Whatever the form or shape of the placenta is, it is always the result of a co-evolution between fetal and maternal structures and processes. This is most obvious in the cotyledonary placenta of ruminants, which consists of tufts of villi that develop in response to and in interaction with the preformed uterine caruncles. Caruncles are permanent uterine structures that interdigitate with the villi of the fetal membrane during pregnancy and thus likely induce the morphology of the cotyledonary placenta. The cotyledonary placenta is not a unitary morphological entity, but a reaction of the extra-embryonic tissues to preformed maternal structures, the caruncles. A similar logic can be applied to the discoidal placenta; if the speculations in the previous section are correct, the discoidal placenta likely evolved in coordination with the origin of a blood-infused placental bed. In either case, the real functional, cell-biological, and evolutionary unit is the emergent fetal-maternal unit (Nuño de la Rosa et al. 2020), where maternal and fetal parts are engaged in a co-evolutionary dynamic; often, if not always, initiated by maternal innovations (Stadtmauer and Wagner 2020). Once the maternal innovations are established, they enable the subsequent elaboration of fetal contributions.

Another important lesson from the above evolutionary analysis of placentation is that "placenta" is not a unitary character. In placental mammals and reptiles, there is homology mediated through the shared origin of the placenta from extra-embryonic tissues. But technically, a placenta is only a relationship between maternal and fetal structures (see above the definitions by Grosser and Mossman). There is an argument to be made that the discoidal placenta (and perhaps the zonary placenta) is a compact, internally structured organ with its own morphological identity. But the discoidal placentae are a subset of all structures that are called "a placenta" in general. The point is that the objective of "explaining the origin of 'the' placenta" is not well defined, similar to explaining the "origin of 'viviparity'," given the variety of ways viviparity can be realized (Chapter 3). Any empirical research program on the origin of the placenta will have to specify what exactly the explanandum is, i.e., the origin of which form of placenta do we want to explain? The evolution of fetal membrane apposition to the uterus? The origin of the discoidal placental organ? Or the ruminant placentome, including novel, i.e., non-homologous, structures such as the caruncle and the cotyledon? In other words, research programs based on premature abstractions risk missing capturing biological reality.

NOTES

1. Page 89 in Grosser 1909: "Als Placentation ist die innige Verbindung (Aneinanderlagerung oder Verwachsung) der Schleimhaut des mütterlichen Genitaltracts mit embryonalen Anhangorganen, in erster Linie mit dem Chorion, zu bezeichnen, zur Ermöglichung des Übergangs von Nährstoffen von der Mutter auf die Frucht" (Engl. Translation by GPW).
2. In German, the human placenta is called "Mutterkuchen" [mother's cake], reflecting the shape similarity with a pie.
3. These uses of the term should not be honored with further discussion.

REFERENCES

Chavan, A. R. and G. P. Wagner (2016). "The fetal-maternal interface of the nine-banded armadillo: endothelial cells of maternal sinus are partially replaced by trophoblast." *Zoological Lett* **2**: 11.

DiFrisco, J., A. C. Love and G. P. Wagner (2020). "Character identity mechanisms: a conceptual model for comparative-mechanistic biology." *Biol Philos* **35**: 43–44.

Elliot, M. G. and B. J. Crespi (2009). "Phylogenetic evidence for early hemochorial placentation in eutheria." *Placenta* **30**(11): 949–967.

Enders, A. C. (1960). "Development and structure of the villous haemochorial placenta of the nine-banded armadillo (Dasypus novemcinctus)." *J Anat* **94**: 34–45.

Enders, A. C., G. D. Buchanan and R. V. Talmage (1958). "Histological and histochemical observations on the armadillo uterus during the delayed and post-implantation periods." *Anat Rec* **130**(4): 639–657.

Furukawa, S., Y. Kuroda and A. Sugiyama (2014). "A comparison of the histological structure of the placenta in experimental animals." *J Toxicol Pathol* **27**(1): 11–18.

Griffith, O. W. and G. P. Wagner (2017). "The placenta as a model for understanding the origin and evolution of vertebrate organs." *Nat Ecol Evol* **1**(4): 72.

Grosser, O. (1909). *Vergleichende Anatomie und Entwicklungsgeschichte der Eihäute und der Placenta.* Vienna, W. Braumüller.

Mess, A. and A. M. Carter (2006). "Evolutionary transformation of fetal membrane characters in Eutheria with special reference to Afrotheria." *J Exp Zool Part B (Mol Dev Evol)* **306B**: 140–163.

Mossman, H. W. (1937). "Comparative morphogenesis of the foetal membranes and accessory uterine structures." *Contr Embyol* **26**: 129–246.

Nuño de la Rosa, L., M. Pavlicev and A. Etxeberria (2020). "Pregnant females as historical individuals: an insight from the philosophy of evo-devo." *Front Psychol* **11**: 572106.

Parker, J. (2024). "Organ evolution: emergence of multicellular function." *Annu Rev Cell Dev Biol* **40**(1): 51–74.

Ramsey, E. M. (1982). *The Placenta. Human and Animal.* Santa Barbara, CA, Praeger Inc.

Seo, H., G. D. Melo, R. V. Oliveira, G. A. Franco-Johannsen, F. W. Bazer, K. G. Pohler and G. A. Johnson (2024). "Immunohistochemical examination of the uteroplacental interface of cows on days 21, 31, 40, and 67 of gestation." *Reproduction* **167**(2): e230444.

Stadtmauer, D. J. and G. P. Wagner (2020). "The primacy of maternal innovations to the evolution of embryo implantation." *Integr Comp Biol.* **60**(3): 742–752

Wildman, D. E., C. Chen, O. Erez, L. I. Grossman, M. Goodman and R. Romero (2006). "Evolution of the mammalian placenta revealed by phylogenetic analysis." *Proc Natl Acad Sci USA* **103**: 3203–3208.

Wooding, F. B. P. and G. J. Burton (2008). *Comparative Placentation.* Berlin and Heidelberg, Springer.

9 The Nature of the Fetal-Maternal Relationship Has Consequences

Menstruation and Cancer

The evolution of the fetal-maternal interface not only impacts reproduction, but, as often in biology, is connected to and has consequences for other aspects of biology. In this chapter, we will briefly visit two areas of mammalian biology that are connected to the mode of female reproduction: menstruation and cancer malignancy. Both topics do not concern the fetal-maternal interface directly but belong to the broader context of female mammalian biology, much of which is entwined with the eutherian-specific mode of female reproduction. Each of these topics would require a more extensive treatment than can be provided here, and there are some reviews published that cover the issues in more depth than is possible here (on menstruation Critchley et al. 2020; on cancer-placenta connection Wagner et al. 2022). Nevertheless, we want to introduce these issues here to ensure that they are recognized for what they are: consequences of the evolutionary cell biology of the fetal-maternal relationship.

THE EVOLUTIONARY ROOTS OF MENSTRUATION

Menstruation is the sloughing off of the superficial layers of the endometrium, called "functionalis," at the end of the luteal phase of the ovarian cycle. It is important to remember this definition to distinguish menstruation from other forms of physiological (i.e., non-pathological) vaginal bleeding, such as that of female dogs at the beginning of the estrus. The biological role of menstruation was and still is a mystery. It is a regular and physiological feature of the life of reproductive-age women with a substantial health burden due to menstruation-related disorders. However, menstruation has only been reported from a limited number of mammals, representing about 5% of extant species. A cursory look at the taxonomic distribution of menstruating species shows that menstruation is a derived character within eutherian mammals and has evolved at least four times independently (Figure 9.1). Menstruation has been found most frequently among primates, in particular apes and Old World monkeys, and some New World Monkeys. Elephant shrews have been known for a long time to menstruate at the end of the last ovarian cycle of the breeding season (Horst and Gillman 1941). Also, a handful of bats have been found to menstruate. Most excitingly, a menstruating rodent species was recently discovered, the spiny mouse *Acomys cahirinus* (Bellofiore et al. 2017, Bellofiore et al. 2018). A few observations about this species are discussed in the latter part of this chapter.

Multiple independent origins of a biological trait are usually understood as a sign that that trait has some adaptive value and is likely evolving due to natural selection under certain ecological circumstances. The problem is, no one has been, to the date of writing this, able to offer such a scenario for menstruation. This does not mean that there is not a plethora of hypotheses offered (some of them discussed below), but to our judgement, none of them is without problems. Of course, it is possible that menstruation evolved for some non-adaptive reason, or that different adaptive scenarios lead to the convergent origin of menstruation in different lineages.

Given the absence of a clearly delineated biological function of menstruation, explanatory narratives have cast a wide net of possible direct or indirect advantages of menstruation to explain why it

 DOI: 10.1201/9781032717777-9

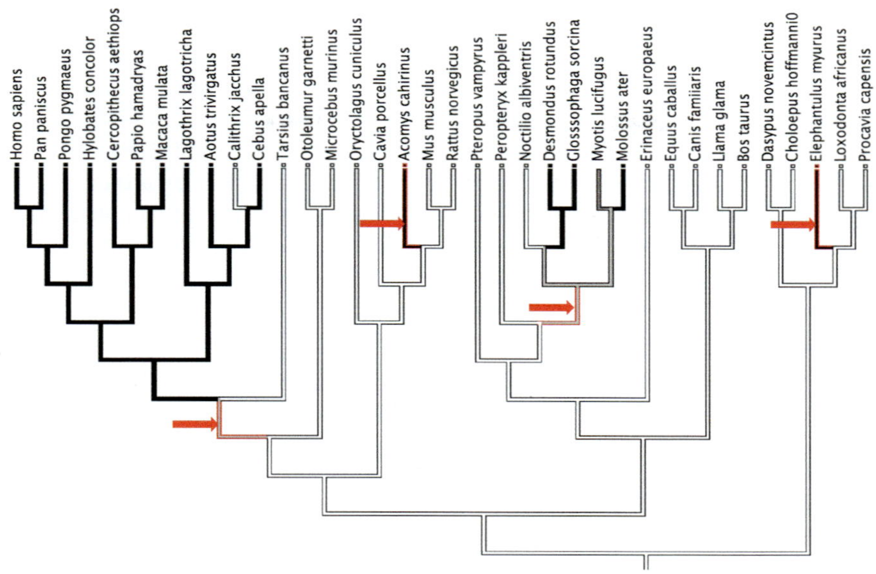

FIGURE 9.1 Simplified eutherian phylogeny showing the distribution of menstruating species. Based on this evidence, menstruation has evolved at least four times in eutherian phylogeny. (Image generated by GPW and published in Critchley et al. (2020) under CC BY-NC-ND 4.0.)

has evolved. This is not the place to offer an evaluation of all or even the main explanations, but we want to mention the best contenders, according to our judgment.

Margie Profet has to be credited with precipitating a broader effort to understand the evolutionary biology of menstruation. Despite academic degrees in political philosophy, physics, and mathematics, Dr. Profet made her impact with theories on the evolution of menstruation (Profet 1993), morning sickness (Profet 1988), and allergies (Profet 1991). Her theory for menstruation posits that menstruation might have evolved to clear the uterus of copulation-introduced pathogens. It is interesting to ask why clearing of pathogens is urgent only in the 5% of eutherian species known to menstruate, and not for the 95% of the other, non-menstruating eutherian species, in particular not in species with intrauterine ejaculation such as armadillo or tenrec. One may also note that clearing pathogens would be much delayed, as menstruation occurs at the end of the luteal phase, whereas copulation would be expected early. Shortly after Profet triggered a broad discussion of the potential benefits of menstruation, Beverly Strassman from the University of Michigan offered a criticism of Profet's theory and, at the same time, her own idea (Strassmann 1996). Dr. Strassman argued that menstruation, and thus the loss of part of the differentiated endometrial mucosa, might have evolved to save energy necessary to maintain the endometrium between luteal phases. This theory also suffers from the same shortcoming as Profet's, namely, it fails to explain the difference between menstruating and the majority of non-menstruating species.

One may note that both of these theories aim at an adaptive explanation of the phenomenon of menstruation itself. In contrast, Collin A. Finn from the University of Liverpool offered a non-adaptive explanation of menstruation (Finn 1986, 1998). Finn's argument makes two points. First, it claims that menstruation itself is not the trait that evolved for its own sake but is a non-adaptive side effect of the evolution of spontaneous decidualization. As mentioned repeatedly in previous chapters, in great apes, some degree of decidualization occurs independently of the presence of an embryo, while in most species with invasive placentation, decidualization only happens during the implantation of the embryo. Decidua, so the argument, cannot be maintained with falling progesterone levels, and thus the decidualized layers of the endometrium have to be disposed of, and menstruation is only the overt manifestation of this process. According to Finn, the real question is why spontaneous decidualization evolved, since, according to his theory, menstruation is just a side effect of the evolution of spontaneous decidualization. One answer is that spontaneous decidualization is a maternal defense against an aggressive conceptus that has the ability for deep implantation (and thus the danger of *placenta accreta*) and has the potential for causing postpartum death of the mother due to unstoppable hemorrhage. Finn's theory is an attractive model, as it explains the evolution of menstruation within a specific biological context that potentially explains its spotty taxonomic distribution, namely the degree of invasiveness of the trophoblast. This theory is supported by an experimental model for menstruation in the laboratory mouse, but it also has difficulties explaining all of the comparative evidence.

The experiment that supports Finn's theory has been done in a variety of ways (Finn and Pope 1984, Rogers et al. 2025), most recently also with transgenic manipulation of the mouse endometrium (Cevrim and colleagues 2025). Here we describe one version that seems to be the most biological, i.e., the one requiring the least amount of intervention (Rudolph et al. 2012) (Figure 9.2). Mice have a very short ovarian cycle of four days, where estrus is soon followed by a new ovulation if no copulation occurs, essentially skipping an extended di-estrus, or luteal phase. In mice, the lifetime of the corpus luteum can be extended through cervical stimulation, as it occurs during copulation. Mating a receptive female with a vasectomized male creates a situation where the luteal phase is extended even in the absence of an embryo. If, in addition, an irritant is placed into the uterus, such as a drop of sesame oil or the endometrium is scratched, we have a model of spontaneous decidualization. In the presence of progesterone and a minimal injury of the endometrium, the endometrium decidualizes, or at least assumes a state closely similar to decidualization, called deciduoma. When

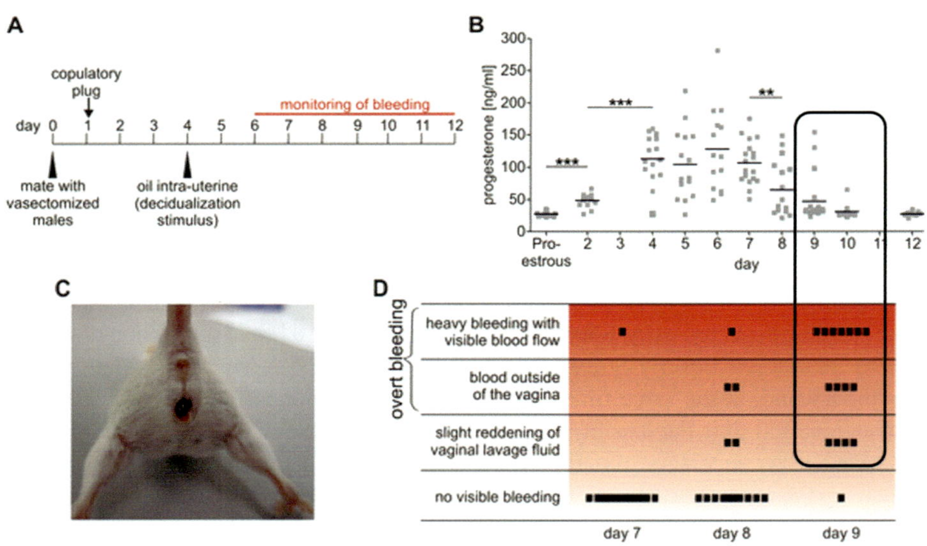

FIGURE 9.2 Experimental design for a mouse model of menstruation. (A) Schedule of experimental manipulations. At day 0, a female is bred with a vasectomized male to induce maintenance of the corpus luteum and thus sustained high progesterone levels. On day 4 pc, the normal day of embryo implantation, a small drop of sesame oil is introduced to induce a decidual reaction, and after that, the mice are monitored for vaginal bleeding, which occurs at and after day 9 pc. (B) Profile of systemic progesterone levels over 12 days. Note the sustained progesterone level up to day 7 pc and the precipitous decline at day 8 pc. (C) Female with vaginal bleeding. (D) Observation of vaginal bleeding from day 7 pc to day 9 pc. Vaginal bleeding is rarely observed on day 7 pc but is frequent and heavy on day 9 pc. This shows that decidual reaction without an embryo and progesterone withdrawal is sufficient to cause menstruation-like vaginal bleeding in an animal that normally does not menstruate. (Image from Rudolph et al. (2012) published under CC BY-NC license.)

eventually the progesterone level decreases because the corpus luteum reaches the end of its lifetime, endometrial breakdown and vaginal bleeding ensue. This is essentially a synthetic model of menstruation in a species that likely never had a menstruating ancestor. This experiment supports Finn's notion that menstruation is a side effect of spontaneous decidualization in conjunction with declining progesterone levels at the end of the luteal phase.

The second part of Finn's model is harder to test, i.e., the question of whether spontaneous decidualization is an adaptation to an aggressively invading blastocyst. In fact, a comparative study of menstruating species brings up several problematic cases. In short, not all species that have been reported to menstruate have good evidence for spontaneous decidualization or evidence of particularly invasive placentation. The most problematic case is the rhesus monkey, which is a menstruating Old World monkey, but has no spontaneous decidualization, and its implantation is not invasive (Carter 2011). In fact, when the embryo attaches to the luminal epithelium, the epithelium forms a plaque rather than being eroded as in other hemochorial mammals (Wislocki and Streeter 1938, Enders et al. 1985, Enders et al. 2001). The hemochorial interface is established not earlier than one month after attachment, and thus, the idea that menstruation is typical for species with spontaneous decidualization and highly invasive implantation is not supported in this species. Table 9.1 gives a list of menstruating species where some information about decidualization is available. A number of species exist where the presence of spontaneous decidualization is not supported or is at least questionable.

Another theory to explain the evolution of spontaneous decidualization is Jan Brosens' theory of embryo selection. This theory agrees with Finn's in that menstruation is a secondary consequence of spontaneous decidualization, but differs in the reason given for spontaneous decidualization. Brosens' theory is based on clinical observations that show a correlation between the frequency of early pregnancy loss and time to clinical pregnancy (Brosens et al. 2014, Macklon and Brosens 2014). Women who conceive quickly are more likely to lose their pregnancy than women who take longer to become clinically pregnant.[1] The interpretation is that under normal conditions, a fraction of the conceptuses fail early, in large part because of genetic reasons, so that pregnancy is not clinically detected. These embryos are lost at about the time of expected menstruation or a little later, perceived by the woman and her physician as "late menstruation". Pregnancy loss occurs together with the menstrual effluence, and pregnancy is thus not detected. In women with frequent early pregnancy loss, according to the theory, the endometrium accepts low-quality embryos

TABLE 9.1
Reproductive Traits of Menstruating Species

Species	Ovarian Cycle [d]	Gestation [d]	Spontaneous Decidualization
Acomys caharinus	10	39	Yes
Elephantulus myurnus	12	49–56	No? (edema and polyp)
Rousettus leschenaulti	33	120	Yes
Molossus ater	?	105	Yes
Glossophaga soricina	22–26	108	No
M. ricketti	?	?	?
Carollia perspicillata	21–27	120	No
Macaca mulatta	23–31	166	No
Papua anubis	23–31	180	No
Ateles geoffroyi	24–27	226–232	Yes?
Cebus sp.	21	180	Yes?

Note: ? means unknown

for implantation, which leads to a clinically detectable pregnancy but later fails to complete pregnancy. These low-quality embryos would otherwise, in women with normal endometrial function, be rejected earlier, i.e., before clinical pregnancy can be detected. Decidua that are formed before the embryo arrives act as a filter that rejects low-quality embryos. Only high-quality embryos can prevent being ejected.

Comparative evidence for the embryo selection model of spontaneous decidualization consists of the fact that menstruating species tend to have either singleton birth or at most two neonates, where the two neonates often come from different uterine horns and thus are "uterine singletons" (summarized in Emera et al. 2011). The reason why this observation supports the embryo-selection model is that quality control of offspring is most important if there is substantial investment in a small number of offspring.

THE SPINY MOUSE, A RODENT MODEL OF MENSTRUATION

A major breakthrough in menstruation research is the discovery of a menstruating rodent species, the Kairo spiny mouse *Acomys cahirinus* (Bellofiore et al. 2017). The spiny mouse is a desert rodent species that has garnered major interest from researchers even before the discovery of menstruation in this species. The first indication that this is a rather strange species came when researchers studying these animals in the field realized that they cannot handle the animal like one would other rodent species, i.e., by pinching the back skin or lifting them up by their tails. If treated this way, the spiny mouse "jumps out of its skin" and the researcher is left with a good part of the back skin in his or her hand, while the animal is scurrying off under the next stone. In fact, the animal that lost its skin is not even bleeding and readily regenerates their back skin in the following weeks. The spiny mouse is thus a major model for skin regeneration (Okamura et al. 2022, Seifert and Temple-Smith 2022, Okamura et al. 2023). The extraordinary regenerative capability of the spiny mouse is not limited to its skin but has also been demonstrated in the kidney and the heart (Okamura et al. 2022). It is also very vulnerable to developing diabetes because, as a desert animal, it is adapted to a very limited diet. Being fed *ad libitum*, as is standard operating procedure in animal laboratories, leads to overeating, metabolic disease, and fatty liver (G. P. Wagner, personal observation). Menstruation is then yet another extraordinary trait discovered in this remarkable species.

In terms of its female reproductive biology, the spiny mouse differs from more familiar rodents in the way one would expect from a menstruating species, based on what we wrote above. The ovarian cycle is much longer than in the laboratory mouse or the rat, including the closest related clade of rodents, the gerbils. The gerbils have a short five-day ovarian cycle similar to that of the mouse and the rat. In contrast, the spiny mouse has a cycle of nine to ten days with a much more extensive luteal phase (Peitz 1981). There are also signs of spontaneous decidualization reported (Bellofiore et al. 2017), and the litter size is small, reported in the literature to be about 1.7, but varies between 1 and 5 (Haughton et al. 2016), and is more developed than lab mouse neonates with open eyes and extensive and pigmented fur (Figure 9.3). In our lab, first pregnancies often produced a litter of two, while subsequent pregnancies of the same female often produced more than two. Average litter size would thus depend on the age and parity state distribution in the population. In any case, it is clear that the spiny mouse has a lower litter size than the mouse and the rat and would thus support the prediction from the embryo selection model: menstruation evolves when the investment in a few neonates becomes high. One may ask, though, whether the spiny mouse has an unusually low litter size for a rodent or whether *Mus musculus* has an unusually high litter size. A literature survey[2] of the litter size of >1,000 rodent species (Figure 9.4) shows a distribution with a mean of 3.5 neonates per litter, while mice and rats with average litter sizes between 5 and 7 are rather on the high side of the distribution. The spiny mouse, on the other hand, belongs to a cohort of species with an average litter size of less than two, which consists of 17% of the species sampled. Hence, the spiny mouse has a smaller-than-average litter size, but not dramatically so. The following question is whether the spiny mouse has suddenly evolved a lower litter size relative to its closest relatives, the gerbils.

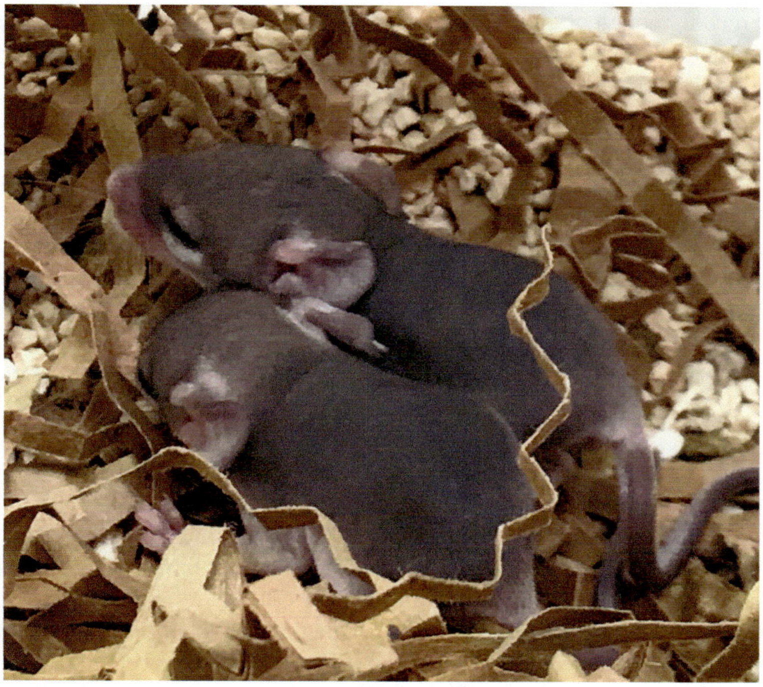

FIGURE 9.3 Two newborn spiny mice, *Acomys cahirinus*. Note the large size, well-developed fur, pigmentation, and open eyelids. (Image by GPW, CC BY-NC.)

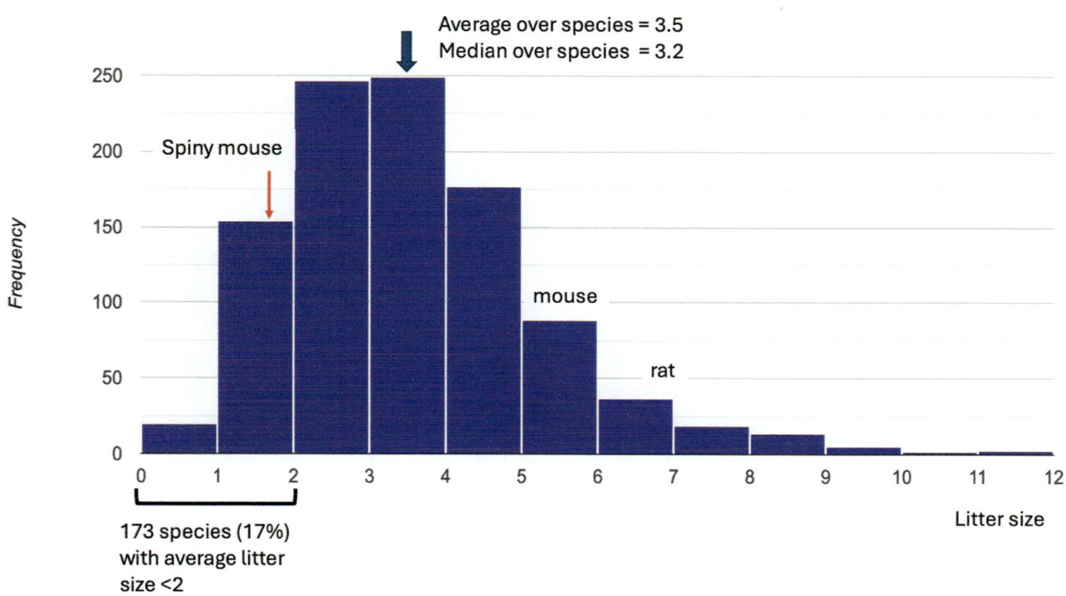

FIGURE 9.4 Distribution of litter sizes from a sample of >1,000 rodent species. Average litter size is 3.5, compared to the spiny mouse between 1 and 2, not very much more. The litter size of the laboratory mouse and rat, with an average of about 6 and 7, respectively, is large compared to the average and thus not typical. (Image generated by GPW, CC BY-NC.)

A phylogenetic reconstruction of ancestral litter sizes estimates that the common ancestor of spiny mice and gerbils had a litter size of 2.2, not much higher than estimated for *Acomys cahirinus*. Gerbils have a litter size between 3.5 and 5.5, depending on species, and thus seem to have evolved a higher litter size than the spiny mice.

It thus seems that, in the evolution of spiny mice, there was no dramatic drop in litter size. The comparison between spiny mice and gerbils rather points to a change in the regulation of the ovarian cycle, re-establishing a more extensive luteal phase, together with a number of other biological traits (see above). At this point, we cannot exclude the possibility that in this species menstruation evolved as a side-effect of other physiological changes, which may be driven by adaptations to extreme environments. The physiological peculiarities of spiny mice in themselves are a biological conundrum. What is driving the evolution of all these derived traits, where menstruation is just one among many? The biology and the evolution of menstruation are still a wide-open field of research.

THE PLACENTA-CANCER CONNECTION

It has been observed for a long time that there are substantial similarities between a malignant tumor spreading from its initial niche and an implanting mammalian embryo (Murray and Lessey 1999). A malignant tumor is breaching the confines of its primary tissue niche and has cells entering the surrounding stoma that eventually can escape to other parts of the body, mostly through the lymph system. The implanted embryo is also damaging the local tissue by breaking through the luminal epithelium of the uterine endometrium and eventually has cells invading the tissue in the form of extravillous (or extra-placental) trophoblast cells in humans as well as in rats and other eutherians. Are these similarities only superficial, or do they point to a deeper biological connection? Do implantation and cancer use the same pathways into the body? Did the evolution of invasive placentation affect the biology of malignant tumors?[3]

A logical way forward is to ask whether eutherian mammals are more vulnerable to malignant cancers than vertebrates without invasive placentation. Data is hard to come by, given that the causes of death in the wild are often not assessable, given how quickly dead animals are consumed or decay. Most data thus come from veterinary records from zoos, which is problematic in itself, since zoo animals are not kept under natural conditions. But as it is, this is our best source of information. So, what is the zoo-data telling us?

Some datasets that include mammalian and non-mammalian amniotes are pretty old. One is from 1933 by Ratcliffe covering mammals and birds from the Philadelphia Zoo (Ratcliffe 1933). Ratcliffe finds a cancer incidence rate of 2.6% for mammals an 1.2% for birds.[4] The other dataset is provided by Effron and colleagues from the San Diego Zoo (Effron et al. 1977). They find a cancer incidence rate for mammals of 2.9% and for birds of 1.9%. Given the two independent studies and different methodologies, the qualitative agreement between these studies is remarkable. A recent extensive study based on over 16,000 necropsies from 292 species confirmed the previous studies (Compton et al., 2025). Compton and colleagues found a median cancer incidence rate for mammals of 12% in contrast to reptiles including birds with a median cancer incidence rate of 4%. Amphibians are even less vulnerable to cancer with a rate of 1.2%.

Mammals are, on average, more vulnerable to cancer than birds and reptiles, consistent with the idea that the evolution of placentation made cancer more likely for mammals.[5] In principle, this result could be caused by a particularly low rate of cancer in birds. It is true that while birds overlap with mammals in size, there are more very large mammals than large birds (especially in zoos), and prolonged growth may contribute to increased cancer rate. What could be the mechanisms underlying this trend?

Cancer, in particular malignant cancer of a solid tumor, is the result of an interaction between tumor cells and their surrounding stroma (non-cancer cells). As a consequence, we have to expect that differences in cancer mortality among species are influenced by factors relating to the biology of the cancer cells themselves as well as those relating to the cancer-associated stroma. We will discuss these two dimensions in turn below.

Cancer is possible in all multicellular lifeforms (Aktipis et al. 2015, Aktipis 2020), and it clearly also happens in birds, reptiles and amphibians as well as fish. So, we need to ask why and how the evolution of mammalian placentation may make mammalian (eutherian) cancer cells more dangerous than those of, say, birds? Let us start by remembering that trophoblast cells are the embryo cells that are in direct contact with the maternal tissue and thus potentially attacked by the maternal immune system. As discussed in Chapter 4, one of the problems for eutherian embryos is to avoid the adaptive immune system of the mother from attacking the trophoblast. This is achieved in part by adaptations of the trophoblast (e.g., downregulation of HLA antigen presentation) as well as the endometrium (e.g., dendritic cell trapping in the mouse endometrium). On the other hand, a tumor also has the same "problem," i.e., to avoid being attacked by the host's immune system. One theory then goes something like this: with the origin of invasive placentation, trophoblast cells evolved cell biological devices to prevent being recognized by the maternal immune system. Cancer cells, in turn, may be able to access these genetic devices due to the mutational decay of the cancer cells' gene regulatory controls (Costanzo et al. 2018). This is the reason why the cancer of a eutherian mammal may be more readily able to evolve an effective way to manipulate the host's immune system, essentially neutralizing the body's ability to fight the cancer. This idea is further supported by the observation that there is a close similarity between the epigenetic landscape of trophoblast cells and cancer cells (Smith et al. 2017). If, by somatic mutation, the cancer cell can access the gene regulatory state of a trophoblast cell, it can protect itself against immune cell attack in the same way as the trophoblast does during pregnancy by coopting part of the trophoblast gene regulatory network.

The second dimension of the cancer-placenta relationship has to do with the evolution of the cellular environment that the mother is providing to the implanting embryo. In species with invasive placentation, the endometrium has the function to both enable implantation as well as limit the invasion by the embryo. As discussed above, in some species, such as the pig, however, the maternal endometrium completely denies entry to the endometrium by evolving mechanisms to prevent invasion. This has been most rigorously shown in the case of the cow endometrial stroma, where it could be shown that cow endometrial fibroblasts prevent the invasion of trophoblast cells also in an *in vitro* invasion assay (Kshitiz et al. 2019). Intriguingly, cow skin fibroblasts are also more resistant to the invasion by cancer cells than human skin fibroblasts, a finding that explains the fact that melanocytoma is turning malignant in cows at much lower rates than in humans (D'Souza and Wagner 2014). Hence, the endometrial resistance to trophoblast invasion in cows is paralleled by resistance to cancer cell invasion of skin fibroblasts. Why should this be the case?

The likely explanation for the parallel increase in invasion resistance of endometrial and skin fibroblasts is that both cell types are fibroblasts and thus evolutionarily related. They share some part of their gene regulatory networks (Musser and Wagner 2015). Mutations that affect the endometrial cells are thus likely to also affect gene expression in skin fibroblasts (Liang et al. 2018). The idea is that the evolution of the epithelio-chorial placenta due to the evolution of endometrial resistance to trophoblast invasion is also affecting fibroblasts in the rest of the body. This has the effect of making skin fibroblasts resist cancer spread more readily in cows than in humans. The idea is based on the concept of correlated selection response from quantitative genetics (Falconer and Mackay 1996). This concept says that, if two quantitative characters are genetically correlated, selection on one of them will lead to a correlated change in the other character. We can apply this idea to gene expression, which is also a quantitative character, such that selection on gene expression in one cell type can lead to a correlated selection response in another cell type. This idea is supported by three lines of evidence. One line of evidence is that evolutionary changes in gene expression in ESF are correlated with gene expression changes in skin fibroblasts (Dighe et al. 2024). Another approach shows that evolutionary changes in the promoter region of genes that affect invasion resistance cause resistance to invasion in both the endometrium and the skin (Suhail et al. 2020). Finally, it has been shown in an experiment that artificial selection on gene expression in skin fibroblasts leads to similar gene expression changes in endometrial fibroblasts (Dighe et al. 2024). The latter is the most direct evidence that the evolution at the fetal-maternal interface, like the evolution of epitheliochorial placentation, is likely affecting the risk of cancer spread in the rest of the body.

Animals, as a multicellular life form, consist of cells that all use, in first approximation, the same genome to direct their activities, with the exception of gene rearrangements in adaptive immune response. Furthermore, cell types arose through specialization from identical cells that make up the soma of primitive multicellular organisms.[6] The main way in which complex animal body plans arose was through the evolution of novel cell types (Arendt 2008, Wagner 2014, Arendt et al. 2016). But nevertheless, cell types are still to various degrees related to each other, as some parts of the genome they use will be shared. As a consequence, the parts of the organism are never completely independent entities. One should expect that the evolution of each and every part of the organism can have consequences for other parts of the organism. While evolvability of complex organisms requires quasi-independent parts (Wagner and Altenberg 1996), arising through differentiation, the *nexus organicus* is never broken, a *nexus* arising from the common evolutionary origin of all cell types in the body.

NOTES

1. The notion of clinical pregnancy acknowledges that pregnancy tests become positive some time after fertilization occurred.
2. This data collection and analysis was performed by Gladys Fang YC'21 as part of her undergraduate thesis.
3. The discussion below summarizes the review in Wagner, G. P., Kshitiz, A. Dighe and A. Levchenko (2022). "The Coevolution of Placentation and Cancer." *Annu Rev Anim Biosci* **10**: 259–279.
4. Meaningful p-values are not available as these species are not independent observations.
5. There are various potential problems with this data, discussed in Wagner et al. 2022. Nevertheless, it is the best we have in terms of comparisons between mammals and birds. Now there are much more extensive datasets available for mammals (e.g., Vincze et al., 2022) but not assessing mammals versus non-mammals.
6. A model for a primitive multicellular organism is Volvox, where the soma consists of only one type of cells.

REFERENCES

Aktipis, A. (2020). *The Cheating Cell: How Evolution Helps Us Understand and Treat Cancer.* Princeton, N.J., Princeton University Press.

Aktipis, C. A., A. M. Boddy, G. Jansen, U. Hibner, M. E. Hochberg, C. C. Maley and G. S. Wilkinson (2015). "Cancer across the tree of life: cooperation and cheating in multicellularity." *Philos Trans R Soc Lond B Biol Sci* **370**(1673): 20140219.

Arendt, D. (2008). "The evolution of cell types in animals: emerging principles from molecualr studies. ." *Nat Rev Genet* **9**: 868–882.

Arendt, D., J. M. Musser, C. V. H. Baker, A. Bergman, C. Cepko, D. H. Erwin, M. Pavlicev, G. Schlosser, S. Widder, M. D. Laubichler and G. P. Wagner (2016). "The origin and evolution of cell types." *Nat Rev Genet* **17**(12): 744–757.

Bellofiore, N., F. Cousins, P. Temple-Smith, H. Dickinson and J. Evans (2018). "A missing piece: the spiny mouse and the puzzle of menstruating species." *J Mol Endocrinol* **61**(1): R25–R41.

Bellofiore, N., S. J. Ellery, J. Mamrot, D. W. Walker, P. Temple-Smith and H. Dickinson (2017). "First evidence of a menstruating rodent: the spiny mouse (Acomys cahirinus)." *Am J Obstet Gynecol* **216**(1): 40.e41–40.e11.

Brosens, J. J., M. S. Salker, G. Teklenburg, J. Nautiyal, S. Salter, E. S. Lucas, J. H. Steel, M. Christian, Y. W. Chan, C. M. Boomsma, J. D. Moore, G. M. Hartshorne, S. Sucurovic, B. Mulac-Jericevic, C. J. Heijnen, S. Quenby, M. J. Koerkamp, F. C. Holstege, A. Shmygol and N. S. Macklon (2014). "Uterine selection of human embryos at implantation." *Sci Rep* **4**: 3894.

Carter, A. M. (2011). "Comparative studies of placentation and immunology in non-human primates suggest a scenario for the evolution of deep trophoblast invasion and an explanation for human pregnancy disorders." *Reproduction* **141**(4): 391–396.

Cevrim, C. and colleagues (2025). Induction of menstruation in mice reveals the regulation of menstrual shedding. bioRxiv preprint.

Compton, Z. T., W. Mellon, V. K. Harris, S. Rupp, D. Mallo, S. E. Kapsetaki, M. Wilmot, R. Kennington, K. Noble, C. Baciu, L. N. Ramirez, A. Peraza, B. Martins, S. Sudhakar, S. Aksoy, G. Furukawa, O. Vincze, M. Giraudeau, E. G. Duke, S. Spiro, E. Flach, H. Davidson, C. I. Li, A. Zehnder, T. A. Graham, B. V. Troan, T. M. Harrison, M. Tollis, J. D. Schiffman, C. A. Aktipis, L. M. Abegglen, C. C. Maley and A. M. Boddy (2025). "Cancer Prevalence across Vertebrates." Cancer Discov 15(1): 227-244.

Costanzo, V., A. Bardelli, S. Siena and S. Abrignani (2018). "Exploring the links between cancer and placenta development." *Open Biol* **8**(6):180081.

Critchley, H. O. D., E. Babayev, S. E. Bulun, S. Clark, I. Garcia-Grau, P. K. Gregersen, A. Kilcoyne, J. J. Kim, M. Lavender, E. E. Marsh, K. A. Matteson, J. A. Maybin, C. N. Metz, I. Moreno, K. Silk, M. Sommer, C. Simon, R. Tariyal, H. S. Taylor, G. P. Wagner and L. G. Griffith (2020). "Menstruation: science and society." *Am J Obstet Gynecol* **223**(5): 624–664.

D'Souza, A. W. and G. P. Wagner (2014). "Malignant cancer and invasive placentation: a case for positive pleiotropy between endometrial and malignancy phenotypes." *Evol Med Public Health* **2014**(1): 136–145.

Dighe, A., J. Maziarz, A. Ibrahim-Hashim, R. A. Gatenby, Kshitiz, A. Levchenko and G. P. Wagner (2024). "Experimental and phylogenetic evidence for correlated gene expression evolution in endometrial and skin fibroblasts." *iScience* **27**(1): 108593.

Effron, M., L. Griner and K. Benirschke (1977). "Nature and rate of neoplasia found in captive wild mammals, birds, and reptiles at necropsy." *J Natl Cancer Inst* **59**(1): 185–198.

Emera, D., R. Romero and G. Wagner (2011). "The evolution of menstruation: a new model for genetic assimilation: explaining molecular origins of maternal responses to fetal invasiveness." *Bioessays* **34**(1): 26–35.

Enders, A. C., T. N. Blankenship, A. T. Fazleabas and C. J. Jones (2001). "Structure of anchoring villi and the trophoblastic shell in the human, baboon and macaque placenta." *Placenta* **22**(4): 284–303.

Enders, A. C., A. O. Welsh and S. Schlafke (1985). "Implantation in the rhesus monkey: endometrial responses." *Am J Anat* **173**(3): 147–169.

Falconer, D. S. and T. F. C. Mackay (1996). *Introduction to Quantitative Genetics*. Essex, England, Longman.

Finn, C. A. (1986). "Implantation, menstruation and inflammation." *Biol Rev Camb Philos Soc* **61**(4): 313–328.

Finn, C. A. (1998). "Menstruation: a nonadaptive consequence of uterine evolution." *Q Rev Biol* **73**(2): 163–173.

Finn, C. A. and M. Pope (1984). "Vascular and cellular changes in the decidualized endometrium of the ovariectomized mouse following cessation of hormone treatment: a possible model for menstruation." *J Endocrinol* **100**(3): 295–300.

Haughton, C. L., T. R. Gawriluk and A. W. Seifert (2016). "The biology and husbandry of the African Spiny Mouse (Acomys cahirinus) and the research uses of a laboratory colony." *J Am Assoc Lab Anim Sci* **55**(1): 9–17.

Horst, C. v. d. and J. Gillman (1941). "The menstrual cycle in Elephantulus." *S Afr J Med Sci* **6**: 27–42.

Kshitiz, K., J. Afzal, J. D. Maziarz, A. Hamidzadeh, C. Liang, E. M. Erkenbrack, H. Nam, J. D. Haeger, C. Pfarrer, T. Hoang, T. L. Ott, T. E. Spencer, M. Pavličev, D. F. Antczak, A. Levchenko and G. P. Wagner (2019). "Evolution of placental invasion and cancer metastasis are causally linked." *Nat Ecol Evol* **3**(12):1743–1753.

Liang, C., J. M. Musser, A. Cloutier, R. O. Prum and G. P. Wagner (2018). "Pervasive correlated evolution in gene expression shapes cell and tissue type transcriptomes." *Genome Biol Evol* **10**(2): 538–552.

Macklon, N. S. and J. J. Brosens (2014). "The human endometrium as a sensor of embryo quality." *Biol Reprod* **91**(4): 98.

Murray, M. J. and B. A. Lessey (1999). "Embryo implantation and tumor metastasis: common pathways of invasion and angiogenesis." *Semin Reprod Endocrinol* **17**(3): 275–290.

Musser, J. M. and G. P. Wagner (2015). "Character trees from transcriptome data: origin and individuation of morphological characters and the so-called 'species signal'." *J Exp Zool B Mol Dev Evol* **324**(7): 588–604.

Okamura, D. M., E. D. Nguyen, D. R. Beier and M. W. Majesky (2022). "Wound healing and regeneration in spiny mice (Acomys cahirinus)." *Curr Top Dev Biol* **148**: 139–164.

Okamura, D. M., E. D. Nguyen, S. J. Collins, K. Yoon, J. B. Gere, M. C. M. Weiser-Evans, D. R. Beier and M. W. Majesky (2023). "Mammalian organ regeneration in spiny mice." *J Muscle Res Cell Motil* **44**(2): 39–52.

Peitz, B. (1981). "The oestrous cycle of the spiny mouse (Acomys cahirinus)." *J Reprod Fertil* **61**(2): 453–459.
Profet, M. (1988). "The evolution of pregnancy sickness as protection of the embryo against pleistogene teratogens." *Evol Theory* **8**: 177–190.
Profet, M. (1991). "The function of allergy: immunological defense against toxins." *Q Rev Biol* **66**(1): 23–62.
Profet, M. (1993). "Menstruation as a defense against pathogens transported by sperm." *Q Rev Biol* **68**(3): 335–386.
Ratcliffe, H. L. (1933). "Incidence and nature of tumors in captive wild mammals and birds." *Am J Cancer* **17**(1): 116–135.
Rogers, L. M., G. E. Lash, G. M. Anderson and J. E. Girling (2025). "Modelling menstruation in the common mouse: a narrative review." *Reprod Fertil Dev* **37**: RD25055.
Rudolph, M., W. D. Docke, A. Muller, A. Menning, L. Rose, T. M. Zollner and I. Gashaw (2012). "Induction of overt menstruation in intact mice." *PLoS One* **7**(3): e32922.
Seifert, A. W. and P. Temple-Smith (2022). "A remarkable rodent: regeneration and reproduction in spiny mice (Acomys)." *Curr Top Dev Biol* **147**: 659–707.
Smith, Z. D., J. Shi, H. Gu, J. Donaghey, K. Clement, D. Cacchiarelli, A. Gnirke, F. Michor and A. Meissner (2017). "Epigenetic restriction of extraembryonic lineages mirrors the somatic transition to cancer." *Nature* **549**(7673): 543–547.
Strassmann, B. I. (1996). "The evolution of endometrial cycles and menstruation." *Q Rev Biol* **71**(2): 181–220.
Suhail, Y., J. D. Maziarz, A. Dighe, G. Wagner and Kshitiz (2020). "Cis-regulatory differences explaining evolved levels of endometrial invasibility in Eutherian mammals." bioRxiv. DOI: https://doi.org/10.1101/2020.09.04.283366.
Vincze, O., F. Colchero, J. F. Lemaitre, D. A. Conde, S. Pavard, M. Bieuville, A. O. Urrutia, B. Ujvari, A. M. Boddy, C. C. Maley, F. Thomas and M. Giraudeau (2022). "Cancer risk across mammals." Nature 601(7892): 263-267.
Wagner, G. P. (2014). *Homology, Genes and Evolutionary Innovation*. Princeton, NJ, Princeton University Press.
Wagner, G. P. and L. Altenberg (1996). "Complex adaptations and the evolution of evolvability." *Evolution* **50**(3): 967–976.
Wagner, G. P., Kshitiz, A. Dighe and A. Levchenko (2022). "The coevolution of placentation and cancer." *Annu Rev Anim Biosci* **10**: 259–279.
Wislocki, G. B. and G. L. Streeter (1938). "On the placentation of the Macaque (Macaca mulatta) from the time of immplantation until the formation of the definite placenta." *Carnegie Institute Contributions to Embryology* **27**: 1–66.

10 Explaining and Interpreting the Eutherian Pregnancy
Evidence, Models, and Metaphors

This book is ostensibly about a specialized issue of biology, the nature of the fetal-maternal relationship in eutherian mammals and its evolutionary origin. But it is also something entirely different. The evolution of eutherian reproduction is a proving ground for ways evolutionary innovations can or should be explained, and the book-length treatment is meant to explore how an understanding of evolutionary innovations can be achieved. This intent was already front and center in the introductory chapter, where different modes of evolutionary explanations have been discussed. In addition, there is the question of how to embed scientific knowledge into an interpretative narrative: is it a war between the fetus and the mother or a harmonious cooperation? Are those the only alternatives, or are there others? Now we want to return to this project and reflect on what has been said about eutherian pregnancy and what it implies for how we may explain and understand evolutionary innovations, as well as how we use scientific knowledge in making sense of the world and our lives.

EXPLAINING EVOLUTIONARY NOVELTIES

In the introduction, we argued that, in evolutionary biology, there are at least three modes of explanation. On the one hand, the familiar model of natural selection, which is the main explanation of what is called an "adaptation," i.e., a trait that increases the fitness of its bearers. Besides that, there is random genetic drift with its outgrowth, constructive neutral evolution (Stoltzfus 1999, Lynch and Conery 2000, Lynch 2007, Stoltzfus 2012). The idea of constructive neutral evolution essentially is an interaction between mechanistic constraints and random genetic drift. Finally, there is the approach taken in this book, specifically employed to explain evolutionary novelties that do not answer to adaptive narratives. The latter is the case because adaptive benefit narratives of viviparity do not address the different forms of viviparity in different lineages, and thus, the special nature of eutherian placentation cannot be accounted for.

The explanatory strategy employed in this book has the following structure. Given a certain outcome of evolution, i.e., mammalian viviparity with invasive placentation, we, and previous investigators (Medawar 1953, Denker 1993), identified a number of obstacles that render the outcome paradoxical (see Chapter 4 for details). Each paradoxon describes a cell biological constraint that should have prevented the origin of a specific evolutionary outcome. These paradoxa define a set of explananda (i.e., what is to be explained). The explanans for each specific explanandum is provided by the evolutionary innovations that overcame the constraint identified by the biological paradoxon. For reference, one can call this form of explanation OC-explanation, standing for "Overcoming Constraints" (see also Müller and Wagner 1991, Wagner and Müller 2002 for the OC conceptualization of evolutionary novelties). This form of evolutionary explanation raises a number of questions that we want to discuss here.

The first issue is that such an explanation has more of the structure of a "how" narrative, for instance, how is it that eutherian mammals do not reject the semi-allogenic fetus via its adaptive immune response? In contrast, evolutionary biology has traditionally focused on answering "why" questions, mostly through invoking natural selection. While knowing the answers to the "how" questions is clearly interesting, it still does not answer the question of why eutherian pregnancy and placentation evolved at all. We will return to this question at the end of this section.

DOI: 10.1201/9781032717777-10

The next issue is whether the OC type of explanation is a scientific explanation at all. One could detect a certain flavor of "just so storytelling" in the OC narratives. It is important to emphasize that recognition (or prediction) of paradoxa is rooted in a deep understanding of mechanisms of tissue integrity, and not simply a leap of faith. Nevertheless, the strategy does involve claims that something that apparently does not occur (e.g., an immune response), logically should. To respond to this issue, one needs to first acknowledge that there is a plethora of types of scientific explanations (Woodward and Ross 2021). A widely accepted mode of explanation is the "nomological deductive" model of Hempel and Oppenheim (1948), where the explanandum is logically derived from a lawlike regularity (also sometimes called a law of nature) plus "boundary conditions" that actuate the law. Clearly, nothing offered in this book on the evolution of eutherian mammals is the logical consequence of a general law of nature. Instead, we are invoking contingent mechanistic necessities encoded in the inferred ancestral conditions (the constraint leading to the paradoxon) and some equally contingent mechanistic workarounds, the explanans. Equally, the "statistical relevance" mode of explanation (see Woodward and Ross 2021, section 3) is of little help given the unique historical nature of evolutionary innovations.

A little more promising is the "unification account" of explanation (Kitcher 1989). Not by coincidence, a philosopher of biology rather than physics proposed this account. According to Kitcher, "Science advances our understanding of nature by showing us how to derive descriptions of many phenomena, using the same pattern of derivation again and again, and in demonstrating this, it teaches us how to reduce the number of facts we have to accept as ultimate" (Kitcher, 1989, page 432). One could argue that OC explanations fall under this umbrella, as understanding the evolutionary innovations does unify our thinking about various phenomena, which, as such, would be "just so" facts of biology and clinical medicine. For instance, understanding the immunological paradoxon leads us to understand the various features at the fetal-maternal interface that are all geared toward preventing an adaptive immune attack against the fetus. The inflammation paradox helps us understand why implantation is associated with quasi-inflammatory processes (Mor et al. 2011) and also the vulnerabilities of human pregnancy against systemic inflammation (Romero et al. 2014). Nevertheless, trying to accommodate the OC narratives in the unification account feels a little forced, given that Kitcher had more lawlike (biological) regularities in mind when he developed his theory, such as the quasi-lawlike rules of Mendelian genetics and population genetics.

If we step back from specific philosophical theories of scientific explanation and assume a broader view, OC narratives feel like explanations. The Wikipedia article on "Explanation"[1] mentions the following characterization: "an explanation is a set of statements which render understandable the existence or occurrence of an object, event, or state of affairs." From that starting point, OC narratives can be accepted as "rendering understandable the existence of invasive placentation in mammals." They provide at least a partial account of what happened during the evolution of the eutherian mammals, without providing a more detailed account of the logical structure of the OC argument. This reproachment, however, leads us back to the issue of "why" questions, usually the domain of evolutionary biology.

Having rejected a straightforward adaptive explanation, based solely on direct natural selection acting on the particular trait, the OC account still leaves unanswered the question of why eutherian pregnancy evolved at the time and in the lineage it did. A plausible way of thinking about an eventual answer is a historical narrative, similar to the ones provided for events in human history: a string of coincidental events shaping the direction of historical change, e.g., a messenger is killed at the wrong time during battle, leading to defeat and subsequently the loss of a whole dynasty; the moral rectitude (or lack thereof) of a political or military leader which determines whether a successful government arises after a revolution (Acemoglu and Robinson 2012) and others more. It is likely that any major transition in evolution resulted from coincidences of ecological needs (e.g., a change in climate) and biological opportunities (whole genome duplications, or transposable element invasion, for instance). This might well be true but raises uncomfortable questions about how to test the validity of such historical narratives. For some evolutionary transitions, such as the origin of tetrapods from sarcopterygian fishes, elaborate narratives have been developed (Clack 2002), but for the evolution of eutherian pregnancy, we are not aware of such an overarching historical narrative. This is probably the case because the mechanistic questions have not been agreed upon by the scientific community, and the hope would be that the current book can contribute toward an agenda for developing a more complete historical narrative. Nevertheless, the question of how to test the validity of such an account remains. The latter point also leads us to raise the question of the validity of the accounts offered here about how the OC scenarios can be validated, and the validity of any EvoDevo scenario proposed. So far, we have relied on plausibility, given current molecular, cell biological, and phylogenetic knowledge. Below, we will argue that this knowledge can be turned into actual evidence.

THE FORENSIC EVIDENCE PRINCIPLE

In the sciences, experimental results are considered the strongest form of evidence. This belief is justified by the falsification principle, which states that if an effect E is derivable (predictable) from a hypothesis H, H→ E, and if E is not found in an experiment, i.e., not-E is true, then it logically follows that H is also wrong (so-called *modus ponens* of propositional logics) (Popper 1935). Hence, hypothesis testing, preferably under controlled experimental conditions, is justified by basic principles of propositional logic.

The experimental approach, though very rigorous and precise, has its limits, not so much in the realm of logical principles but in the realm of the physical world of earthly science. Experiments need to be done under the control of an investigator with an experimental setup in a laboratory or a field site. The experimental setup can be small, fitting into an Eppendorf tube, or rather large, like the Large Hadron Collider (LHC) of CERN, with its 27 km long tunnels 175 meters below the surface of the earth. But even the LHC is no match for processes that govern our weather systems, the movement of the earth's crust, or the dynamics of the planetary system, not to speak of galaxies. Yet, for all these, weather, geology, and astronomy, we claim scientific knowledge, which certainly cannot only flow from laboratory experiments. This shows that there have to be other sources of valid scientific evidence and knowledge.

Another limitation of the experimental method is temporal. Experiments can be a means of investigating processes that are happening now and here, or can be reproduced in the present. This limits the usefulness of the experimental method for testing statements regarding events in the remote past, for instance, in the case of evolutionary events in deep time. Is there a way to know or at least test what happened in the distant past, short of time travel? Of course, these limitations have not kept scientists, historians, and philosophers from speculating about past events, such as the chemical processes that eventually led to the origin of life, or the demise of the dinosaurs. The question, however, is this: if not with experiments directly, can such inferences about the evolutionary and geological past be justified as rigorously as the principle of experimental falsification, in some other way? We see two ways forward, each with its own limitations based on technical feasibility and the available resources.

One way to solve this problem is to recreate some biological entities in the lab that existed in the evolutionary past. This has been done successfully with DNA and even proteins. Using phylogenetic methods, one can, under favorable circumstances, computationally reconstruct the amino acid sequence of an ancestral protein. This is a routine task in molecular evolution. Adding to the computational reconstructions, the actual synthesis of these predicted ancestral proteins allows us to investigate the biochemistry of extinct biomolecules and test ideas about their evolution. Examples are the reconstitution of ancestral opsins to determine their spectral sensitivities and thus infer the light environment in which an ancestral species lived (Chang and Donoghue 2000, Chang et al. 2002). Another example is reconstructing the amino acid changes that were responsible for a change in ligand-binding specificity of nuclear receptors (Thornton 2001, Bridgham et al. 2010). Finally, reconstruction of ancestral transcription factor proteins allowed us to determine the amino acid changes responsible for the evolution of new allosteric activities (Brayer et al. 2011, Lynch et al. 2011, Nnamani et al. 2016). This approach is possible because we can synthesize DNA of any sequence in the laboratory and express it in a cell to harvest these proteins for further analysis. This shows that "partial time travel" is indeed possible. For developmental evolutionary biology, it would be ideal if we could expand this approach to other levels of biological organization, such as gene regulatory networks and cell types. There is some hope that this might be possible in the not-too-distant future with advances in "synthetic biology," but for now, this approach is out of reach for most biologists.

Another approach with broader applicability is what we call the forensic evidence principle (Larsson and Wagner 2012). In brief, the method relies on the fact that different causes for a particular outcome, say the death of a person, leave different traces in the resulting phenomenon; either a bullet hole in the skull, water or smoke particles in the lung, etc. Of course, this principle has been used not only in forensic science, but informally also in all branches of inquiry dealing with historical events, like archeology, paleontology, geology, and comparative evolutionary biology as well. But how does the forensic evidence-principle work, and can it be justified as rigorously as the logic of experimental falsification?

An articulation of this principle, as applied to theories about the origin of modern metabolism from hypothesized ribozyme life forms, was provided by Maynard-Smith and Szathmáry (Maynard-Smith and Szathmary 1995). The question was whether some features of modern metabolism could have originated from catalytic RNA. They suggest the following lines of evidence in support of such a claim (from Maynard-Smith and Szathmáry 1995, page 108, modified):

- The trait must be found at least in some outgroup of the focal taxon (e.g., bacteria).
- There should be some aspects of the process present in modern metabolism that serve no selected function in extant biochemistry, and which therefore can best be explained as relics of an ancestral condition.

The most important point here is in the second bullet point: the past leaves some features, i.e., "traces," that cannot be explained by current utility. This is one instantiation of the forensic evidence principle in biology.

A simple example from developmental evolution is the question of which digits were lost during the evolution of the bird wing. Generically, bird wings have three or fewer ossified digits, and a long-standing controversy raged for more than a century over which digits are retained in birds from the ancestral pentadactyl configuration. The solution is found in the fact that, in evolution, endochondral skeletal elements do not just disappear. Long after the skeletal element is lost in the adult, there are still developmental precursor states retained in the embryo. Endochondral elements arise from a sequence of developmental events, starting with mesenchymal condensations, i.e., aggregation of mesenchymal cells, which later chondrify and finally ossify. Long after a bone is lost in evolution, either cartilaginous precursors (Burke and Feduccia 1997) or pre-chondrogenic condensations can be found (Kundrát et al. 2001, Kundrát et al. 2002, Larsson and Wagner 2002, Welten et al. 2005, Larsson et al. 2010). Hence, there remains a trace of the historical loss of anatomical elements, which objectively answers the question of which digit got lost.[2]

An example relevant to the topic of this book is the fact that decidual cell differentiation is going through a phase where the cells express the hallmarks of activated fibroblasts (see Chapter 6). This can count as evidence that decidual cells evolved from the wounding response during embryo implantation, including fibroblast activation. It is a facet of the decidualization process that meets the criterion of Maynard-Smith and Szathmáry of a feature that seems to serve no function in extant biology (see above), and "which therefore can best be explained as a relic of an ancestral condition."

But what is the principled justification that these inferences actually represent scientific evidence? An argument can be made based on the so-called symmetry principle of theoretical physics: the effect has to have the same symmetries as the cause. In less abstract form, the principle is that different kinds of causes of a particular effect must lead to differences in the "microstructure" of the effect[3] (Rosen 1983). Once articulated, the forensic evidence principle for developmental evolution can be cast into a specific rule, set for providing evidence of past events (Larsson and Wagner 2012). The point is that the forensic evidence principle, if applied in a rigorous and disciplined way, is as valid as any other form of scientific evidence, be it experimental or otherwise.

METAPHORS AND NARRATIVES ABOUT THE FETAL-MATERNAL RELATIONSHIP

When one aims at understanding the evolution and function of the fetal-maternal relationship, it is helpful to reflect upon the potential nature of this interaction. Shall we think of this relationship as we do for any other physiological exchange surface, like the lung or the nephric glomeruli? Or is the evolution of placentation the origin of a novel unit, the fetal-maternal unit, that reflects a two-way integration? If one allows the second possibility, the answer will still depend on the taxon considered, with less integration in, for instance, viviparous lizards and marsupials, and more integration in primates and rodents. The conceptual consequences of these questions are more relevant for evolutionary considerations, since they pertain to the question of whether the fetal-maternal integration leads to a new unit of evolutionary change, similar to a new body part (e.g., the evolution of the insect wing). Alternatively, the fetal and maternal parts of the placenta could be understood as separate evolutionary units, each evolving according to the evolutionary interests of the corresponding individual, the fetus or the mother. This question has deep philosophical implications (Nuño de la Rosa et al. 2020). It also touches upon the question of where and how genetic conflict theory is appropriate.

Childbirth and pregnancy have been of central importance to humans as long as we existed. Not surprisingly, each culture has developed ideas and stories around pregnancy and childbirth to give meaning to what is happening. This "storytelling" has not stopped with the advent of scientific knowledge. It changed in character as it reflects upon scientific discoveries about pregnancy and the fetal-maternal relationship. As we will see, a short survey of these "interpretative narratives" (iN) convinces us that there is no straightforward and unique connection between a scientific discovery and the iN attached to it. Here we want to reflect upon the iNs that relate to our scientific understanding of pregnancy and embryo implantation.

The empirical investigation of pregnancy and placentation started, as so much else, in the Renaissance, as exemplified by Leonardo da Vinci's famous sketch of a human fetus in the uterus (Figure 10.1), even though he endowed the human fetus with a ruminant placenta with cotyledons, rather than a human placenta.[4] This accident of artistic license also shows that the study of animals was always integral to the study of reproduction. The history of placental research is long and full of twists and turns due to limited technical resources and misinterpretations, although the true results were also often arrived at more because of the dedication and ingenuity of the investigators, rather than due to the sophistication of their investigative tools. For our purpose, three steps in the discovery of the structure of the fetal-maternal interface are relevant: the discovery of separate blood circulation of the fetus and the mother, the discovery of the decidua, and the correct identification of fetal and maternal cells in the uterus.

The modern understanding of placental biology was cemented with observations obtained on the body of a young pregnant woman who died close to term in May of 1754. John Hunter (1718–1783) was called to examine the woman's body after the uterine vessels were injected with colored wax, both the arteries and the veins. Dissecting the placenta and the placental bed revealed the extent of the maternal blood spaces, expanded at the contact zone with the placenta, but no indication of a direct connection to fetal circulation. Together with later examinations of placentas injected with wax through the umbilical blood vessels established the fact that the fetus has its own closed circulatory system. Hunter, however, was not the first to "discover"[5] that fact. As far as can be reconstructed, the first to come to the correct conclusion was Julius Caesar Aranzi (1529/30–1589), a leading Italian anatomist of the 16th century (deWitt 1959). He based his conclusions on detailed

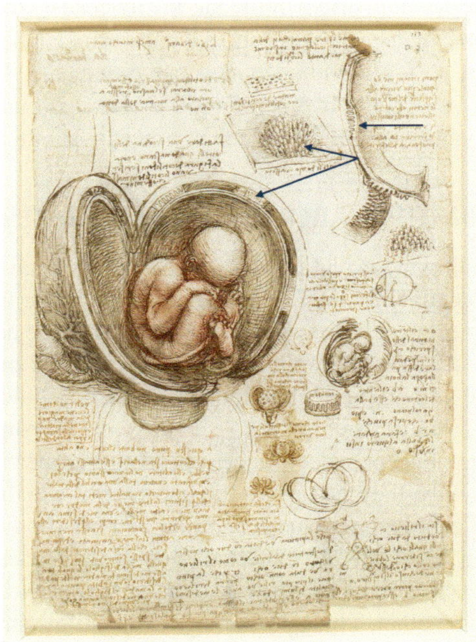

FIGURE 10.1 Leonardo da Vinci's sketch of an advanced human fetus in utero. What is remarkable about this sketch is that Leonardo drew a cotyledonary placenta, see arrows showing cotyledons, instead of a human placenta, suggesting that he also, or maybe primarily, studied pregnant animals rather than a human. (Image by Leonardo da Vinci, public domain via Wikimedia and modified by GPW.)

dissections of the placenta. Aranzi's idea was experimentally confirmed more than a century later by Camillis Falconet (1671–1762) by bleeding a pregnant dog and showing that the fetus retained its blood even after the mother was completely exsanguinated.

The significance of this discovery for our story is that the separate circulation between mother and fetus suggests that they are different individuals, an interpretation that will play an outsized role in the development of later interpretative narratives. In particular, the idea that the woman is the container for the incubation of another individual, the fetus, has its scientific root in this fact. Interestingly, this is also relevant for the much later debate about Paul Medawar's interpretation of the embryo as a "xeno-transplant," an idea that was the starting point for the field of reproductive immunology. However, as pointed out by Ashley Moffett and Norman Shreeve, the problem with this interpretation is that transplants usually become vascularized by the host organism, while nothing of that sort is happening with the embryo (Moffett and Shreeve 2023).

The next discovery adding to the interpretation of pregnancy and the fetal-maternal relationship was that of the decidua, i.e., the transformation of the uterine mucosa in animals with hemochorial placentation. The term decidua was introduced by William Hunter in his 1774 monograph "*Anatomia uteri humani gravidi tabulis illustrate*" (Pijnenborg and Vercruysse 2008). The description of decidualized endometrium, however, goes back to William's brother John Hunter (1728–1793) (deWitt 1959). The theorized role of the decidua is a prime example of how a scientific discovery can inspire divergent interpretations. For Ernst Gräfenberg (1881–1957), the formation of the decidua was a defensive reaction of the mother against an invasive embryo (Gräfenberg 1910, cited after Haig 2015). This interpretation was supported by the discovery of the invasive nature of the human embryo based on the examination, performed by Hubert Peters, of a suicide victim who took her life three days after missing her period in 1897. This study made clear that the human embryo is actively embedding itself into the uterine mucosa and is thus not a passive "seed" protected by the uterine "soil." Further evidence of the active invasion of the uterine mucosa by the placenta was found when Gräfenberg demonstrated that first-trimester human placentae harbor proteolytic activity while late-gestation placentae do not. From these observations, Gräfenberg suggested that the decidua secretes protease inhibitors to control embryo invasion. All of these observations and others more inspired a militaristic interpretation of the fetal-maternal interface as a line of contact between an invasive embryo and a defending uterus. A more extensive discussion of this narrative and its background can be found in an essay by David Haig (Haig 2015). It is notable, though, that "[n]one of the authors who described the maternal-fetal boundary as a battleground offered well-articulated reasons for why mother and offspring should be at war" (Haig 2015, page 168). That task fell to David Haig himself with his theory of fetal-maternal conflict (Haig 1993).

In contrast, Otto Grosser (1873–1951) took the same set of observations and concluded that the decidua is a "fertile soil" to nourish the embryo (Grosser 1927). Interestingly, he already pointed out that the war metaphor is out of place in the case of the fetal-maternal relationship. The trophoblast and the decidua stand in a mutually interdependent relationship with the purpose of forming the next generation of the species and thus cannot be in the business of destroying each other, as is the case in war. Along the same lines, L. B. Arey argued that the relationship between trophoblast and decidua is a "nicely worked out cooperation to produce a definite harmonious end" (Arey 1933, cited after Haig 2015). In fact, one should remember that the "antagonism" between proteolytic activity by the placenta and the inhibitory activity of the decidua can also be seen as a form of physiological regulation, if fetus and mother are seen as an integrated physiological system (Nuño de la Rosa et al. 2020).

WHAT IS THE ROLE OF THE SCIENTIST IN SHAPING INTERPRETATIVE NARRATIVES?

At this point, it is worth reflecting on whether a scientist should at all engage in discussing or providing such interpretations as discussed above. Neither the war narrative nor the cooperation narrative contributes anything essential to the scientific facts. At least it is questionable whether they do, given the divergent narratives offered by knowledgeable researchers on either side of the debate. Simple, unadorned reporting of the experimental and descriptive facts should, in principle, be sufficient. However, this point of view ignores the fact that human reproduction, and by implication also research on animal sexuality and reproduction, will always attract interpretative narratives. The human need for "stories" to give meaning to important junctures in life is just too strong to ignore. How then preserve the integrity of science when interpretative narratives are unavoidable? We think science can and should be part of the conversation about the nature and interpretation of reproductive biology, if some guidelines are respected. Here we want to briefly discuss what these should be, before we return to the question of how an interpretative narrative can look like, given what we think today.

An interpretative narrative should always be open to challenge by scientific facts. If an interpretative narrative is offered that does not accord with all empirical findings, it loses its validity. In other words, an interpretative narrative can never justify the deformation of the scientific record or ignore facts. For the individual scientist, this can be hard, since scientists, as most people, once they are committed to a particular narrative, have a hard time letting it go in the face of new or previously ignored empirical facts.

It also has to be clear that all the psychological and ethical implications of a particular interpretative narrative are the responsibility of the scientist, historian, philosopher, or theologian forging or propagating such an interpretative narrative. Nobody can hide behind scientific facts, because the interpretative narrative does not logically follow from objective facts. There will always be ethical or psychological implications attached to an interpretative narrative, but since the facts do not necessitate a particular interpretative narrative, the creation or propagation of an interpretative narrative is a human construct of the scholar and thus an act that carries with it ethical responsibilities. When two or more interpretative narratives, consistent with all we know, are available, then the scholar is called upon to choose the one that is consistent with his or her ethical beliefs. But doing so and expressing the choice in public also reflects upon the speaker's ethical stance, which itself can be challenged based on its ethical consequences. Offering an interpretative narrative shifts the conversation from the scientific to the ethical, and the debate will have to be conducted accordingly. Note, however, that such debate is about the acceptance of a particular interpretative narrative, not about the validity of scientific facts.

BEYOND CONFLICT AND COOPERATION

Returning to the history of human and mammalian reproductive biology, we see a situation where the majority of the discoveries up to the early 20th century supported the notion that the mother and fetus are two different individuals. That was the discovery of separate circulatory systems of the fetus and the mother, as well as the active role of the embryo in establishing the placenta, and the counteracting activities of the uterus, limiting the invasion of the mucosa by the embryo. Assuming the "two-individuals perspective" allows a range of possible interpretations of the nature of these individuals from container (=mother) -cake (=embryo) model, the conflict models, with the war narrative as an extreme, all the way to cooperation narratives, which also assume that fetus and mother need to be conceptualized as different individuals engaging in a transaction of some sort. In contrast to this tradition, we want to support here a novel approach that abandons the two-individuals assumption and instead recognizes the pregnant eutherian female as an emergent individual in itself (Nuño de la Rosa et al. 2021); see also Kingma's theory for a step in a similar direction (Kingma 2020). The motivation to move in this direction comes from reflecting upon the ideas extensively discussed in this book, namely the primacy of female innovations in the evolution of eutherian placentation, and the mutual integration and interdependencies found between female and fetal physiological and immunological relationships.

The concept of a biological individual is complex and has at least three dimensions: the physiological, evolutionary, and ecological dimensions. Notions of individuality along those lines have been discussed in depth in the paper by Nuño de la Rosa and colleagues (2021) and shall not be repeated here. Instead, we want to offer an additional narrative that supports the notion of an emerging individuality of the eutherian pregnant female. In doing so, we want to offer an evolutionary narrative that complements the arguments forwarded by Nuño de la Rosa and colleagues (2021) as well as Elselijn Kingma (2020). Our argument proposes that the evolution of eutherian pregnancy is a transition between two structural process types in place during female reproduction. One is what could be called a vectorial process from ovulation to free living individuals, the other assumes that the vectorial process is interrupted by the evolution of a self-maintaining stage, pregnancy, that is ended by perturbations from outside the process itself. We thus contrast here the process, which is a chain of brief transient states, each with a goal to reach the next one (vectorial process), with the temporally extended process, which has strong self-maintaining properties.

In biology, a vectorial process type is often called a cascade. Event A causes the next event B, which in turn triggers event C, etc.

$$A \rightarrow B \rightarrow C \rightarrow \ldots$$

Here, we argue that the ancestral and most widely distributed forms of female reproduction in vertebrates are vectorial processes:

Oviparity

ovulation→ oviposition→ external fertilization→ development→ hatching

ovulation→ internal fertilization→ vesting of the ovum→ oviposition→ development→ hatching

Ovoviviparity

…→ vesting of the ovum→ egg retention→ internal hatching→ "birth"

Opossum-style viviparity:

… →egg retention→ internal hatching→ attachment & inflammation→ birth

All of these processes have the character of a cascade; none of them has actively self-maintaining stages, as far as is known, and thus are vectorial in nature. In asserting this, we assume, for instance, that egg-retention is due to a slowing of the otherwise vectorial process of oviposition rather than a self-maintaining stage of gestation, which is an empirical question to be investigated.

In contrast, there are processes where a vectorial process is punctuated by stable self-maintaining stages, which only progress to later stages when perturbed by factors outside itself.

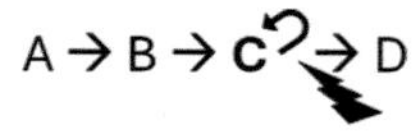

In his cartoon, state C is reached via a cascade A→ B→ C. But instead of directly triggering "D," the process C feeds back onto itself, rendering it a stable state. Progression to the next stage must be caused by a process that interrupts the self-maintaining feedback, either entirely from the outside (seasonal changes) or from some secondary consequence of the processes themselves (e.g., increasing energy demand from the growing fetus, uterine stretch, etc.).[6]

The proposed distinction between entirely vectoral processes and those processes punctuated by a self-maintaining stage is structurally analogous to the distinction between an ecological succession and a climax community. For instance, after a glacier recedes, the open landscape goes through a series of vegetation types, where each step in the succession sets the stage for the next: bare rock is colonized by lichens, later joined by grass and other small annual plants, followed by shrubs and shade intolerant trees, progressing toward what is called a climax community, which is a stable assembly of species where the ecological processes actively maintain a community.[7]

For the case of eutherian viviparity, the state "C" in the above cartoon would correspond to the stage where the implantation and nidatory inflammation are suppressed by the action of the decidual and allied cell types, leading to the "climax state" of mid-pregnancy (Mor et al. 2011). The self-maintaining nature of the process includes the stability of the fetal-maternal interface, which is reached via the re-establishment of tissue stability due to the integration of the trophoblast into the cell-cell communication network of the endometrium (see Chapter 6). While this state at the FMI is maintained, as is also the general stability of the feto-maternal unit due to numerous modifications of the maternal physiology to support this new feto-maternal unit, some vectorial processes continue. These are the development and growth of the embryo/fetus, the gradual erosion of the decidua, and secondary consequences of fetal growth, such as uterine wall stretch. Eventually, some of these vectorial processes lead to the perturbation of the stable equilibrium at the placental-endometrium unit, such as the maturation of the lung, where surfactants contribute to triggering the demise of the decidua, a process called decidual activation (Casey and MacDonald 1988), and initiating the parturition cascade.

The evolutionary origin of a self-maintaining state of the FM unit makes this part of the reproductive process a quasi-independent unit of the lifecycle. It is an evolutionary novelty in the sense of Wagner (2014), with its own evolvability relative to other life stages. The independent evolvability manifests itself in the explosive increase of morphological and physiological diversity of eutherian mammalian placentae (Ramsey 1982), and the diversity of mechanisms regulating pregnancy length (Basanta and Pavlicev 2025). It is this uniqueness that justifies the interpretation of the eutherian pregnant females as a novel evolutionary individual, though transient, as all things in biology, and life in general, are. The placental-endometrial unit initiates a physiological integration between mother and fetus that renders narratives based on the two-individual model, be it conflict, war, or cooperation, inapplicable. The maternal-fetal unit instantiates the pregnant eutherian female as a historical individual (sensu Wagner and Tomlinson 2022), as it has its quasi-independent evolvability, making pregnancy-related adaptations and innovations in both the female and the placental/fetal side inevitable.

This is the alternative to fetal-maternal conflict narratives as they arose in the early 20th century and still affect the thinking about the fetal-maternal relationship: cellular interactions at the fetal-maternal interface, that establish and maintain the placental-endometrial unit, are physiological regulatory feedback circuits rather than exploitative attacks of the fetus on the integrity of the mother. Yes, the female changes her entire physiological state in order to accommodate the growing fetus, but this situation is fully analogous to feedback regulation, like those regulating the glucose or oxygen levels in the blood. The fetus is, in this view, physiologically no more an intruder than the heart or liver is.

Let us finally explain, metaphorically, how we conceive the relationship between the developmental evolution approach to the evolution of viviparity in contrast to conflict theory, based on population genetic theory. If we allow an analogy between the evolutionary origin of a novel phenotypic unit of integration (functionally, developmentally, as well as evolutionarily) with the historical origin of social organizations, like families, churches, and universities, it is clear that any unit of organization contains the seed for internal conflict between its members. But the potential for conflict is rarely, if ever, the reason and explanation for the origin of any one of these organizations. The university owes its historical origin to the need to organize the education of clergy or other "servants of the realm" such as doctors, administrators, and lawyers. Is the further development of the University free of internal conflict between different parts of the University? Of course not, but the potential for conflict of the kind playing out (unfortunately) in universities is a consequence of the existence of the university, not the motive force for its creation. In analogy, eutherian viviparity as a mode of reproduction originated for ecological and physiological reasons, and once established, also provided the stage for fetal/paternal-maternal conflict to play out. For these reasons, we think that conflict theory is relevant to understanding the diversification of forms of viviparity but plays no role in explaining its origin.

NOTES

1. Retrieved on April 6, 2025, from the English instantiation of Wikipedia.
2. The situation is more complicated because the evidence discussed here only answers the question of which digit precursors have been abandoned in evolution. A deeper complication arises from the fact that digit identity can shift in location, such that an adult digit morphology can develop from a precursor that, in the pentadactyl hand, develops in another digit. It is pretty well documented that the most anterior avian wing digit is morphologically and developmentally a digit I but developing out of the precursor of digit: Stewart, T. A., C. Liang, J. L. Cotney, J. P. Noonan, T. J. Sanger and G. P. Wagner (2019). "Evidence against tetrapod-wide digit identities and for a limited frame shift in bird wings." *Nat Commun* **10**(1): 3244. Vargas, A. and J. F. Fallon (2005). "Birds have dinosaur wings: the molecular evidence." *J Exp Zool Part B (Mol Dev Evol)* **304B**: 86–90, Wang, Z., R. L. Young, H. Xue and G. P. Wagner (2011). "Transcriptomic analysis of avian digits reveals conserved and derived digit identities in birds." *Nature* **477**(7366): 583–586.
3. A more extensive discussion of the interpretation of the symmetry principle is given in Larssen and Wagner (2012).
4. It does not help that even today the villi of the human placenta are sometimes called cotyledons, even though by now it is clear that ruminant cotyledons and primate villi are not the same.
5. This story highlights the fact that it is not clear what "discovery" really means, as the creation of a scientific fact is an extended process, not a singular event (see also Ludwig Fleck, 1935).
6. Embryonic diapause can, by the way, also be described that way, although it is interesting to ask whether it is an actively self-maintaining process or a stalled cascade.
7. This abbreviated summary follows the explanation at the University of Chicago website https://news.uchicago.edu/explainer/what-is-ecological-succession.

REFERENCES

Acemoglu, D. and J. A. Robinson (2012). *Why Nations Fail: The Origins of Power, Prosperity and Poverty.* New York, Crown Publ.

Arey, L. B. (1933). Placentation, fetal membranes and deciduae. *Obstetics and Gynecology.* A. H. Curtis. Philadelphia, PA, W. B. Saunders.

Basanta, S. and M. Pavlicev (2025). "The shifting role and regulation of the Corpus Luteum in vertebrate reproduction: a synthetic review." *Q Rev Biol* 100(3): 189–231.

Brayer, K. J., V. J. Lynch and G. P. Wagner (2011). "Evolution of a derived protein-protein interaction between HoxA11 and Foxo1a in mammals caused by changes in intramolecular regulation." *Proc Natl Acad Sci U S A* 108(32): E414–420.

Bridgham, J. T., G. N. Eick, C. Larroux, K. Deshpande, M. J. Harms, M. E. Gauthier, E. A. Ortlund, B. M. Degnan and J. W. Thornton (2010). "Protein evolution by molecular tinkering: diversification of the nuclear receptor superfamily from a ligand-dependent ancestor." *PLoS Biol* 8(10): e1000497.

Burke, A. C. and A. Feduccia (1997). "Developmental patterns and the identification of homologies in the avian hand." *Science* 278: 666–668.

Casey, M. L. and P. C. MacDonald (1988). "Biomolecular processes in the initiation of parturition: decidual activation." *Clin Obstet Gynecol* 31(3): 533–552.

Chang, B. S. and M. J. Donoghue (2000). "Recreating ancestral proteins." *Trends Ecol Evol* 15(3): 109–114.

Chang, B. S., K. Jonsson, M. A. Kazmi, M. J. Donoghue and T. P. Sakmar (2002). "Recreating a functional ancestral archosaur visul pigment." *Mol Biol Evol* 19(9): 1483–1489.

Clack, J. A. (2002). *Gaining Ground: The Origin and Evolution of Tetrapods.* Bloomington, IN, Indiana University Press.

Denker, H. W. (1993). "Implantation: a cell biological paradox." *J Exp Zool* 266(6): 541–558.

deWitt, F. (1959). "An historical study on theories of the placenta." *J Hist of Med and Allied Sci* 14(3): 360–374.

Fleck, L. (1935). Entstehung und Entwicklung einer wissenschaftlichen Tatsache: Einführung in die Lehre vom Denkstil und Denkkollektiv. Benno Schwabe und Co., Basel, Schweiz.

Grosser, O. (1927). *Fruhentwicklung, Eihautbildung und Placentatsion des Menschen und der Saugetiere.* Munchen, J. F. Bermann.

Haig, D. (1993). "Genetic conflicts in human pregnancy." *Q Rev Biol* 68(4): 495–532.

Haig, D. (2015). Fertil soil or no man's land: cooperation and conflict in the placental bed. *Placental Bed Disorders.* R. Rijneborg, I. Brosens and R. Romero. Cambridge, Cambridge University Press: 165–173.

Hempel, C. G., and P. Oppenheim (1948). "Studies in the logic of explanation." *Phil Sci* 15: 135-175.

Kingma, E. (2020). "Bioplogical individuality, pregnancy, and (mammalian) reproduction." *Phil Sci* 87: 1037–1048.

Kitcher, P. (1989). Explanatory unification and the causal structure of the world. *Scientific Explanation.* P. Kitcher and W. Salmon. Minneapolis, MN, University of MInnesota Press: 410–505.

Kundrát, M., V. Seichert and A. Russell (2001). "Developmental remnants of the first avian metacarpus." *J Morph* 248: 252A.

Kundrát, M., V. Seichert, A. P. Russell and K. SmetanaJr (2002). "Pentadactyl pattern of the avian wing autopodium and pyramid reduction hypothesis." *J Exp Zool (Mol. Dev. Evol.)* 294: 152–159.

Larsson, H. C. E., A. C. Heppleston and R. M. Elsey (2010). "Pentadactyl ground state of the manus of Alligator mississippiensis and insight into the evolution of digit reduction in Archsauria." *J Exp Zool (Mol. Dev. Evol.)* 314B: 571–579.

Larsson, H. C. E. and G. P. Wagner (2002). "The pentadactyl ground state of the avian wing." *J Exp Zool (Mol. Dev. Evol.)* 294: in press.

Larsson, H. C. E. and G. P. Wagner (2012). "Testing inferences in develomental evoultion: the forensic evidence principle." *J Exp Zool (Mol. Dev. Evol.)* 318: 489–500.

Lynch, M. (2007). *The Origins of Genome Architecture.* Sunderland, MA, Sinauer Associates.

Lynch, M. and J. S. Conery (2000). "The evolutionary fate and consequences of duplicate genes." *Science* 290: 1151–1155.

Lynch, V. J., G. May and G. P. Wagner (2011). "Regulatory evolution through divergence of a phosphoswitch in the transcription factor CEBPB." *Nature* 480(7377): 383–386.

Maynard-Smith, J. and E. Szathmary (1995). *The Major Transitions in Evolution.* Oxford, UK, Oxford University Press.

Medawar, P. B. (1953). Some immunological and endocrinological problems raised by the evolution of viviparity in vertebratges. *Evolution.* R. Brown and J. F. Danielli. New York, NY, Academic Press: 320–338.

Moffett, A. and N. Shreeve (2023). "Local immune recognition of trophoblast in early human pregnancy: controversies and questions." *Nat Rev Immunol* 23(4): 222–235.

Mor, G., I. Cardenas, V. Abrahams and S. Guller (2011). "Inflammation and pregnancy: the role of the immune system at the implantation site." *Ann N Y Acad Sci* 1221: 80–87.

Müller, G. B. and G. P. Wagner (1991). "Novelty in evolution: restructuring the concept." *Ann Rev Ecol Syst* 22: 229–256.

Nnamani, M. C., S. Ganguly, E. M. Erkenbrack, V. J. Lynch, L. S. Mizoue, Y. Tong, H. L. Darling, M. Fuxreiter, J. Meiler and G. P. Wagner (2016). "A derived allosteric switch underlies the evolution of conditional cooperativity between HOXA11 and FOXO1." *Cell Rep* 15(10): 2097–2108.

Nuno de la Rosa, L., M. Pavlicev and A. Etxeberria (2021). "Pregnant females as historical individuals: an insight from the philosophy of evo-devo." *Front Psychol* 11: 572106.

Pijnenborg, R. and L. Vercruysse (2008). "Shifting concepts of the fetal-maternal interface: a historical perspective." Placenta 29 Suppl A: S20-25.

Popper, K. R. (1935). *Logik der Forschung: zur Erkenntnistheorie der modernen Naturwissenschaft*. Vienna, Austria, Springer Wien.

Ramsey, E. M. (1982). *The Placenta. Human and Animal*. Santa Barbara, CA, Praeger Inc.

Romero, R., S. K. Dey and S. J. Fisher (2014). "Preterm labor: one syndrome, many causes." *Science* 345(6198): 760–765.

Rosen, J. (1983). *A Symmetry Primer for Scientists*. New York, NY, Wiley & Sons.

Stewart, T. A., C. Liang, J. L. Cotney, J. P. Noonan, T. J. Sanger and G. P. Wagner (2019). "Evidence against tetrapod-wide digit identities and for a limited frame shift in bird wings." *Nat Commun* 10(1): 3244.

Stoltzfus, A. (1999). "On the possibility of constructive neutral evolution." *J Mol Evol* 49(2): 169–181.

Stoltzfus, A. (2012). "Constructive neutral evolution: exploring evolutionary theory's curious disconnect." *Biol Direct* 7: 35.

Thornton, J. W. (2001). "Evolution of vertebrate steroid receptors from an ancestral estrogen receptor by ligand exploitation and serial genome expansions." *Proc Natl Acad Sci U S A* 98(10): 5671–5676.

Vargas, A. and J. F. Fallon (2005). "Birds have dinosaur wings: the molecular evidence." *J Exp Zool Part B (Mol Dev Evol)* 304B: 86–90.

Wagner, G. P. (2014). Homology, Genes and Evolutionary Innovation. Princeton, NJ, Princeton University Press.

Wagner, G. P. and G. B. Müller (2002). "Evolutionary innovations overcome ancestral constraints: a re-examination of character evolution in male sepsid flies (Diptera: Sepsidae)." *Evol Dev* 4(1): 1–6; discussion 7–8.

Wagner, G. P. and G. Tomlinson (2022). "Extending the explanatory scope of evolutionary theory: the origination of historical kinds in biology and culture." *Philos Theor Pract Biol* 14: 1–25.

Wang, Z., R. L. Young, H. Xue and G. P. Wagner (2011). "Transcriptomic analysis of avian digits reveals conserved and derived digit identities in birds." *Nature* 477(7366): 583–586.

Welten, M. C. M., F. J. Verbeek, A. H. Mijer and M. K. Richardson (2005). "Gene expression and digit homology in the chicken embryo wing." *Evol Dev* 7: 18–28.

Woodward, J. and L. Ross (2021). Scientific explanation. *Standord Encyclopedia of Philosophy*. E. N. Zalta and Uri Nodelman (eds.). https://plato.stanford.edu/archives/win2012.

Index

For Product Safety Concerns and Information please contact our
EU representative GPSR@taylorandfrancis.com Taylor & Francis
Verlag GmbH, Kaufingerstraße 24, 80331 München, Germany